Monographs on Pathology of Laboratory Animals

Sponsored by the
International Life Sciences Institute

The following volumes have appeared so far

Endocrine System
1983. 346 figures. XV, 366 pages. ISBN 3-540-11677-X

Respiratory System
1985. 279 figures. XV, 240 pages. ISBN 3-540-13521-9

Digestive System
1985. 352 figures. XVIII, 386 pages. ISBN 3-540-15815-4

Urinary System
1986. 362 figures. XVIII, 405 pages. ISBN 3-540-16591-6

Genital System
1987. 340 figures. XVII, 304 pages. ISBN 3-540-17604-7

The following volumes are in preparation

Integument and Mammary Gland
Hemopoietic System
Musculoskeletal System
Cardiovascular System
Special Sense

T. C. Jones U. Mohr R. D. Hunt (Eds.)

Nervous System

With 242 Figures and 12 Tables

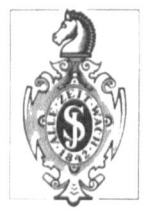

Springer-Verlag Berlin Heidelberg GmbH

Thomas Carlyle Jones, D.V.M., D.Sc.
Professor of Comparative Pathology, Emeritus
Harvard Medical School
New England Regional Primate Research Center
One Pine Hill Drive, Southborough, MA 01772, USA

Ulrich Mohr, M.D.
Professor of Experimental Pathology
Medizinische Hochschule Hannover
Institut für Experimentelle Pathologie
Konstanty-Gutschow-Strasse 8
3000 Hannover 61, Federal Republic of Germany

Ronald Duncan Hunt, D.V.M.
Professor of Comparative Pathology
Harvard Medical School
New England Regional Primate Research Center
One Pine Hill Drive, Southborough, MA 01772, USA

ISBN 978-3-642-83518-6   ISBN 978-3-642-83516-2 (eBook)
DOI 10.1007/978-3-642-83516-2

Library of Congress Cataloging-in-Publication Data.
Nervous system / T.C.Jones, U.Mohr, R.D.Hunt (eds.).
p. cm. - (Monographs on pathology of laboratory animals)
Includes bibliographies and index.
ISBN 0-387-19416-9 (U.S.)
1. Nervous system - Diseases - Animal models. I. Jones, Thomas Carlyle.
II. Mohr, U. (Ulrich) III. Hunt, Ronald Duncan. IV. Series.
[DNLM: 1. Animals, Laboratory. 2. Nervous System Diseases - pathology.
3. Nervous System Diseases - veterinary. 4. Nervous System Neoplasms -
pathology.   WL 100   N4561]
RC337.N46   1988   616.8'0072'4 - dc19   DNLM/DLC   88-24760

© Springer-Verlag Berlin Heidelberg 1988
Softcover reprint of the harcover 1st edition 1988

Typesetting, Printing, and Binding: Appl, Wemding

Foreword

The International Life Sciences Institute (ILSI) was established in 1978 to stimulate and support scientific research and educational programs related to nutrition, toxicology, and food safety, and to encourage cooperation in these programs among scientists in universities, industry, and government agencies to assist in the resolution of health and safety issues.

To supplement and enhance these efforts, ILSI has made a major commitment to supporting programs to harmonize toxicological testing, to advance a more uniform interpretation of bioassay results worldwide, to promote a common understanding of lesion classifications, and to encourage wide discussion of these topics among scientists. The *Monographs on the Pathology of Laboratory Animals* are designed to facilitate communication among those involved in the safety testing of foods, drugs, and chemicals. The complete set will cover all organ systems and is intended for use by pathologists, toxicologists, and others concerned with evaluating toxicity and carcinogenicity studies. The international nature of the project – as reflected in the composition of the editorial board and the diversity of the authors and editors – strengthens our expectations that understanding and cooperation will be improved worldwide through the series.

Alex Malaspina
President
International Life Sciences Institute

Preface

This book, on the nervous system, is the sixth volume of a set prepared under the sponsorship of the International Life Sciences Institute (ILSI). One aim of this set on the Pathology of Laboratory Animals is to provide information which will be useful to pathologists, especially those involved in studies on the safety of foods, drugs, chemicals, and other substances in the environment. It is expected that this and future volumes will contribute to better communication, on an international basis, among people in government, industry, and academia who are involved in protection of the public health.

The arrangement of this volume is based, in part, upon the philosophy that the first step toward understanding a pathologic lesion is its precise and unambiguous identification. The microscopic and ultrastructural features of a lesion that are particularly useful to the pathologist for definitive diagnosis, therefore, are considered foremost. Diagnostic terms preferred by the author and editors are used as the subject heading for each pathologic lesion. Synonyms are listed, although most are not preferred and some may have been used erroneously in prior publications. The problems arising in the differential diagnosis of similar lesions are considered in detail. The biologic significance of each pathologic lesion is considered under such headings as etiology, natural history, pathogenesis, and frequency of occurrence under natural or experimental conditions.

Comparison of information available on similar lesions in man and other species is valuable as a means to gain broader understanding of the processes involved. Knowledge of this nature is needed to form a scientific basis for safety evaluations and experimental pathology. References to pertinent literature are provided in close juxtaposition to the text in order to support conclusions in the text and lead toward additional information. Illustrations are an especially important means of nonverbal communication, especially among pathologists, and therefore constitute important features of each volume.

The subject under each heading is covered in concise terms and is expected to stand alone, but in some instances it is important to refer to other parts of the volume. A comprehensive index is provided to enhance the use of each volume as a reference.

Some omissions are inevitable and we solicit comments from our colleagues to identify parts which need strengthening or correcting. We have endeavored to include important lesions which a pathologist might encounter in studies involving the rat, mouse, or hamster. Newly recognized lesions or better understanding of old ones may make revised editions necessary in the future.

The editors wish to express our deep gratitude to all of the individuals who have helped with this enterprise. We are indebted to each author and member of the Editorial Board whose names appear elsewhere in the volume. We are especially grateful to the Officers and Board of Trustees of the International Life Sciences Institute for their support and understanding. Several people have worked directly on important details in this venture. These include Mrs. Nina Murray,

Executive Secretary; Mrs. Ann Balliett, Editorial Assistant; Mrs. June Armstrong, Medical Illustrator; Mrs. Katie A. Parker, Secretary; and Mrs. Virginia Werwath, Administrative Assistant. Ms. Sharon K. Coleman, ILSI Coordinator for External Affairs, Ms. Karen A. Taylor, ILSI Manager, Publications, and Ms. Sharon Senzik, Administrator of the ILSI Washington office, were helpful on many occasions.
We are particularly grateful to Dr. Dietrich Götze and his staff at Springer-Verlag for the quality of the published product.

June 1988   THE EDITORS

                                             T. C. Jones
                                             U. Mohr
                                             R. D. Hunt

Table of Contents

List of Contributors

Hisashi Aikawa, M.D.
Chief, Neuroanatomy & Neuropathology Section
National Institute of Neuroscience
Tokyo, Japan

Roger H. Alison, BVSc, MRCVS
National Toxicology Program
Research Triangle Park, North Carolina, USA

Holger Altenkirch, M.D.
Associate Professor of Neurology
Department of Neurology, Freie Universität Berlin
Berlin, Federal Republic of Germany

Stephen W. Barthold, D.V.M., Ph.D.
Associate Professor, Yale University School of Medicine
New Haven, Connecticut, USA

Michael J. Buchmeier, B.S., M.S., Ph.D.
Associate Member, Department of Immunology
Scripps Clinic and Research Foundation
La Jolla, California, USA

Heinrich Ernst, D.V.M.
Hannover Medical College
Hannover, Federal Republic of Germany

Robert H. Garman, B.S., D.V.M.
Senior Research Scientist, Carnegie-Mellon Institute of Research
Bushy Run Research Center
Export, Pennsylvania, USA

Susan M. Hall, B.Sc., Ph.D.
Senior Lecturer, Department of Anatomy
United Medical and Dental Schools
London Bridge, England

Jerry F. Hardisty, D.V.M.
Director, Experimental Pathology Laboratories
Research Triangle Park, North Carolina, USA

Toshiaki Hasegawa, B.S.
Senior Investigator, Shionogi Research Laboratories
Osaka, Japan

Yuzo Hayashi, M.D., Ph.D.
Chief, Department of Pathology
National Institute of Hygienic Sciences
Tokyo, Japan

Asao Hirano, M.D.
Head, Division of Neuropathology,
Montefiore Hospital & Medical Center
Professor, Department of Pathology & Neuroscience,
Albert Einstein College of Medicine
New York, New York, USA

Fusahiro Ikuta, M.D.
Professor and Chairman
Department of Pathology, Niigata University
Niigata, Japan

Robert O. Jacoby, D.V.M., Ph.D.
Professor and Chairman
Section of Comparative Medicine, Yale University
New Haven, Connecticut, USA

Bernard S. Jortner, V.M.D.
Professor of Pathology
Virginia-Maryland Regional College of Veterinary Medicine
Blacksburg, Virginia USA

Michael W. Kalichman, Ph.D.
Assistant Professor of Anesthesiology, University of California
San Diego, California, USA

Makoto Koga, D.M.Sc., M.D.
Associate Professor of Neuropathology
Neurological Institute, Faculty of Medicine, Kyushu University
Fukuoka, Japan

Georg J. Krinke, MVDr
Research Associate
Department of Toxicological Pathology, CIBA-GEIGY AG
Basel, Switzerland

Akihiko Maekawa, M.D., Ph.D.
Chief, Department of Chemical Pathology
National Institute of Hygienic Sciences
Tokyo, Japan

Robert Maronpot, D.V.M., M.S., M.P.H.
Head, Experimental Pathology
National Toxicology Program
Research Triangle Park, North Carolina, USA

Yasuhiko Matsuki, Ph.D.
Chief, Pharmacokinetic Laboratory
Hatano Research Institute, Food and Drug Safety Center
Kanagawa, Japan

Kunitoshi Mitsumori, D.V.M., Ph.D.
National Toxicology Program
Research Triangle Park, North Carolina, USA

Ulrich Mohr, M.D.
Professor of Experimental Pathology
Hannover Medical College
Hannover, Federal Republic of Germany

Kevin T. Morgan, B. V. Sc., Ph. D., M. R. C. Path.
Chemical Industry Institute of Toxicology
Research Triangle Park, North Carolina, USA

Robert R. Myers, Ph. D.
Associate Professor, Anesthesiology and Neurosciences
School of Medicine, University of California
La Jolla, California, USA

Henry C. Powell, M. D., B. Ch., M. R. C. Path.
Professor of Pathology
School of Medicine, University of California
La Jolla, California, USA

Karen S. Regan, D. V. M.
Teaching and Research Associate in Pathology
College of Veterinary Medicine
Urbana, Illinois, USA

Kenneth R. Reuhl, Ph. D.
Associate Professor
Department of Pharmacology & Toxicology
School of Pharmacy, Rutgers University
New Jersey, USA

Jerry M. Rice, Ph. D.
Chief, Laboratory of Comparative Carcinogenesis
National Institutes of Health, National Cancer Institute
Frederick, Maryland, USA

Bernhard Ryffel, M. D.
Assistant Professor, Pharmacology Division, SANDOZ
Pratteln, Switzerland

Dr. Yuji Sato
Department of Neuropathology, Kyushu University
Fukuoka, Japan

John A. Shadduck, D. V. M., Ph. D.
Professor and Head
Department of Veterinary Pathobiology
College of Veterinary Medicine
Urbana, Illinois, USA

Winslow G. Sheldon, D. V. M.
Pathology Associates, Inc.
Jefferson, Arkansas, USA

Masayuki Shintaku, M. D.
Assistant Professor
Department of Pathology, Kansai Medical University, Japan
Visiting Fellow, Division of Neuropathology
Montefiore Medical Center
Bronx, New York, New York, USA

Steven A. Stefanski, D. V. M., M. S.
Staff Pathologist, National Toxicology Program-NIEHS
Research Triangle Park, North Carolina, USA

Gisela Stoltenburg-Didinger, M.D.
Associate Professor of Neuropathology
Freie Universität Berlin
Berlin, Federal Republic of Germany

Kinuko Suzuki, M.D.
Professor Department of Pathology
University of North Carolina
Chapel Hill, North Carolina, USA

James A. Swenberg, D.V.M., Ph.D.
Head, Department of Biochemical Toxicology and Pathobiology
Chemical Industry Institute of Toxicology
Research Triangle Park, North Carolina, USA

Michihito Takahashi, M.D., Ph.D.
Chief, Department of Pathology
National Institute of Hygienic Sciences
Tokyo, Japan

Jun Tateishi, D.M.Sc., M.D.
Chairman, Department of Neuropathology
Neurological Institute, Faculty of Medicine, Kyushu University
Kyushu, Japan

Dale M. Walker, D.V.M.
Staff Pathologist, Experimental Pathology Laboratories, Inc.
Research Triangle Park, North Carolina, USA

Vernon E. Walker, D.V.M.
Chemical Industry Institute of Toxicology
Research Triangle, Park North Carolina, USA

Jerrold M. Ward, D.V.M., Ph.D.
Chief, Tumor Pathology and Pathogenesis Section
Laboratory of Comparative Carcinogenesis, National Cancer Institute
Frederick, Maryland, USA

Kathryn E. Wright, B.A., M.A., M.Sc., Ph.D.
Post-doctoral Research Fellow, Canadian Arthritis Society
Scripps Clinic and Research Foundation
La Jolla, California, USA

Yasuji Yoshida, M.D.
Department of Neuropathology
Brain Research Institute, Niigata University
Niigata, Japan

Shinsuke Yoshimura, D.V.M.
Hatano Research Institute, Food and Drug Safety Center
Kanagawa, Japan

Microvasculature in Experimental Glioma and Developing Brain, Rat

Yasuji Yoshida and Fusahiro Ikuta

Introduction

In this report we describe the microvascular morphology of the experimental astrocytoma (2 mm or less in diameter) produced in nude mice (Yoshida 1983) and compare the architectural characteristics of the microvasculature with that of the developing rat cerebellum (Yoshida et al. 1985).

Experimental Methods

Experimental gliomas in the rat brain (astrocytoma, oligodendroglioma, ependymoma, mixed glioma, and/or undifferentiated glioma) may be induced by transplacental exposure to ethylnitrosourea (ENU) (Jänisch and Rath 1979). In general, these neoplasms develop in the cerebral parenchyma and form solid tumors with whitish or semitranslucent, gelatinous appearance and with borders relatively well demarcated from cerebral tissue. When the size of the tumor reaches 4-5 mm in diameter, it is often accompanied by multiple hemorrhagic foci around blood vessels and in necrotic areas of the tumor. The growth of these neoplasms to the point when clinical signs are evident requires several months after exposure.

Similar gliomas may also be produced in the brains of nude mice by intracerebral inoculation of viable cells of the rat glioma, C-6. This is a glioma cell line established in vitro, after induction by ENU (Benda et al. 1968). In the brain of the nude mouse, the tumor grows rapidly for 15-20 days after inoculation (Fig. 1). These transplanted tumors have some advantages as experimental models for studying the vascular system in the neoplasm because an expected size of growing tumor is reached by a specific time following transplantation, and the histology of the tumor is consistently of an anaplastic astrocytoma. In gross appearance, the tumor tissue is eas-

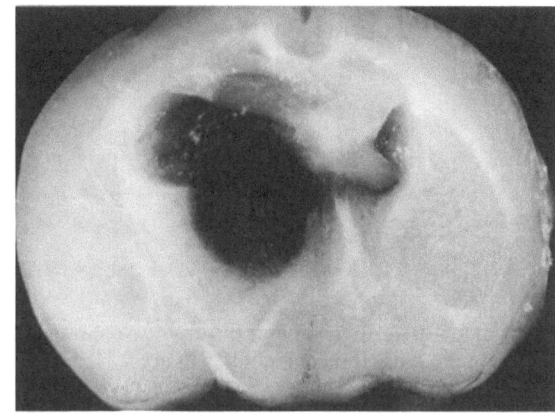

Fig. 1. Experimental glioma in a nude mouse cerebrum. A large tumor grown in the left basal ganglia and stained by Evans' blue, ×10

ily discerned by staining with Evan's blue administered intravenously before sacrifice. This staining indicates leakage of the dye from the vascular bed because of an impaired blood-brain barrier.

Microscopic Features

Induced Gliomas. The tumor grown in the mouse cerebral parenchyma is made up of a solid mass which displaces the cerebral cortex or basal ganglia, but, at the border, tumor cells usually infiltrate into the cerebral parenchyma with no capsule formation. In animals employed in this study, the maximal diameter of the tumor is less than 2 mm, and necrotic or hemorrhagic foci are not recognized in the tumor. Histologically, tumor cells are diffusely arranged and frequently include mitotic figures (Fig. 2).

Their nuclei are pleomorphic, contain prominent nucleoli, and their cytoplasm is spindle- or star-shaped, containing some fine glial fibrillary acidic protein. No mixture of oligodendroglial or immature cell components is evident. Thus, this

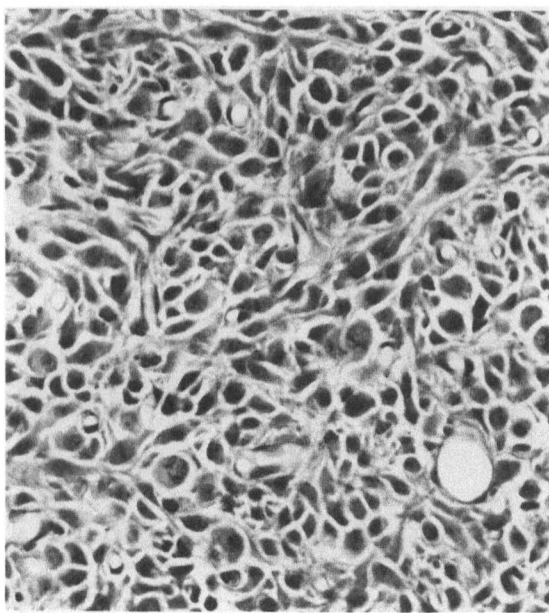

Fig. 2. Anaplastic astrocytoma in the brain. Note nuclear pleomorphysm and frequent mitotic figures. H and E, ×340

tumor is considered to be an anaplastic astrocytoma.

Under the light microscope the vascular density of this astrocytoma is seen to be definitely increased in comparison to that of surrounding cerebral cortex.

The blood vessels with conspicuously thin walls vary in diameter from 8 to 20 µm in size. However, the vascular structure of "glomerular tuft," which can be seen frequently in human gliomas, is not usually observed. However, we have observed structures of the glomerular tuft in the ENU-induced glioma in rats which survived more than 8–10 months.

Fetal Rat Cerebellum. It is well known that the cerebellum has a specific pattern of cell growth and kinetics during its normal development (Altman 1972). The matrix cell layer which produces neuroblasts is formed on the outermost layer of the cerebellum. During the first 4 postnatal days, this layer grows rapidly by division of the external granule cells. Many irregularly shaped vascular lumina with thin walls can be observed during this period at the subarachnoid space covering the external granular layer, although only a few penetrating vessels are recognizable in the external granular layer or other parts of the cerebellar parenchyma (Yoshida et al. 1985).

Ultrastructure

Microvasculature of Glioma and Adjacent Brain. Scanning electron-microscopic (SEM) studies of vascular casts (Kessel and Kardon 1979; Yoshida and Ikuta 1984) of the tumor were undertaken to obtain three-dimensional views of the vasculature. At the border zone between the cerebral cortex and glioma, apparently normal capillaries of relatively uniform diameter (5–7 µm) and constant arborizing patterns were seen to connect directly with vessels in the tumor (Fig. 3). Within the tumor the diameters of the blood vessels were definitely increased, the majority of them were 15–20 µm, and their pattern also became irregular and tortuous.

In the central portion of the tumor, the complex vascular architecture was indicated by multiple nodular protrusions on the casts (Fig. 4), and septum formation within the casts and ring structures (Figs. 5, 6). Some of the nodular protrusions were elongated and anastomosed frequently with each other, resulting in increased vascular density (Fig. 5). Although these casts do not always demonstrate the detail of vascular sproutings at the pre-existing terminals, which have been shown by rapid Golgi preparations (Marin-Padilla 1985), we must consider from the endothelial cell kinetics that DNA synthesis is not confined to the pre-existing terminals, but is also widely distributed within endothelial cells of microvessels in the tumors. Evidence for this was provided by the immunohistochemical demonstration of bromodeoxyuridine, an analog of thymidine, incorporated into the endothelial cells. Therefore, the three-dimensional architecture of neovascularization in the glioma was demonstrated by our SEM findings.

The fine structures of the blood vessels in the glioma differ in some respects from that of adult normal brain capillaries. The endothelial cells in the glioma usually have immature nuclei with larger and more irregular shape and numerous mitotic figures. Their abundant cytoplasm is rich in intracytoplasmic organellae and frequently contains Weibel-Palade bodies (Hirano and Matsui 1975). Increased numbers of pinocytic vesicles and endothelial pores have also been observed.

Although it is still in controversy whether these endothelial cells are neoplastic or reactive as a part of the mesenchymal stroma in the glioma, these vascular findings are not specific to the tumor because similar structures are also observed during developing stages of other blood vessels.

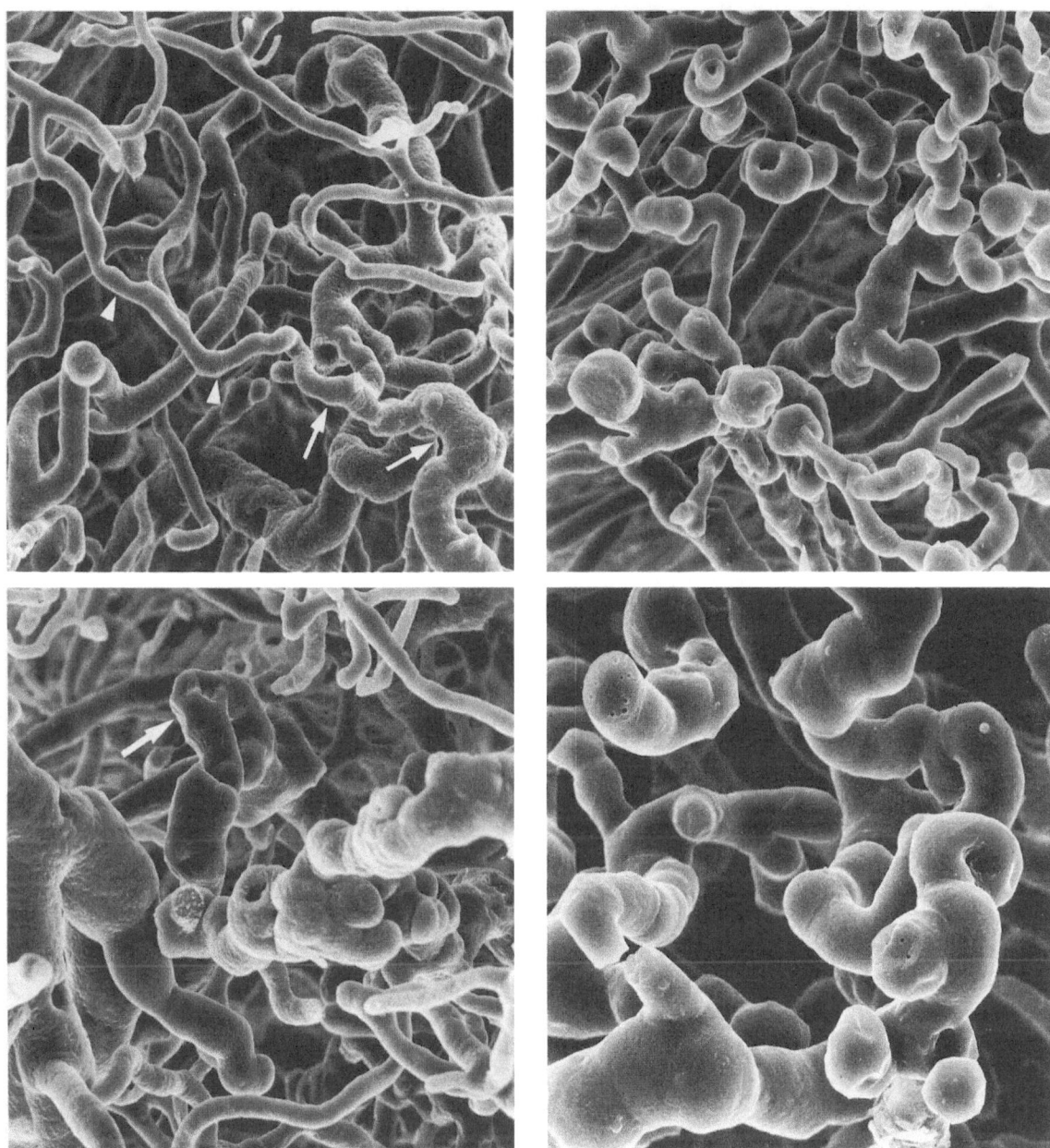

Fig. 3 *(upper left)*. Vascular architecture of corrosion casts at the border zone of the astrocytoma. Capillaries with normal appearance *(arrow heads)* in the surrounding brain are connected with dilated and tortuous vessels in the neoplasm *(arrows)*. SEM, × 330

Fig. 4 *(lower left)*. Corrosion casts of blood vessels within the tumor. Note many nodular protrusions on the casts and a ring structure of the vessels *(arrow)*. SEM, × 440

Fig. 5 *(upper right)*. Corrosion cast of the tumor. Note polymorphic microvascular architecture of the tumor, nodular protrusions of the casts and their elongation and intricate network causing increased vascular density. SEM, × 420

Fig. 6 *(lower right)*. Corrosion cast of the tumor. Note ring structures of the small vessels. SEM, × 840

4   Yasuji Yoshida and Fusahiro Ikuta

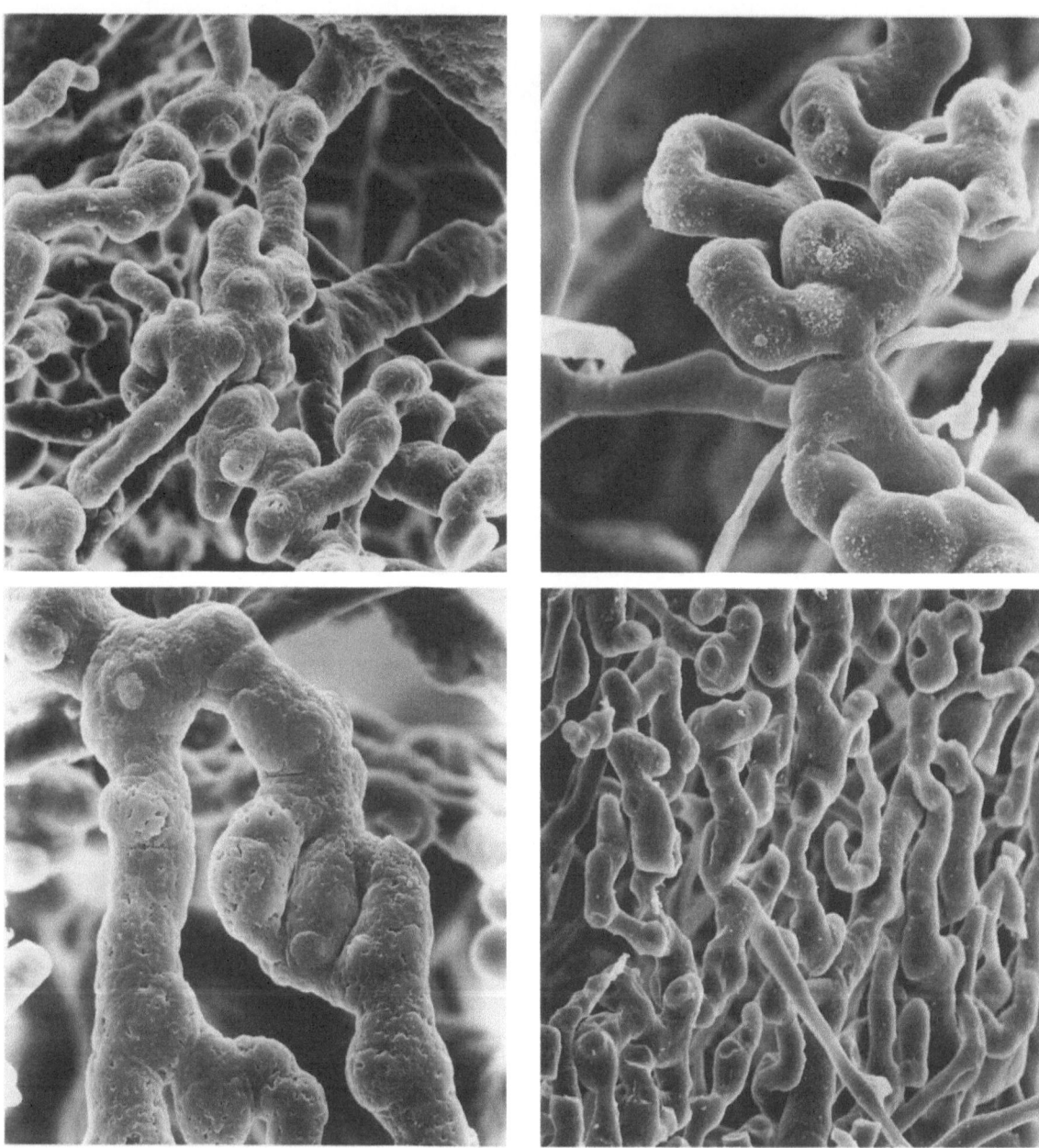

Fig. 7 *(upper left)*. Normal rat cerebellum at the 2nd postnatal day. Note vascular architecture in the subarachnoid space with nodular protrusions on the casts and their elongation. SEM, × 390

Fig. 8 *(lower left)*. Septum formations within the dilated vessels at the same developing stage of Fig. 7. SEM, × 680

Fig. 9 *(upper right)*. Ring structures of the vessels at the same developing stage of Fig. 7. SEM, × 720

Fig. 10 *(lower right)*. Increased number of small vessels in the subarachnoid space at the 4th postnatal day, rat. SEM, × 450

Microvasculature of the Fetal Cerebellum. The developing microvascular architecture of the rat cerebellum during the first 4 postnatal days, observed by using the casting method combined with SEM, was revealed to be essentially analogous with that of the glioma. Similarities were

evident in the multiple nodular protrusions on the casts, some of which were elongated (Fig. 7), septum formation within the dilated portion of the casts (Fig. 8), and ring structures of the casts (Fig. 9). These structural alterations, widely observed on the vessels of the cerebellar surface

Discussion and Conclusions

The blood vessels in the human glioma are known to play an important role in the clinical and biologic behavior of the tumor (Folkman and Cotran 1976; Hossmann et al. 1979; Vick 1980). In addition to the expansive growth of the glioma, accompanied by intensified blood supply and increased density of the vascular bed, the impaired blood-brain barrier in the glioma produces intractable but biologically ingenious brain edema for neoplastic cell motility in the extracellular space and surrounding cerebral tissue (Ikuta et al. 1979). Furthermore, chemotherapeutic measures against the glioma are partly dependent on this pathophysiology of the impaired blood-brain barrier (Vick 1980). Morphologic details concerning the neovascularization in the glioma are essential features in understanding its biologic properties. In fine structural studies previously reported, most attention has been paid to disclosing the specificity of the blood vessels in the glioma.

In this experimental study, we demonstrated the three-dimensional microvasculature of the intricate network in the glioma. Cerebral capillaries surrounding the neoplasm were found to be directly connected with the microvessels in the tumor. Corrosion cast of these vessels in the tumor revealed alterations in morphology involving diameter, pattern, and anastomosing channels. Among these vascular networks some of the principal microvascular architecture was considered as the profile of neovascularization. These consisted of nodular protrusions on the casts, septum formation within the lumina, and small ring formations of the vessels. All of these seemed to possess a close interrelationship of alternative structures during vascular proliferation. The most interesting point in this study is that these features are not confined to the glioma, but normal brain contains similar structures during its neonatal vascular development. This means that vascular proliferation in both the glioma and developing brain has analogies in the architectural pattern, although the underlying mechanism is unknown.

Acknowledgements. The authors wish to thank Dr. K. Yamazaki, and Dr. M. Yamada for their assistance. We are also grateful to Mr. T. Ichikawa, Mr. K. Kobayashi, Mr. S. Egawa, Miss S. Sekimoto, Mrs. Y. Tanahashi, Miss K. Murayama, and Mrs. A. Sasaki for their kind cooperation. This work was supported in part by Grants No.

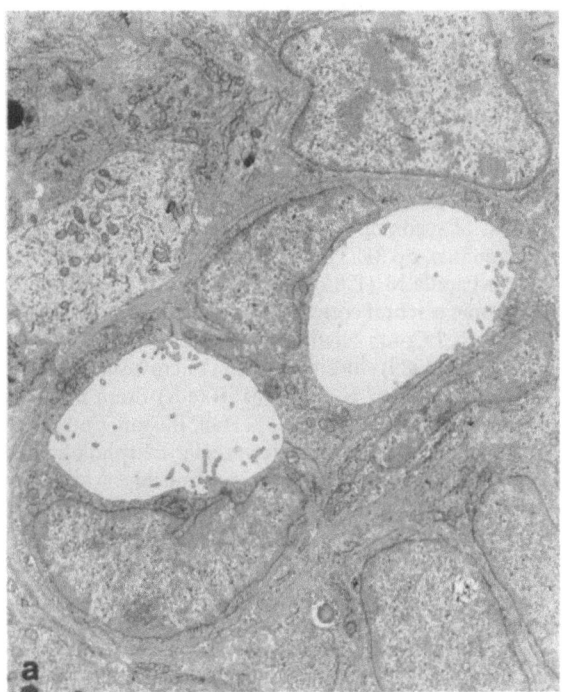

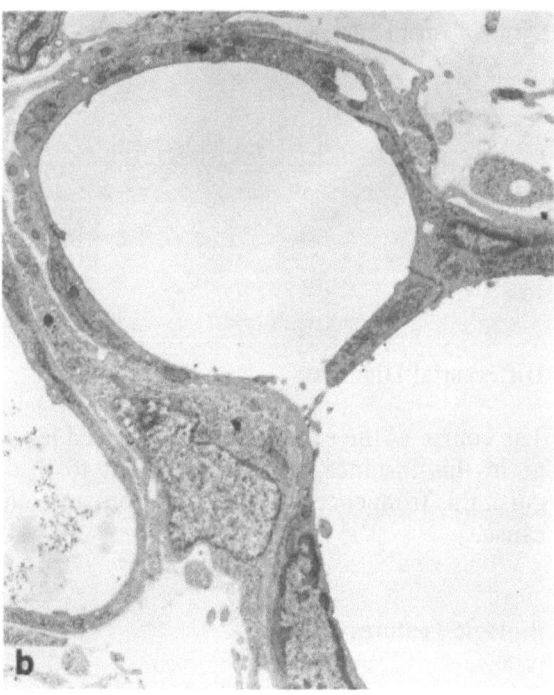

Fig. 11 a, b. Endothelial septation of the vascular lumina in the tumor (**a**) and developing cerebellum at the 2nd postnatal day (**b**). TEM, **a** x 5500, **b** × 6300

and often on the same tributaries, may indicate a close interrelationship of these structures. Several days after the 4th perinatal day, intricate networks of microvessels were formed to result in increased microvascular density (Figs. 10, 11 a, b).

60015024, 60440046, and 61570693 from the Ministry of Education, Science and Culture, Japan.

References

Altman J (1972) Postnatal development of the cerebellar cortex in the rat. I. The external germinal layer and the transitional molecular layer. J Comp Neurol 145: 353–397

Benda P, Lightbody J, Sato G, Levine L, Sweet W (1968) Differentiated rat glial cell strain in tissue culture. Science 161: 370–371

Folkman J, Cotran R (1976) Relation of vascular proliferation to tumor growth. In: Richter GW, Epstein MA (eds) International review of experimental pathology, vol 16. Academic, New York, pp 207–248

Hirano A, Matsui T (1975) Vascular structures in brain tumors. Hum Pathol 6: 611–621

Hossmann KA, Wechsler W, Wilmes F (1979) Experimental peritumorous edema. Morphological and pathophysiological observations. Acta Neuropathol (Berl) 45: 195–203

Ikuta F, Ohama E, Yamazaki K, Takeda S, Egawa S, Ichikawa T (1979) Morphology of migrating glial cells in normal development, neoplasia and other disorders. In: Zimmerman HM (ed) Progress in neuropathology, vol 4. Raven, New York, pp 377–405

Jänisch W, Rath FW (1979) Early stages of brain tumor development in experimental chemical carcinogenesis. In: Zimmermann HM (ed) Progress in neuropathology, vol 4. Raven, New York, pp 215–233

Kessel RG, Kardon RH (1979) Tissue and organs: a text-atlas of scanning electron microscopy. Freeman C, San Francisco, pp 35–310

Marin-Padilla M (1985) Early vascularization of the embryonic cerebral cortex. Golgi and electron microscopic studies. J Comp Neurol 241: 237–249

Vick NA (1980) Brain tumor microvasculature. In: Weiss L, Gilbert HA, Posner JB (eds) Brain metastasis, a monograph series; V2. GK Hall, Boston, pp 115–133

Yoshida Y (1983) Stereotoxic vascular morphology in experimental gliomas and its relationship with normal vascularization in the developmental stage. No To Shinkei 35: 619–627 (in Japanese; English abstr.)

Yoshida Y, Ikuta F (1984) Three-dimensional architecture of cerebral microvessels with a scanning electron microscope: a cerebrovascular casting method for fetal and adult rats. J Cereb Blood Flow Metab 4: 290–296

Yoshida Y, Ikuta F, Watabe K, Nagata T (1985) Developmental microvascular architecture of the rat cerebellar cortex. Anat Embryol (Berl) 171: 129–138

Experimental Allergic Encephalomyelitis, Rat

Bernhard Ryffel

Gross Appearance

At the injection site in the foot pad a chronic ulcerative lesion develops due to the adjuvant, and the regional popliteal lymph node is grossly enlarged. If supportive care is provided, most animals recover from acute experimental allergic encephalomyelitis and the extent of the central inflammatory process decreases gradually.

Microscopic Features

The histopathologic changes consist of perivascular inflammation mainly in the brain stem and spinal cord (Brosnan and Wisniewski 1980). In Fig. 12 one can see typical perivascular infiltrate in the brain stem consisting of monocytes and lymphocytes. At later stages slight demyelination and reactive gliosis are present. Similar lesions also occur in the spinal cord (Fig. 13).

Differential Diagnosis

The course of the experimentally induced lesions is, in this instance, usually sufficient to distinguish this from encephalomyelitis from any other cause.

Biologic Features

Etiology. A common method of inducing autoimmunity is to introduce an autoantigen together with complete Freund's adjuvant to break tolerance by by-passing various immunoregulatory pathways. These conditions can be induced in most normal strains of animals. However, in most cases, these diseases resemble the normal immune responses to heterologous antigens in that they are self-limiting due to homeostatic mechanisms in the immune system. To maintain a state of autoimmunity, there must be some inherent (e.g., the susceptibility of only certain

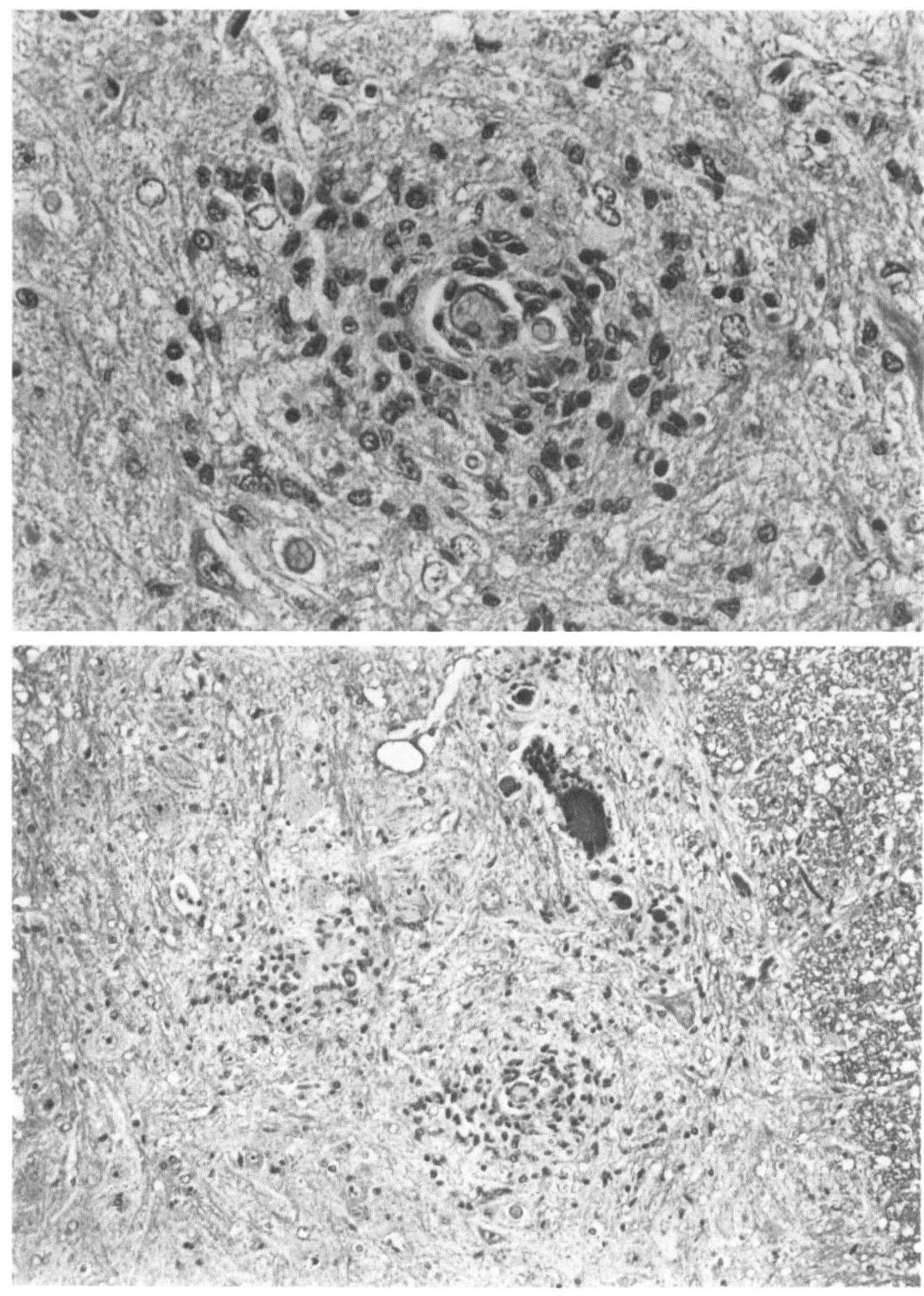

Fig. 12 *(above).* Perivascular infiltration in the brain stem in Lewis rat (14 days after immunization). H and E, × 400

Fig. 13 *(below).* Perivascular infiltration in the spinal cord in Lewis rat (14 days after immunization). H and E, × 210

strains of animals to various diseases) or induced (e.g. thymectomy and whole body irradiation) abnormalities in the immune system.

Experimental allergic encephalomyelitis is an autoimmune inflammatory disease of the central nervous system. It is induced in a variety of laboratory animals by a single injection of whole central nervous tissue or myelin basic protein in complete Freund's adjuvant. In adult animals, the disease is usually monophasic with clinical signs of weight loss, paralysis of hindquarters and incontinence occurring 10-14 days after sensitization. Depending on the adjuvant, which determines the severity of the disease, the animals either die or recover spontaneously within 1-2 weeks. Recovered animals of the adult age group usually have no relapse and are resistant to induction of a second disease. The main pathologic change in this monophasic disease is perivascular inflammation in the central nervous system with little demyelination. In contrast, sensitization of juvenile animals, especially immunodeficient strain 13 guinea pigs, leads to a relapsing-remitting form with extensive demyelination and formation of confluent plaques. In this respect experimental allergic encephalomyelitis bears several features in common with postinfectious encephalomyelitis and multiple sclerosis in man. Since the immunologic regulating mechanisms have been extensively investigated, there is a rational basis for specific intervention with several immunosuppressive agents (for general review, see Paterson 1978; Weigle 1980; Raine 1984; Vandenbark and Raus 1984).

Pathogenesis in Rats. Active experimental allergic encephalomyelitis is induced in the Lewis rat by a single injection of central nervous tissue in complete Freund's adjuvant, whereas passive disease is achieved by cellular transfer of specific reactive cells. The active acute paralytic disease appears about 10 days after sensitization and the rats recover within 7 days. The passive transfer of 10^7 cultured spleen cells (2-3 days culture in the presence of mitogen or myelin basic protein) from actively sensitized donor rats results in clinical disease within 5 days.

Immunoregulation of Experimental Allergic Encephalomyelitis. The immunologic mechanisms responsible for induction, expression and recovery of the disease have been studied extensively (Weigle 1980; Vandenbark and Raus 1984) and will be summarized.

Neuroantigens. Experimental allergic encephalomyelitis is usually induced by injection of crude nervous tissue extract emulsified in complete Freund's adjuvant, which is essential for actively induced disease. Neuroantigens given in incomplete Freund's adjuvant do not cause clinical signs but confer resistance to the animals upon a second immunization. The neuroantigens have been characterized as myelin basic proteins with a molecular weight of 18 Kd, and the structural requirement for disease induction and/or prevention has been identified (Arnon 1981).

Cell-Mediated Immune Reaction. The mononuclear cell infiltrate, consisting mainly of T lymphocytes with the helper cell phenotype, and antigen-presenting cells are typical of a cell-mediated immune reaction (Hickey and Gonatas 1984). Circumstantial evidence supports the view that the lesions are mediated by lymphocytes of the T_{DTH} subset. Conclusive evidence for a cell-mediated immune response is derived from adoptive cell transfer experiments: serum from diseased animals does not cause encephalomyelitis in recipients, but transfer of lymph node cells from diseased animals causes paralysis in recipient rats (Peters and Hinrichs 1982). The immune reaction against the relevant antigen depends on antigen presentation. Antigen presentation is mediated by macrophages in the draining lymph nodes after local sensitization. Recently, an antigen-presenting function of astrocytes in the central nervous system has been proposed since astrocytes have the capability to activate myelin basic protein-specific T cell lines in vitro (Fontana et al. 1984; Schnyder et al. 1986). Furthermore, cerebral vascular endothelial cells express class II histocompatibility antigens and present antigen as shown by elegant in vitro techniques (McCarron et al. 1986). Evidence for the importance of an intact B-lymphocytic compartment for the induction of active disease in rats was reported by Willenborg et al. (1986). Immunoglobulin-deficient rats did not develop the disease after sensitization with myelin basic protein in complete Freund's adjuvant.

Suppressor Cells. After recovery of actively induced encephalomyelitis the animals are resistant to a second active disease induction. Resistance after recovery of actively induced encephalomyelitis was shown to be mediated by T suppressor cells. Furthermore, adoptive transfer of these suppressor cells conferred resistance to naive recipient animals (Adda et al. 1977).

Cellular Transfer of Experimental Allergic Encephalomyelitis. Direct transfer of a large number of lymph node cells from paralyzed animals results in disease in recipient animals. The adoptive transfer is only possible between inbred animals indicating genetic restriction of the immune reaction. Direct transfer experiments need large cell numbers ($> 10^8$ cells), but adoptive transfer of cells after a short incubation in vitro are possible with lower cell numbers. In this culture-enhanced transfer system, lymph node or spleen cells from paralyzed rats are cultured in vitro in the presence of myelin basic protein or a polyclonal activator. This step allows the proliferation and differentiation of T effector cells (Peters and Hinrichs 1982; Hinrichs et al. 1981). The cell number required for adoptive transfer of the disease can even be reduced by the use of specifically committed T effector cell lines or clones against myelin basic protein (Ben-Nun et al. 1981; Ben-Nun and Cohen 1982; Hayosh and Swanborg 1986).

In addition to these cellular transfer studies in rats, several groups have reported induction of chronic relapsing, demyelinating disease in mice by the transfer of myelin basic protein specific L3T4+ lymphocytes or clones (Mokhtarian et al. 1984; Zamvil et al. 1985; Lemire and Weigle 1986). In recent studies, it was shown that acute encephalomyelitis was also elicited in the absence of the thymus by specific T cells (Saka et al. 1986).

Recurrence of the disease is rare in young rats, but occurs more frequently in older animals and in females (McFarlin et al. 1974; Keith 1978). A chronic, relapsing form of experimental allergic encephalomyelitis was recently described as being produced by modifying the composition of the adjuvants (Feurer et al. 1985). Similarly, increasing the dose of *Bordetella pertussis* in the adjuvant mixture may result in a peracute form of the disease (Linthicum et al. 1982). Generally, rats which have recovered from acute allergic encephalomyelitis are resistant to active disease induction. By contrast, passive disease may be caused in these rats by passive transfer of reactive cells (see below).

Reinduction of Allergic Encephalomyelitis. Suppressor cells produced in animals recovering from active disease provide the control point that prevents antigen-dependent disease reinduction. The concept of immunoregulation by suppressor cells is strengthened by the transfer of suppression and radiosensitivity of suppressor cell activi-

Table 1. Development of allergic encephalomyelitis in rats. Actively induced disease compared with adoptively transferred disease

Primary treatment	Result	Secondary treatment	Result
BP-FCA	Disease, recovery	BP-FCA	No disease, resistance
BP-IFA	No disease	BP-FCA	No disease, resistance
BP-FCA	Disease, recovery	Cultured activated spleen cells	Disease, recovery
Cultured activated spleen cells	Disease, recovery	BP-FCA	Disease, recovery
Cultured activated spleen cells	Disease, recovery	Cultured activated spleen cells	Disease, recovery

BP, myelin basic protein; *FCA*, complete Freund's adjuvant; *IFA*, incomplete Freund's adjuvant.

ty. Specific suppression can also be demonstrated in recovered animals (Adda et al. 1977; Holda and Swanborg 1981; Hickey and Gonatas 1984).

Whereas antigen-induced disease is generally followed by resistance, the situation for the adoptive transfer of allergic encephalomyelitis is different. Table 1 summarizes the development of disease after primary or secondary induction with antigen or with culture-enhanced cell transfer. As shown, disease mediated by culture-enhanced transfer cells confers no resistance to a second challenge by either antigen or adoptive cell transfer. It appears that the suppressor cell development is dependent on antigen-driven events; recovery from adoptively transferred disease is not associated with regulatory responses (Hinrichs et al. 1981; Vandenbark and Raus 1984).

Requirements for Effector Cell Production. Priming of T cells from naive animals with the relevant antigen basic protein results in the emergence of a population of precursor cells reactive to basic protein. This precursor population does not cause the disease. After in vivo sensitization of animals with basic protein and complete Freund's adjuvant, the precursor cell population proliferates, differentiates, and matures in an effector cell population which most likely belongs to a subpopulation of T_{DTH}. The activated precursor cell population may also reach a final maturation state with effector function under appropriate culture conditions in the presence of basic protein. Added interleukin 2 to the in vitro culture accelerates the production of effector cells (Schluesener and Lassmann 1985). The need of antigen-presenting cells for the generation of reactive precursor and effector cells has been shown repeatedly. It is assumed that effector cells are short lived, which may explain the rapid recovery after adoptive transfer of allergic encephalomyelitis. Recovery from active disease is mediated by the emergence of suppressor T cells which inhibit the antigen-driven recruitment of precursor cells, decreased availability of precursor cells and rapid decay of effector cells (Hinrichs, cited in Vandenbark and Raus 1984).

Comparison with Other Species

Mice. A delayed and often-relapsing encephalomyelitis has been described especially for the female SJL strain after sensitization with murine spinal cord emulsion (with *B. pertussis* and complete Freund's adjuvant). In addition to the perivascular infiltration by mononuclear cells and acute demyelination, areas of chronic demyelination (plaques) are also observed (Lublin et al. 1981; Fritz et al. 1983). This model (with a relapsing course and morphologic lesions) reflects more closely the condition seen in human multiple sclerosis. The neuropathology of this model, in the absence of *B. pertussis* in complete Freund's adjuvant, has been described by Brown et al. (1982) in great detail. The same group of investigators also demonstrated the adoptive transfer of chronic relapsing allergic encephalomyelitis in the murine model (Raine et al. 1984).

Guinea Pigs. Chronic relapsing allergic encephalomyelitis may be produced, especially in juvenile guinea pigs of immunodeficient strain 13. The disease is characterized by delayed onset and a protracted course with spontaneous relapses. The histopathologic changes consist of perivascular infiltrates and extensive areas of demyelination (Raine and Stone 1977; Traugott et al. 1979). The perivascular infiltrates consist of T lymphocytes and, to a lesser extent, B lymphocytes (Sobel et al. 1984; Traugott et al. 1982). Although immunocompetent strain 2 guinea pigs do not develop clinical disease, distinct morphologic changes can be observed (Stone et al. 1983). A chronic progressive form of the disease has been described in adult guinea pigs given a high dose of neuroantigen (Wisniewski and Madrid 1983).

Similar lesions have been described in other species, including monkeys and dogs, after sensitization with neuroantigen.

Pharmacologic Modification of Experimental Allergic Encephalomyelitis

The knowledge of the immunologic and inflammatory mechanisms regulating this experimental disease allows the study of pharmacologic and immunologic interventions. Major therapeutic approaches are possible at the level of: (a) monocytes/macrophages; (b) lymphocytes; (c) vessels/endothelium. Although this distinction may be an oversimplification, it will facilitate an ordered discussion of the available data, which are by no means complete.

Inhibition at the Monocyte Level. Based on the assumption that tissue damage may be nonspecific due to products of mononuclear cells, Brosnan et al. (1981) investigated the effect of monocyte/macrophage depletion on the development of allergic encephalomyelitis in rats. Silica quartz dust, which has a selective toxicity for macrophages, given 8 or 11 days after sensitization, produced a significant delay of the disease. As functional reactive lymphocytes against myelin basic protein could be demonstrated, the results support the conclusion that cellular products from the monocyte/macrophage series function as mediators of tissue damage.

In support of an effector role of inflammatory cells are the studies using proteinase inhibitors: inhibition of the synthesis of plasminogen activator and other neutral proteinases give significant protection against allergic encephalomyelitis (Brosnan et al. 1980).

Activated macrophages liberate, among other factors, hydrogen peroxide and superoxide, which, in the presence of free iron, is converted to the highly toxic hydroxyl radical. Using desferroxamine B mesylate, which has iron-chelating properties, Bowern et al. (1984) reported suppression of clinical signs and lesions of allergic encephalomyelitis. Thus, prevention of toxic hydroxyl radical formation by reducing free iron concentration may inhibit nonspecific effector cell function. Inhibition of the antigen-presenting cell function with antibodies blocking recognition of class II histocompatibility antigens represents a further possible mechanism for modulation of the disease (Steinmann et al. 1981).

Inhibition at the Level of Lymphocytes. Modulation of antigen recognition, differentiation, and maturation of effector lymphocytes are possible by a variety of chemical immunosuppressants. The main drawback of this approach is the lack of tissue specificity, i. e., all proliferating cells are affected or destroyed. More specific interventions, e. g., selective effects on lymphocytes, including antibodies against T lymphocytes, vaccination, and the use of cyclosporine, will be discussed separately.

Chemical Immunosuppressants. Several chemotherapeutic agents, such as cyclophosphamide, methotrexate, and 6-mercaptopurine, have been investigated experimentally in allergic encephalomyelitis. Cyclophosphamide at a dose of 5 mg/kg prevented the development of the disease in rats (Paterson and Drobish 1969; Paterson and Hanson 1969). Administration of cyclophosphamide at the onset of the paralytic disease improved the clinical condition within 2–3 days and prevented the formation of perivascular infiltrates in the central nervous system. Furthermore, cyclophosphamide treatment of sensitized donors inhibited the adoptive lymphoid transfer of encephalomyelitis in syngeneic recipient rats. Finally, cyclophosphamide treatment of recipients of lymphoid cells from sensitized donors abrogated the development of the disease. Methotrexate, the folic acid antagonist, inhibited the development of lesions in guinea pigs (Brandriss 1963). Similar results were described for 6-mercaptopurine in rabbits and guinea pigs (Hoyer et al. 1962).

Radiation. Whole body X-radiation in rats prior to sensitization suppressed allergic encephalomyelitis whereas X-radiation after sensitization was without any effect (Paterson and Beisaw 1963). Whole body ultraviolet radiation of SJL/J mice prevented allergic encephalomyelitis, but had no effect after the disease was ongoing (Hauser et al. 1984). The preventive effect of ultraviolet irradiation most likely occurred at the level of antigen-presenting cells.

Vaccination. Immunization with a variety of peptides of the basic protein series may prevent the experimental disease. Another approach involves the immunization of rats with attenuated cell lines reactive against basic protein. Single inoculation of irradiated anti-basic protein cell lines conferred significant protection of rats against actively induced allergic disease, whereas no protection was found to be mediated by passive transfer of anti-basic protein cell lines (Ben-Nun and Cohen 1981).

Monoclonal Antibodies. Prior to the era of monoclonal antibodies, polyspecific sera were used successfully as immunosuppressants. The advent of monoclonal antibodies against selective immune cell subpopulations allows specific blockade and/or elimination of T cells or antigen-presenting cells. For example, the monoclonal antibody against L3T4+ lymphocytes (helper cells) prevented the development of allergic encephalomyelitis in mice (Waldor et al. 1985).

Steroids. In view of the potent immunosuppressive effect of glucocorticosteroids and adrenocorticotropic hormone (ACTH), the preventive effect by this agent was tested a long time ago (Kabat et al. 1952).

Inhibition at the Level of Small Vessels. The acute phase of experimental allergic encephalomyelitis is characterized by recruitment and entry of mononuclear cells into the central nervous system. A variety of mediators are released which facilitate the perivascular transit of inflammatory cells.
Depletion or inhibition of vasoactive amines were shown to modulate the course of allergic encephalomyelitis (Linthicum et al. 1982; Waxman et al. 1984). Alteration of the vascular tone by alpha-1 adrenergic receptor antagonists, e. g., prazosin, suppressed the disease (Brosnan et al. 1985). The effect observed with alpha-1 blockade is due to suppression of increased vascular permeability (Goldmuntz et al. 1986; Brosnan et al. 1986).

Effects of Cyclosporine on Experimental Allergic Encephalomyelitis. With the advent of cyclosporine, which is a noncytotoxic immunosuppressant with potent effects on T cell-mediated immune responses (Borel and Lafferty 1983; Borel 1986), a new wave of investigations on chemical immunosuppression of allergic encephalomyelitis was initiated. In the initial publication on biologic effects of cyclosporine, Borel et al. (1976) reported a preventive effect on induction of allergic encephalomyelitis in rats. These results agree with effects of cyclosporine on T cell functions and the importance of cellular mechanisms in allergic encephalomyelitis. The reader is referred to excellent reviews on this topic by Bolton et al. (1982a, b, c).

Table 2. Effect of cyclosporine on actively induced encephalomyelitis in Lewis rats

Preventive

Cyclosporine[a] (mg/kg/day)	Number of paralyzed rats per group[b]	EAE average grade		Delayed expression of EAE[c]
		Clinical	Histologic	
0	19/20	2.8	2.7	5/5
5	5/5	2.6	2.6	–
10	3/5	1.7	2.1	–
15	0/5	0	0.4	–
20	0/15	0	0	5/5
50	0/20	0	0	10/10

Therapeutic

Start of CS administration[d]	Number of paralyzed rats per group	EAE average grade	
		Clinical	Histologic
4	0/4	0	0
6	0/4	0	0.3
10	1/6	0.5	1.2
No CS	6/6	2.6	2.7

EAE, experimental allergic encephalomyelitis; *CS*, cyclosporine; *CNS*, central nervous system; *CFA*, complete Freund adjuvant.

[a] Cyclosporine was given orally concurrently with the CNS-CFA injection for 20 days.

[b] EAE incidence at days 10–15 post sensitization.

[c] EAE incidence after cessation of CS administration.

[d] CS treatment (50 mg/kg daily) was delayed by 4–10 days post sensitization.

Prevention of Experimental Allergic Encephalomyelitis by Cyclosporine. The effects of cyclosporine on the induction of allergic encephalomyelitis in Lewis rats sensitized with guinea pig spinal cord in suspended complete Freund adjuvant is shown in Table 2. Animals given cyclosporine at the rate of > 15 mg/kg daily did not develop the disease during the period of drug administration. Lower doses (10 and 5 mg/kg daily) had little or no effect on the disease. These results essentially confirm earlier published data (Borel et al. 1976; Ryffel et al. 1982; Hinrichs et al. 1983). The perivascular inflammatory changes were prevented by a dose of 20 mg/kg daily.

Delayed or Therapeutic Intervention with Cyclosporine in Allergic Encephalomyelitis. If administration of cyclosporine was delayed by 4, 6 or 8 days after sensitization, the disease was still prevented. In the therapeutic group (day 10, early signs of encephalomyelitis) the duration and severity of the paralytic disease was greatly reduced with cyclosporine at the rate of 50 mg/kg daily. The extent of the central nervous system changes were also attenuated (Table 2). Thus, cyclosporine affected later stages of allergic encephalomyelitis and had a beneficial effect when used therapeutically. These results are corroborated by other published data (Bolton et al. 1982a, b, c; Cammisuli and Feurer 1984).

Cyclosporine Inhibits Passive Allergic Encephalomyelitis. Upon intravenous transfer of $1-2 \times 10^7$ reactive cells conditioned in vitro from previously sensitized donors, recipient rats developed clinical disease within 5 days. Administration of cyclosporine (50 mg/kg daily) to recipients, commencing concurrently with the cellular transfer, inhibited the development of the passive allergic encephalomyelitis (Bolton et al. 1982a; Ryffel et al. 1982). However, inhibition was only observed at this high dose since lower doses of cyclosporine failed to inhibit the adoptively transferred disease (Hinrichs et al. 1983).

Suppression of Allergic Encephalomyelitis Depends on the Availability of Cyclosporine. As already reported (Ryffel et al. 1982), all sensitized rats developed the disease after termination of cyclosporine treatment (Table 2). Encephalomyelitis occurred on days 28–33, i.e., 8–13 days after the last dose of cyclosporine. Prolonged administration of cyclosporine (25 mg/kg daily for 40 days) did not prevent the development of disease upon cessation of drug administeration, indicating that this drug does not eliminate T effector precursor cells, and the disease may develop as long as the neuroantigen is available in lymphoid tissues.

Effect of Cyclosporine on Suppressor Mechanisms. Recovery after an actively induced disease results in resistance to rechallenge with the neuroantigen which is mediated by suppressor T cells. Similarly, rats developing encephalomyelitis after cessation of administration of the drug and after recovery are resistant to reinduction of the disease, indicating that cyclosporine did not impair this suppressive mechanism. The results also indicate that concomitant treatment with the drug does not allow the induction of suppressor T cells since all the rats treated preventively developed the disease after withdrawal of the drug. This may be due to the fact that the mechanism which inhibits the induction of encephalomyelitis effector T cells is also operative for the induction of suppressor T cells (Hinrichs et al. 1981).

Thus, prevention of the disease at this level of the immune system will not result in resistance to it. Resistance may, however, be obtained by cytotoxic drugs which eliminate all functional T cells (Paterson and Drobish 1969).

Cyclosporine Inhibits the Development of Encephalomyelitis-Reactive T Cells In Vitro. Since cyclosporine inhibits mitogen- and antigen-induced proliferation, it was of interest to determine whether it would have an effect on the in vitro conditioning step required for passive transfer of the disease with immune spleen cells. Cyclosporine at concentrations of 100–1000 ng/ml completely prevented the development of active cells which transfer allergic encephalomyelitis (Ryffel et al. 1982; Bolton et al. 1982b; Hinrichs et al. 1983). If the drug was added 24 or 48 hours after the initiation of the mitogen- or antigen-stimulated culture, the cells transferred the disease. This result agrees with the established finding that cyclosporine suppresses an in vitro immune response only if present from the start of culture (Wiesinger and Borel 1980).

Effects of Cyclosporine on Experimental Allergic Encephalomyelitis in Other Animal Species

Guinea Pigs. Davison and Cuzner (1980) reported the effects of cyclosporine in the acute model of guinea pigs. Administration of the drug commencing with the antigen injection conferred almost a complete protection, especially in females. A significant therapeutic effect was shown when administration was started at the onset of disease.

Relapsing-Remitting Experimental Allergic Encephalomyelitis. This form, which closely reflects the lesions observed in human multiple sclerosis, may be induced in young animals, especially in strain 13 guinea pigs and in SJL mice. No information on the effects of cyclosporine in chronic allergic encephalomyelitis of guinea pigs is available. The chronic disease in SJL mice (Schuller-Levis et al. 1986) is inhibited by cyclosporine. The occurrence of chronic and/or relapsing encephalomyelitis in rats has been reported sporadically in the literature. In an attempt to study the effect of cyclosporine in a chronic progressive form of the disease with marked demyelination in splenectomized or thymectomized Lewis rats (Ben-Nun et al. 1980), the model was not reproducible (unpublished observation).

Rhesus Monkeys. Acute disease developing in rhesus monkeys after injection of nervous tissue in complete Freund's adjuvant can be inhibited by administration of cyclosporine (Borel 1981).

Summary of Experiments with Cyclosporine. This drug inhibits the development of encephalomyelitis in actively immunized Lewis rats, the minimal daily dose being 15 mg/kg daily. It also exerts a protective effect in other species and has an inhibitory effect in spite of delayed treatment. Furthermore, a therapeutic effect on the duration and/or severity of this disease is observed in several species.

The culture of encephalomyelitis-reactive cells with mitogen or antigen resulting in passive transfer of the disease depends, among other factors, on interleukin 2. Since cyclosporine effectively inhibits production of interleukin 2, the inability of cells cultured in the presence of cyclosporine to transfer the disease passively may be due to deficient interleukin 2 production.

The protection by cyclosporine lasts only as long as the compound is administered. All rats develop acute disease within 10–14 days after administration of the drug ceases. Suppressor mechanisms are present in rats recovered from actively induced disease. Cyclosporine does not affect this state of resistance. However, the failure to induce suppressor cells in the presence of cyclosporine may be due to the fact that the development of suppressor cells depends on a similar mechanism to that of T effector cells. Thus, the data do not necessarily indicate that cyclosporine has a detrimental effect on T suppressor cells, as recently suggested in the guinea pig model (Fredane et al. 1983). Passive encephalomyelitis may be inhibited by treatment of recipient rats by high doses of cyclosporine.

Conclusion. Experimental allergic encephalomyelitis is an interesting model of autoimmune disease of the central nervous system. Of particular interest are the chronic and recurring – remitting variants of the disease, which have some resemblance to pathologic lesions in the human central nervous system, especially multiple sclerosis. The pathogenesis of the latter disease, however, is still elusive (McFarlin and McFarland 1982; McKhann 1982). Recent reports from patients suffering from multiple sclerosis indicate that defective regulation of interleukin 2 receptors and modulation of T cell differentiation antigens on lymphocytes may represent a basic immunologic defect in multiple sclerosis (Antel et

14   Bernhard Ryffel

al. 1982; De Freitas et al. 1986). Progress in understanding of immunologic mechanisms regulating the experimental disease allowed an intervention with a variety of immunosuppressant agents of which cyclosporine is particularly interesting. Whether this latter drug will be useful in multiple sclerosis and related diseases of the central nervous system, for which presently no established therapy exists (Hommes et al. 1980), awaits further clinical trials.

References

Adda DH, Beraud E, Depieds R (1977) Evidence for suppressor cells in Lewis rats' experimental allergic encephalomyelitis. Eur J Immunol 7: 620–623

Antel J, Oger JJ, Jackevicius S, Kuo HH, Arnason BGW (1982) Modulation of T-lymphocyte differentiation antigens: potential relevance for multiple sclerosis. Proc Natl Acad Sci USA 79: 3330–3334

Arnon R (1981) Experimental allergic encephalomyelitis: susceptibility and suppression. Immunol Rev 55: 5–30

Ben-Nun A, Cohen IR (1981) Vaccination against autoimmune encephalomyelitis (EAE): attenuated autoimmune T lymphocytes confer resistance to induction of active EAE but not to EAE mediated by the intact T lymphocyte line. Eur J Immunol 11: 949–952

Ben-Nun A, Cohen IR (1982) Experimental autoimmune encephalomyelitis (EAE) mediated by T cell lines: process of selection of lines and characterization of the cells. J Immunol 129: 303–308

Ben-Nun A, Ron Y, Cohen IR (1980) Spontaneous remission of autoimmune encephalomyelitis is inhibited by splenectomy, thymectomy or ageing. Nature 288: 389–390

Ben-Nun A, Wekerle H, Cohen IR (1981) The rapid isolation of clonable antigen-specific T lymphocyte lines capable of mediating autoimmune encephalomyelitis. Eur J Immunol 11: 195–199

Bolton C, Borel JF, Cuzner ML, Davison AN, Turner AM (1982a) Immunosuppression by cyclosporin A of experimental allergic encephalomyelitis. J Neurol Sci 56: 147–153

Bolton C, Allsopp G, Cuzner ML (1982b) The effect of cyclosporin A on the adoptive transfer of experimental allergic encephalomyelitis in the Lewis rat. Clin Exp Immunol 47: 127–132

Bolton C, Borel JF, Cuzner ML, Davison AN, Turner AM (1982c) Autoimmunity: cyclosporin A therapy in experimental allergic encephalomyelitis. In: White DJG (ed) Cyclosporin A. Elsevier Biomedical, Amsterdam, pp 135–142

Borel JF (1981) Pharmacology and pharmacokinetics of cyclosporin A. In: Touraine JL et al. (eds) Transplantation and clinical immunology, vol 13. Excerpta Medica, Amsterdam, pp 3–6

Borel JF (ed) (1986) Cyclosporin. Prog Allergy 38: 9–18

Borel JF, Lafferty KJ (1983) Cyclosporine: speculation about its mechanism of action. Transplant Proc 15: 1881–1885

Borel JF, Feurer C, Gubler HU, Stahelin H (1976) Biological effects of cyclosporin A: a new antilymphocytic agent. Agents Actions 6: 468–475

Bowern N, Ramshaw IA, Clark IA, Doherty PC (1984) Inhibition of autoimmune neuropathological process by treatment with an iron-chelating agent. J Exp Med 160: 1532–1543

Brandriss MW (1963) Methotrexate: suppression of experimental allergic encephalomyelitis. Science 140: 186–187

Brosnan CF, Wisniewski HM (1980) Immunopathology of allergic encephalomyelitis. In: Batistin L, Hashim G, Lajtha A (eds) Neurochemistry and clinical neurology. Liss, New York, pp 379–390 (Progress in clinical and biological research series, vol 39)

Brosnan CF, Cammer W, Norton WT, Bloom BR (1980) Proteinase inhibitors suppress the development of experimental allergic encephalomyelitis. Nature 285: 235–237

Brosnan CF, Bornstein MB, Bloom BR (1981) The effects of macrophage depletion on the clinical and pathologic expression of experimental allergic encephalomyelitis. J Immunol 126: 614–620

Brosnan CF, Goldmuntz EA, Cammer W, Factor SM, Bloom BR, Norton WT (1985) Prazosin, an (alpha)₁-adrenergic receptor antagonist, suppresses experimental autoimmune encephalomyelitis in the Lewis rat. Proc Natl Acad Sci USA 82: 5915–5919

Brosnan CF, Sacks HJ, Goldschmidt RC, Goldmuntz EA, Norton WT (1986) Prazosin treatment during the effector stage of disease suppresses experimental autoimmune encephalomyelitis in the Lewis rat. J Immunol 137: 3451–3456

Brown A, McFarlin DE, Raine CS (1982) Chronologic neuropathology of relapsing experimental allergic encephalomyelitis in the mouse. Lab Invest 46: 171–185

Cammisuli S, Feurer C (1984) The effect of cyclosporin-A and dihydrocyclosporin-D on the therapy and prophylaxis of experimental allergic encephalomyelitis. Prog Clin Biol Res 146: 415–421

Davison AN, Cuzner ML (1980) The suppression of experimental allergic encephalomyelitis and multiple sclerosis. Academic, London

DeFreitas EC, Sandberg-Wollheim M, Schonely K, Boufal M, Koprowski H (1986) Regulation of interleukin 2 receptors on T cells from multiple sclerosis patients. Proc Natl Acad Sci USA 83: 2637–2641

Feurer C, Prentice DE, Cammisuli S (1985) Chronic relapsing experimental allergic encephalomyelitis in the Lewis rat. J Neuroimmunol 10: 159–166

Fontana A, Fierz W, Wekerle H (1984) Astrocytes present myelin basic protein to encephalitogenic T-cell lines. Nature 307: 273–276

Fredane LM, Hashim GA, McCabe RE (1983) The effect of cyclosporine on lymphocyte subsets in experimental allergic encephalomyelitis. Functional loss of disease-suppressing cells in vivo. Transplant Proc (Suppl) 15: 2909–2913

Fritz RB, Chou CHJ, McFarlin DE (1983) Relapsing murine allergic encephalomyelitis induced by myelin basic protein. J Immunol 130: 1024–1026

Goldmuntz EA, Brosnan CF, Norton WT (1986) Prazosin treatment suppresses increased vascular permeability in both acute and passively transferred experimental autoimmune encephalomyelitis in the Lewis rat. J Immunol 137: 3444-3450

Hauser SL, Weiner HL, Che M, Shapiro ME, Gilles F, Letvin NL (1984) Prevention of experimental allergic encephalomyelitis (EAE) in the SJL/J mouse by whole body ultraviolet irradiation. J Immunol 132: 1276-1281

Hayosh NS, Swanborg RH (1986) Autoimmune effector cells. VII. Cells isolated from thymus and spinal cord of rats with experimental allergic encephalomyelitis transfer disease. Am J Pathol 122: 218-222

Hickey WF, Gonatas NK (1984) Suppressor T-lymphocytes in the spinal cord of Lewis rats recovered from acute experimental allergic encephalomyelitis. Cell Immunol 85: 284-288

Hinrichs DJ, Roberts CM, Waxman FJ (1981) Regulation of paralytic experimental allergic encephalomyelitis in rats: susceptibility to active and passive disease reinduction. J Immunol 126: 1857-1862

Hinrichs DJ, Wegmann KW, Peters BA (1983) The influence of cyclosporin A on the development of actively induced and passively transferred experimental allergic encephalomyelitis. Cell Immunol 77: 202-209

Holda JH, Swanborg RH (1981) Regulation of experimental allergic encephalomyelitis. III. Demonstration of effector cells in tolerant rats. Eur J Immunol 11: 338-340

Hommes OR, Lamers KJB, Reekers P (1980) Effect of intensive immunosuppression on the course of chronic progressive multiple sclerosis. J Neurol 223: 177-190

Hoyer LW, Good RA, Condie RM (1962) Experimental allergic encephalomyelitis: the effect of 6-mercaptopurine. J Exp Med 116: 311-327

Kabat EA, Wolf A, Bezer AE (1952) Studies on acute disseminated encephalomyelitis produced experimentally in rhesus monkeys. VII. Effect of cortisone. J Immunol 68: 265-275

Keith AB (1978) Sex difference in Lewis rats in the incidence of recurrent experimental allergic encephalomyelitis. Nature 272: 824-825

Lemire JM, Weigle WO (1986) Passive transfer of experimental allergic encephalomyelitis by myelin basic protein-specific L3T4+ T cell clones possessing several functions. J Immunol 137: 3169-3174

Linthicum DS, Munoz JJ, Blaskett A (1982) Acute experimental autoimmune encephalomyelitis in mice. I. Adjuvant action of *Bordetella pertussis* is due to vasoactive amine sensitization and increased vascular permeability of the central nervous system. Cell Immunol 73: 299-310

Lublin FD, Maurer PH, Berry RG, Tippett D (1981) Delayed, relapsing, experimental allergic encephalomyelitis in mice. J Immunol 126: 819-822

McCarron RM, Spatz M, Kempski O, Hogan RN, Muehl L, McFarlin DE (1986) Interaction between myelin basic protein-sensitized T lymphocytes and murine cerebral vascular endothelial cells. J Immunol 137: 3428-3435

McFarlin DE, McFarland HF (1982) Multiple sclerosis. N Engl J Med 307: 1183-1188, 1246-1251

McFarlin D, Blank SE, Kibler RF (1974) Recurrent experimental allergic encephalomyelitis in the Lewis rat. J Immunol 113: 712-715

McKhann GM (1982) Multiple sclerosis. Annu Rev Neurosci 5: 219-239

Mokhtarian F, McFarlin D, Raine CS (1984) Adoptive transfer of myelin basic protein-sensitized T cells produces chronic relapsing demyelinating disease in mice. Nature 309: 356-359

Paterson PY (1978) Autoimmune neurological disease: experimental animal systems and implications for multiple sclerosis. In: Talal N (ed) Autoimmunity: genetic, immunologic, virologic and clinical aspects. Academic, New York, pp 644-691

Paterson PY, Beisaw NE (1963) Effect of whole body x-irradiation on induction of allergic encephalomyelitis in rats. J Immunol 90: 532-539

Paterson PY, Drobish DG (1969) Cyclosphosphamide. Effect on experimental allergic encephalomyelitis in Lewis rats. Science 165: 191-192

Paterson PY, Hanson MA (1969) Cyclophosphamide inhibition of experimental allergic encephalomyelitis and cellular transfer of the disease in Lewis rats. J Immunol 103: 1311-1316

Peters BA, Hinrichs DJ (1982) Passive transfer of experimental allergic encephalomyelitis in the Lewis rat with activated spleen cell: differential activation with mitogens. Cell Immunol 69: 175-185

Raine CS (1984) Biology of disease. Analysis of autoimmune demyelination: its impact upon multiple sclerosis. Lab Invest 50: 608-635

Raine CS, Stone SH (1977) Animal model for multiple sclerosis: chronic experimental allergic encephalomyelitis in inbred guinea pigs. NY State J Med 77: 1693-1696

Raine CS, Mokhtarian F, McFarlin DE (1984) Adoptively transferred chronic relapsing experimental autoimmune encephalomyelitis in the mouse. Neuropathologic analysis. Lab Invest 51: 534-546

Ryffel B, Feurer C, Heuberger B, Borel JF (1982) Immunosuppressive effect of cyclosporin A in two lymphocyte transfer models in rats: comparison of in vivo and in vitro treatment. Immunobiology 163: 470-483

Saka K, Namikawa T, Kunishita T, Yamanouchi K, Tabira T (1986) Studies of experimental allergic encephalomyelitis by using encephalitogenic T cell lines and clones in euthymic and athymic mice. J Immunol 137: 1527-1531

Schluesener HJ, Lassmann H (1985) Recombinant interleukin 2 (IL-2) promotes T cell line-mediated neuro-autoimmune disease. J Neuroimmunol 11: 87-91

Schnyder B, Weber E, Fierz W, Fontana A (1986) On the role of astrocytes in polyclonal T cell activation. J Neuroimmunol 10: 209-218

Schuller-Levis GB, Kozlowski PB, Wisniewski HM (1986) Cyclosporin A treatment of an induced attack in a chronic relapsing model of experimental allergic encephalomyelitis. Clin Immunol Immunopathol 40: 244-252

Sobel RA, Blanchette BW, Bhan AK, Colvin RB (1984) The immunopathology of experimental allergic encephalomyelitis. I. Quantitative analysis of inflammatory cells in situ. J Immunol 132: 2393-2401

Steinman L, Rosenbaum JT, Sriram S, McDevitt HO (1981) In vivo effects of antibodies to immune response gene products: prevention of experimental allergic encephalitis. Proc Natl Acad Sci USA 78: 7111-7114

Stone SH, Traugott U, Raine CS (1983) Chronic experimental allergic encephalomyelitis in strain 2 guinea pigs: absence of resistance to nervous system changes and sex dependence of clinical disease. J Neuroimmunol 4: 187-199

Traugott U, Stone SH, Raine CS (1979) Chronic relapsing experimental allergic encephalomyelitis. Correlation of circulating lymphocyte fluctuations with disease activity in suppressed and unsuppressed animals. J Neurol Sci 41: 17-29

Traugott U, Shevach E, Chiba J, Stone SH, Raine CS (1982) Chronic relapsing experimental allergic encephalomyelitis: identification and dynamics of T and B cells within the central nervous system. Cell Immunol 68: 261-275

Vandenbark AA, Raus JCM (eds) (1984) Immunoregulatory processes in experimental allergic encephalomyelitis and multiple sclerosis. Research monographs in immunology. Elsevier, Amsterdam

Waldor MK, Sriram S, Hardy R, Herzenberg LA, Herzenberg LA, Lanier L, Lim M, Steinman L (1985) Reversal of experimental allergic encephalomyelitis with monoclonal antibody to a T-cell subset marker. Science 227: 415-417

Waxman FJ, Taguiam JM, Whitacre CC (1984) Modification of the clinical and histopathologic expression of experimental allergic encephalomyelitis by the vasoactive amine antagonist cyproheptadine. Cell Immunol 85: 82-93

Weigle WO (1980) Analysis of autoimmunity through experimental models of thyroiditis and allergic encephalomyelitis. Adv Immunol 30: 159-273

Wiesinger D, Borel JF (1980) Studies on the mechanism of action of cyclosporin A. Immunology 156: 454-463

Willenborg DO, Sjollema P, Danta G (1986) Immunoglobulin deficient rats as donors and recipients of effector cells of allergic encephalomyelitis. J Neuroimmunol 11: 93-103

Wisniewski HM, Madrid RE (1983) Chronic progressive experimental allergic encephalomyelitis (EAE) in adult guinea pigs. J Neuropathol Exp Neurol 42: 243-255

Zamvil S, Nelson P, Trotter J, Mitchell D, Knobler R, Fritz R, Steinman L (1985) T-cell clones specific for myelin basic protein induce chronic relapsing paralysis and demyelination. Nature 317: 355-358

Neurotoxic Effects of Pyridoxine (Megavitaminosis B6), Rat

Georg J. Krinke

Synonyms. Primary sensory neuronopathy; peripheral sensory neuronal neuropathy.

Gross Appearance

No macroscopic alterations are obvious in the nervous system of intoxicated rats. Individuals with advanced sensory paralysis appear emaciated.

Microscopic Features

The lesions are confined to the primary sensory neurons: the nerve cell bodies in the dorsal root and sensory trigeminal ganglia and their processes in the spinal cord and the peripheral nerves. Large neurons are more susceptible than small ones.

Exposure to extremely large amounts of vitamin B_6 is followed by the initial changes which occur in the cytons (nerve cell bodies) after 1–2 days (Krinke et al. 1985); they show remodeling in the form of an eccentric displacement of the nucleus, folding of that portion of the nuclear membrane which faces the center, and rearrangement of the Nissl bodies into a ring-shaped zone at the periphery (Fig. 14a). Focal cytoplasmic clearing or larger vacuoles may occur in occasional cytons (Fig. 14b).

Prominent bundles of neurofilaments appear in the form of streaks of pale material adjacent to the Nissl bodies 2–3 days after treatment (Fig. 14c); residual clumps of pale neurofilamentous material are still present at the end of the 1st week. The occurrence of coarse granular material in the cyton center indicates the presence of mitochondria and dense bodies. The satellite cells surrounding the large cytons appear to increase in number (Fig. 14d).

Degeneration of the nerve cell processes becomes apparent 2–3 days after treatment. The first areas affected are those containing the terminal portions of the largest and longest sensory neurons: the spinal cervical Goll's tract and the peripheral plantar nerve. The breakdown of the peripheral nerve fibers, with initial fragmentation in the central portion of their internodal segments (Fig. 15), follows the pattern of secondary, wallerian-like degeneration (Krinke et al. 1986). The affected spinal cord fibers show initial distention of the myelin sheath with either swelling or shrinkage of the axon, followed by collapse of the myelin sheath in the absence of the axon (Fig. 16).

Degeneration of the nerve fibers progresses retrogradely toward the nerve cell body. In occasional isolated peripheral nerve fibers the initial damage is restricted only to their distal segments (Fig. 15), whereas the more advanced lesion involves the proximal segments as well; moreover, the spinal Goll's tract appears to be damaged earlier in time at the distal (cervical) level than at the proximal (lumbar) level. A few of the degenerated nerve fibers seen early on at the proximal level probably originate from the most severely, irreversibly damaged cytons.

In most neurons, changes such as the remodeling of cyton and probably also the distal degeneration of the peripheral nerve fibers may revert to normal when the administration of excessive vitamin B_6 is discontinued (Krinke et al. 1985; Windebank et al. 1985). There is no evidence, however, that the damaged central processes in the spinal cord can regenerate.

Continuous and prolonged exposure to excessively large amounts of vitamin B_6 results in severe damage of large dorsal root cytons; this change may be heralded by cytoplasmic vacuolation. The destroyed cytons are substituted by the proliferation of satellite cells; these are arranged in groups called "nodules of Nageotte" (Fig. 17) and they indicate irreversible damage to the spinal and peripheral primary sensory nerve fibers.

18   Georg J.Krinke

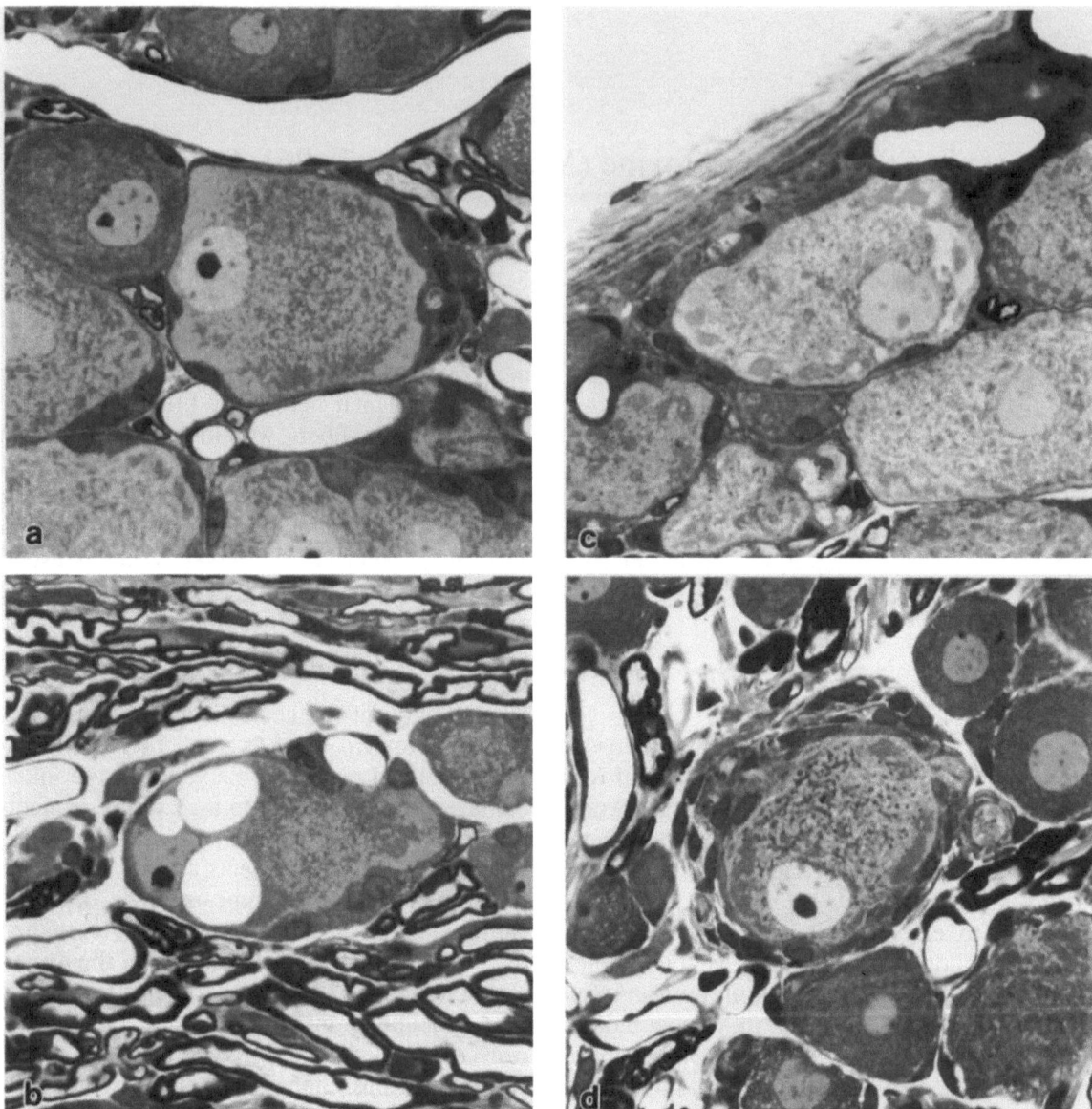

Fig. 14a–d. Alterations in lumbar dorsal root cytons of male rats treated with pyridoxol hydrochloride 1200 mg/kg i.p. twice daily for 1 day. **a** One day after treatment; a cyton in the initial stage of remodeling exhibits nuclear eccentricity and rearrangement of Nissl bodies at the periphery. **b** Another cyton, at the same time, shows addi-tional cytoplasmic vacuolation. **c** Three days after treat-ment the Nissl bodies are surrounded by pale streaks in-dicating the presence of neurofilaments. **d** Six days after treatment, a remodeled cyton surrounded by numerous satellite cells contains coarse granular organelles in the cyton center. Toluidine blue, ×575

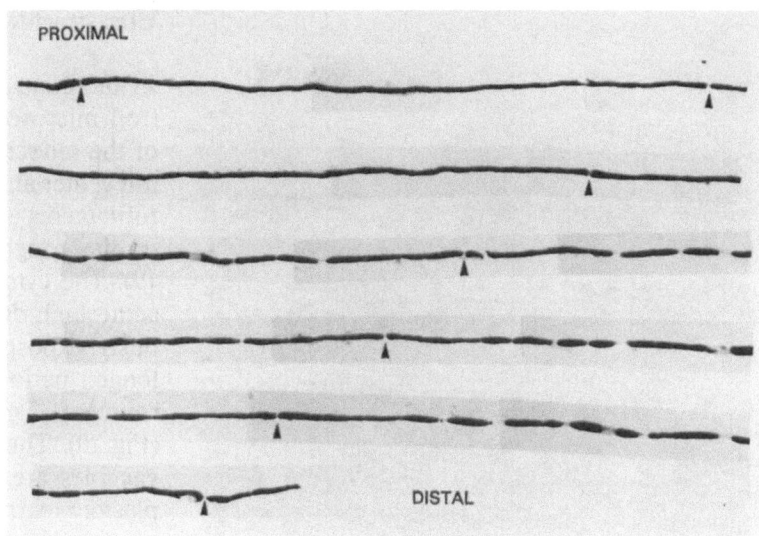

Fig. 15. A myelinated nerve fiber isolated from the plantar nerve of a male rat treated as in Fig. 14 and examined 3 days after treatment. The nodes of Ranvier are indicated with *arrowheads*. The first two proximal segments are still intact, while the following distal segments show fragmentation of their central portion. Sudan black, × 130

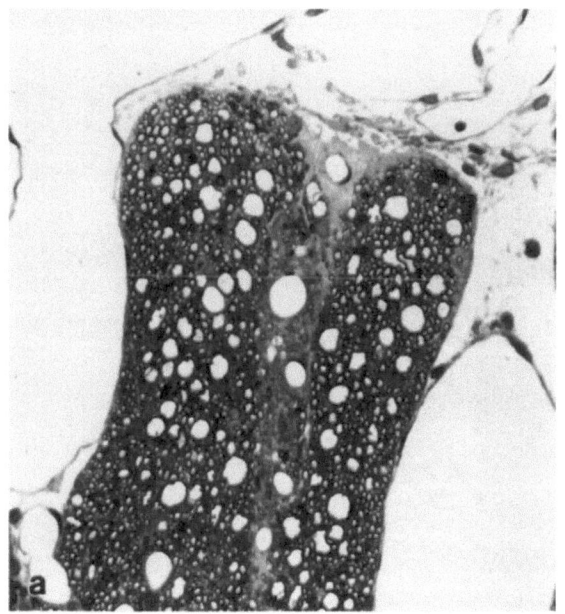 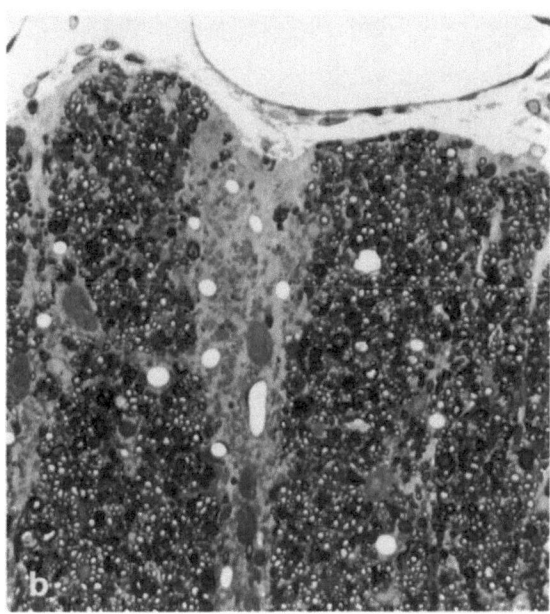

Fig. 16a, b. Transverse section of the upper cervical Goll's tract, from animals treated as in Fig. 14. **a** Two days after treatment, numerous myelinated nerve fibers are distended. **b** Many collapsed myelin sheaths are present 6 days after treatment. Toluidine blue, × 370

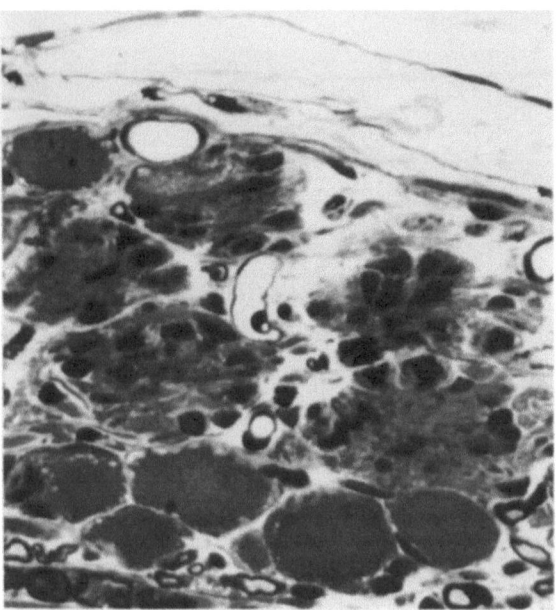

Fig. 17. Lumbar dorsal root ganglion from a male rat treated twice daily with 600 mg/kg i.p. pyridoxol hydrochloride for 14 days. Nodules of Nageotte replace the destroyed cytons. Toluidine blue, × 575

Ultrastructure

In the course of remodeling of the cyton, electron microscopy demonstrates an accumulation of the mitochondria and dense bodies in the cyton center and also of prominent bundles of neurofilaments adjacent to the more peripheral areas of the rough endoplasmic reticulum (Figs. 18, 19). The cytoplasm of cytons recuperating from acute high-dose exposure and of those continuously exposed to a low toxic dose for a prolonged period of time contains unusually large, rounded mitochondria (megamitochondria) (Fig. 20). The focal cytoplasmic clearing and the vacuoles are caused by rarefaction of the cytoplasmic matrix; they appear to be especially frequent in the area of the axon hillock or the initial axon segment and may contain fragments of disrupted membranes (Krinke et al. 1985).

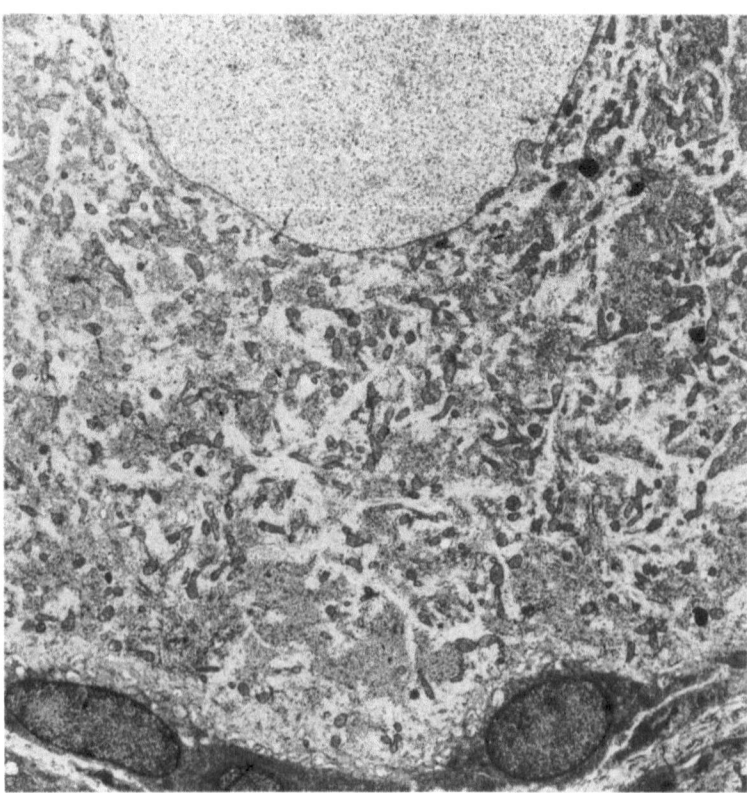

Fig. 18. Large lumbar dorsal root cyton of a control male rat. Clusters of rough endoplasmic reticulum (with light microscope they appear as the Nissl bodies) are regularly distributed in the cytoplasm intermingled with other organelles. Uranyl acetate and lead citrate, × 4065

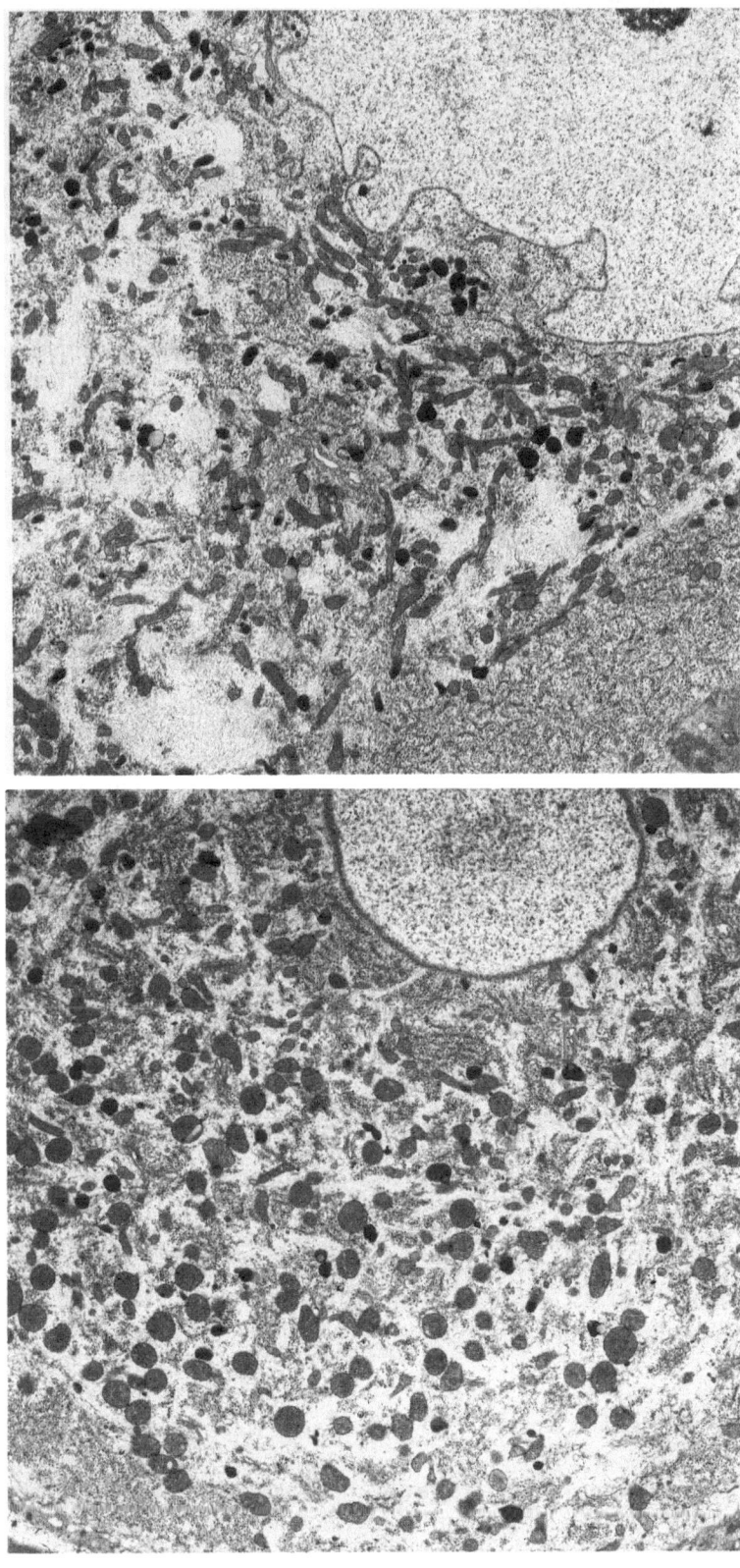

Fig. 19 *(above).* A large remodeled lumbar dorsal root cyton from a rat treated as in Fig. 14. Three days after treatment the nuclear membrane is folded, mitochondria and dense bodies are concentrated in the cyton center, and bundles of neurofilaments surround the rough endoplasmic reticulum. Uranyl acetate and lead citrate, × 5213

Fig. 20 *(below).* Large lumbar dorsal root cyton from a rat treated as in Fig. 14. Six days after treatment, prominent rounded megamitochondria occur in the cytoplasm. Uranyl acetate and lead citrate, × 4193

Differential Diagnosis

The light- and electron-microscopic alterations induced by vitamin B_6 are quite nonspecific; they are very similar to the changes that occur following mechanical injury such as transection or crushing of a peripheral nerve, called the "axon reaction" (Liebermann 1971) or "retrograde reaction" (Zelená 1971) of the cyton, and "secondary degeneration" of the severed distal nerve cell processes. Unlike mechanical trauma, which may damage all the neurons present at one site, vitamin B_6 selectively affects only the primary sensory neurons; in addition, it damages the cyton initially before affecting the nerve fibers formed by its distal processes, a reversal of the events that follow trauma.

Chemically induced damage to the primary sensory neurons has been observed with a number of agents. For instance, isoniazid and acrylamide induce remodeling of the cyton similar to that occurring with vitamin B_6 or following mechanical injury. Particular features of this reaction, however, appear to be related to specific insults. Unlike vitamin B_6, mechanical injury and isoniazid affect the small cytons more rapidly and more severely than the large ones (Jones and Cavanagh 1981); in acrylamide intoxication the neurofilaments become severely depleted (Jones and Cavanagh 1986), while with vitamin B_6 they form prominent bundles. Moreover, the effects of isoniazid and acrylamide are not restricted to primary sensory neurons. Adriamycin, in contrast to vitamin B_6, produces initial changes in the neuronal nucleus; cell types other than the primary sensory neurons, e.g., the autonomic neurons, are also susceptible to its toxicity (Cho et al. 1980). The effects of mercury are characterized by degranulation and disintegration of the rough endoplasmic reticulum; other areas of the nervous system, especially the cerebellum, are susceptible to its effects (Chang 1980), but not to those of vitamin B_6.

Biological Features

Natural History. The presence of biologically active derivatives of vitamin B_6 [pyridoxine, adermine, 2-methyl-3-hydroxy-4,5-bis-(hydroxymethyl)-pyridine] is essential for the metabolism of amino acids, proteins, carbohydrates, lipids, nucleic acids, hormones, and other vital substances. The naturally occurring derivatives, pyridoxol, pyridoxal, and pyridoxamine, are supplied in the diet and phosphorylated after absorption to become biologically active phosphates (Ebadi 1981). The physiologic dietary requirement for healthy individuals amounts to several milligrams a day.

The signs of deficiency in the rat include anemia and dermatitis ("rat acrodynia"); in humans, a "peripheral neuritis" may occur in addition to these changes.

Synthetic vitamin B_6 has been widely used in the treatment of human diseases such as pyridoxine-dependent seizures, autism, schizophrenia, carpal tunnel syndrome, premenstrual syndrome, hyperemesis gravidarum, restless legs, and others. This therapy appears to be benefical, and a patient may tolerate a daily intake of hundreds of milligrams without developing toxicity. In view of the risk of damaging the nervous system, the consumption of extremely large quantities - grams (e.g., by food faddists and body builders) - would appear to be inadvisable; a risk-benefit assessment is, however, acceptable when considering the administration of such large quantities of vitamin B_6 as an antidote to isoniazid toxicity (Sievers and Herrier 1984).

Although vitamin B_6 toxicity is an improbable hazard to domestic or experimental animals, it offers an interesting model for studying the functional defects (Alder and Zbinden 1973) as well as the spectrum of pathologic changes in the primary sensory neurons. It further demonstrates the relativity of "toxicity" in relation to a compound that is essential in small quantities for the maintenance of good health, but harmful when administered in massive amounts.

Etiology and Frequency. Among the natural vitamin B_6 derivatives only pyridoxol and pyridoxol phosphate are neurotoxic. The absence of neurotoxicity with pyridoxamine and pyridoxic acid (the major excretion product of vitamin B_6) indicates that excessive pyridoxol may be converted to a neurotoxic agent independently of the physiologic biocatalytic action. A chemical-model reaction has demonstrated the generation of an alkylating metabolite from pyridoxol; this may bind to biopolymers in the nervous tissue and damage them (Frater-Schröder et al. 1976).

The exact biochemical site of the toxic action is uncertain; but, since vitamin B_6 is engaged in a number of enzymatic reactions as a coenzyme, the toxic agent could damage the apoenzymes, in this way acting as a vitamin B_6 antagonist. The similarity between the lesions observed in experimental studies on vitamin B_6 deficiency (Victor

Table 3. Neurotoxic effects of various dose regimens of pyridoxine in the laboratory rat

Regimen	Effect	Reference
Various doses s.c. and p.o.	s.c. LD_{50} 3.1 g/kg B6 base s.c. LD_{50} 3.7 g/kg B6 HCl p.o. LD_{50} 5.5 g/kg B6 HCl	Unna (1940)
4–6 g/kg	Tonic convulsions, opisthotonus, convulsive seizures over 1 or 2 weeks	
3–7 g/kg p.o.	Sensory neuropathy (transient with small, and persistent with large doses); damage of posterior spinal columns, dorsal roots, their ganglia, and peripheral nerves	Antopol and Tarlov (1942)
100 mg/kg i.p. twice daily	Slight neuropathy after 18–20 days	Alder and Zbinden (1973)
250 mg/kg i.p. twice daily	Slight neuropathy after 7 days	
500 mg/kg i.p. twice daily	Severe neuropathy after 7–10 days	
300 and 600 mg/kg p.o., initially once, then twice daily for up to 49 days	Distally accentuated sensory neuropathy affecting primary sensory neurons and sensory nerve endings	Krinke et al. (1978a, b)
600 mg/kg i.p. twice daily for 1–14 days	Initial, reversible changes in the dorsal root cytons; secondary degeneration of nerve fibers	Krinke et al. (1985)
200 mg/kg i.p. for up to 6 or 8 weeks	Sensory neuropathy without loss of dorsal root cytons; clinical recovery 12 weeks after withdrawal	Windebank et al. (1985)
1200 mg/kg i.p. twice daily for 1 day	Early damage of dorsal root cytons; secondary, distally accentuated degeneration of nerve fibers	

and Adams 1956; Yonezawa et al. 1969) and those occurring in toxicity indicate a common target mechanism.

Pyridoxol hydrochloride is generally used to induce neurotoxicity in animals. Table 3 shows a summary of experiments on rats. No strain- or sex-related differences in susceptibility are known.

Pathogenesis. Unlike the central nervous system, the dorsal root ganglia are not protected against excessively high levels of circulating vitamin B_6 by either a blood-nerve barrier or a saturable uptake mechanism. This fact, however, does not explain the selective vulnerability of dorsal root cytons because other nervous system areas directly exposed to the circulating agents are not susceptible (Krinke et al. 1980). The greater metabolic demand of the large primary cytons maintaining very long axonal processes could account for their preferential damage.

The probable target site for the neurotoxic effects of vitamin B_6 is located in the axon hillock or the initial axon segment (Krinke et al. 1985); this would explain the promptness of cyton remodeling in comparison to the much slower changes in response to peripheral nerve damage (Zelená 1971). The accumulation of neurofilaments within the affected cytons may indicate a (direct or indirect) disturbance in anterograde axonal transport, which is required for axonal integrity. The absence of specific primary changes in the peripheral nerve fibers (Windebank et al. 1985) is in accordance with the direct early effects of excessive levels of vitamin B_6 on the nerve cell bodies.

Behavioral Observations. Disturbances of neuromuscular function has been demonstrated in intoxicated rats by means of the "rotating rod test" prior to the development of overt signs of peripheral neuropathy (Alder and Zbinden 1973). Rats exposed to low toxic levels become unsteady, first in the hindlimbs and then in all four limbs; when the treatment is discontinued they recover and appear normal (Windebank et al. 1985). Animals receiving massive toxic doses develop severe sensory paralysis with preserved muscle force (Krinke et al. 1985).

Comparison with Other Species

The rat, the dog, man, and probably many other species are susceptible. The dog appears to be more sensitive than the rat: sensory neuropathy occurs in dogs treated with 150 mg/kg daily (Hoover and Carlton 1981) while this dose is tolerated by rats; exposure to 300 mg/kg daily will produce greater damage, especially vacuolation and death of the dorsal root cytons, in dogs than in rats (Krinke et al. 1978a, 1980). This difference in susceptibility between the two species may be related to the different rate of excretion: over 80% of the vitamin B_6 administered is excreted within 24 h in rats compared with only 20% in dogs (Phillips et al. 1978).

Reversible sensory dysfunctions has occurred in humans at dose levels varying between 2 and 6 g daily for 2–34 months (Schaumburg et al. 1983); other reports describe similar effects at lower dose levels, between 200 mg and 5 g daily for 1–36 months (Berger and Schaumburg 1984; Parry and Bredesen 1985). Sural nerve biopsy performed on two of these patients produced evidence of degeneration and loss of nerve fibers (Schaumburg et al. 1983).

References

Alder S, Zbinden G (1973) Use of pharmacological screening tests in subacute neurotoxicity studies of isoniazid, pyridoxine HCl and hexachlorophene. Agents Actions 3: 233–243

Antopol W, Tarlov IM (1942) Experimental study of the effects produced by large doses of vitamin B_6. J Neuropathol Exp Neurol 1: 330–336

Berger A, Schaumburg HH (1984) More on neuropathy from pyridoxine abuse. N Engl J Med 311: 986–987

Chang LW (1980) Mercury. In: Spencer PS, Schaumburg HH (eds) Experimental and clinical neurotoxicology. Williams and Wilkins, Baltimore, pp 508–526

Cho ES, Spencer PS, Jortner BS (1980) Doxorubicin. In: Spencer PS, Schaumburg HH (eds) Experimental and clinical neurotoxicology. Williams and Wilkins, Baltimore, pp 430–439

Ebadi M (1981) Regulation and function of pyridoxal phosphate in CNS. Neurochem Int 3: 181–206

Frater-Schröder M, Alder S, Zbinden G (1976) Neurotoxic effects of pyridoxine and analogs in rats. In: Duncan WAM, Leonard BJ, Brunaud M (eds) The prediction of chronic toxicity from short term studies, vol XVII. Proceedings of the European Society of Toxicology. Elsevier Scientific, New York, pp 277–284

Hoover DM, Carlton WW (1981) The subacute neurotoxicity of excess pyridoxine HCl and clioquinol (5-chloro-7-iodo-8-hydroxyquinoline) in beagle dogs. II. Pathology. Vet Pathol 18: 757–768

Jones HB, Cavanagh JB (1981) Comparison between the early changes in isoniazid intoxication and the chromatolytic response to nerve ligation in spinal ganglion cells of the rat. Neuropathol Appl Neurobiol 7: 489–501

Jones HB, Cavanagh JB (1986) The axon reaction in spinal ganglion neurons of acrylamide-treated rats. Acta Neuropathol (Berl) 71: 55–63

Krinke G, Krüger L, Heid J, Bittiger H, Hess R (1978a) Das neurohistologische Läsionsmuster der Pyridoxol-neuropathie der weißen Ratte. Schweiz Med Wochenschr 108: 466

Krinke G, Heid J, Bittiger H, Hess R (1978b) Sensory denervation of the plantar lumbrical muscle spindles in pyridoxine neuropathy. Acta Neuropathol (Berl) 43: 213–216

Krinke G, Schaumburg HH, Spencer PS, Suter J, Thomann P, Hess R (1980) Pyridoxine megavitaminosis produces degeneration of peripheral sensory neurons (sensory neuronopathy) in the dog. Neurotoxicology 2: 13–24

Krinke G, Naylor DC, Skorpil V (1985) Pyridoxine megavitaminosis: an analysis of the early changes induced with massive doses of vitamin B_6 in rat primary sensory neurons. J Neuropathol Exp Neurol 44: 117–129

Krinke G, Grieve AP, Schnider K (1986) The role of Schmidt-Lanterman incisures in Wallerian degeneration. Acta Neuropathol (Berl) 69: 168–170

Lieberman AR (1971) The axon reaction: a review of the principal features of perikaryal responses to axon injury. In: Pfeiffer CC, Smythies JR (eds) International review of neurobiology, vol 14. Academic, Orlando, pp 49–124

Parry GJ, Bredesen DE (1985) Sensory neuropathy with low-dose pyridoxine. Neurology 35: 1466–1468

Phillips WE, Mills JH, Charbonneau SM, Tryphonas L, Hatina GV, Zawidzka Z, Bryce FR, Munro IC (1978) Subacute toxicity of pyridoxine hydrochloride in the beagle dog. Toxicol Appl Pharmacolal 44: 323–333

Schaumburg HH, Kaplan J, Windebank A, Vick N, Rasmus S, Pleasure D, Brown MJ (1983) Sensory neuropathy from pyridoxine abuse. A new megavitamin syndrome. N Engl J Med 309: 445–448

Sievers ML, Herrier RN (1984) Sensory neuropathy from pyridoxine abuse (Letter). N Engl J Med 310: 198

Unna K (1940) Studies on the toxicity and pharmacology of vitamin B_6 [2-methyl-3-hydroxy-4,5-bis-(hydroxymethyl)-pyridine]. J Pharmacol Exp Ther 70: 400–407

Victor M, Adams RD (1956) The neuropathology of experimental vitamin B_6 deficiency in monkeys. Am J Clin Nutr 4: 346–353

Windebank AJ, Low PA, Blexrud MD, Schmelzer JD, Schaumburg HH (1985) Pyridoxine neuropathy in rats: specific degeneration of sensory axons. Neurology 35: 1617–1622

Yonezawa T, Mori T, Nakatani Y (1969) Effects of pyridoxine deficiency in nervous tissue maintained in vitro. Ann NY Acad Sci 166: 146–157

Zelená J (1971) Neurofilaments and microtubules in sensory neurons after peripheral nerve section. Z Zellforsch Mikrosk Anat 117: 191–211

Neurotoxic Effects of Doxorubicin, Rat

Bernhard S. Jortner

Synonym. Adriamycin neurotoxicity.

Gross Appearance

Gross lesions have not been noted. Doxorubicin (Adriamycin) is a glycosidic anthracycline antibiotic comprised of a tetracycline ring structure with the sugar daunosamine attached by a glycosidic linkage. Neurotoxicity has been demonstrated in young rats (250–350 g) given 10 mg/kg doxorubicin intravenously. These rats develop progressive limb ataxia and dyssynergia at about 11–12 days. Involvement of hindlimbs occurs earlier and is the more prominent sign (Fig. 21) (Cho 1977).

Microscopic Features and Ultrastructure

Lesions within the peripheral nervous system ganglia form the pathologic basis for the signs. Lesions are best developed in dorsal root ganglia (Cho 1977; Cho et al. 1980 a, b), more slowly developing and less severe in trigeminal ganglia, and minimal in autonomic ganglia. Initial lesions observed in dorsal root ganglia involve neuronal nuclei (Cho et al. 1980 a, b) and consist of local loss of chromatin manifest as focal regions of nuclear clearing. Development of lesions begins within 3 h of doxorubicin administration and is well delineated by day 4 (Fig. 22). The early onset of nuclear change is correlated with the intranuclear presence of the drug as demonstrated by fluorescence (Sahenk and Mendell 1979). Segregation of normally interspersed nucleolar granular and fibrillary components with subsequent progressive loss of stainable nuclear material occurs by experimental day 6, resulting in pale staining and sometimes displaced neuronal nuclei (Eddy and Nathaniel 1982). Such neurons susequently undergo necrosis and contain cytoplasmic dense bodies, neurofilament masses, and vacuoles (Fig. 23). The latter may derive from smooth endoplasmic reticulum (Eddy and Nathaniel 1982). Nuclear changes consist of pyknosis and karyolysis. Local aggregates of phagocytic satellite cells become progressively more prominent, surrounding and eventually replacing devitalized neuronal cell bodies (forming nodules of Nageotte). Initial necrotic neurons are noted by day 9. By days 15 and 34 an estimated 40% and 50%, respectively, of the neuronal population is so affected. Smaller neurons appear less affected by the process than larger ones. Wallerian degeneration of nerve fibers involving peripheral nerves, dorsal roots, and dorsal columns of the spinal cord, accompanies the neuronal necrosis.

Younger rats appear more susceptible to the neurotoxic effects of doxorubicin. Administration of 10 mg/kg subcutaneously to 1-week-old animals results in lesions in 67.7% of the neurons in dorsal root ganglia and loss of 60.2% of these cells

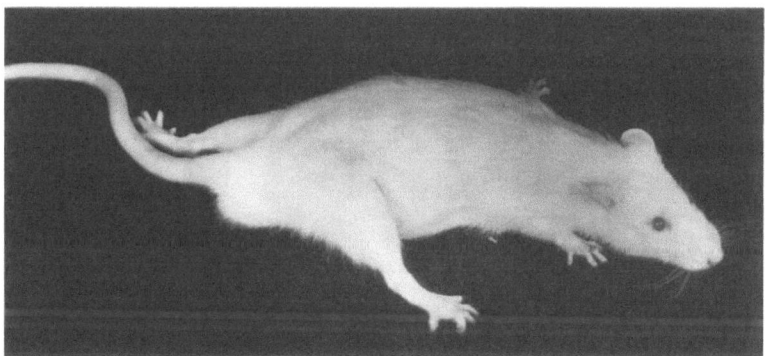

Fig. 21. Ataxia in a rat manifest by abdomen placed on the floor and asymmetric splaying of rear legs; 19 days after 10 mg/kg doxorubicin intravenously. (From Cho 1977)

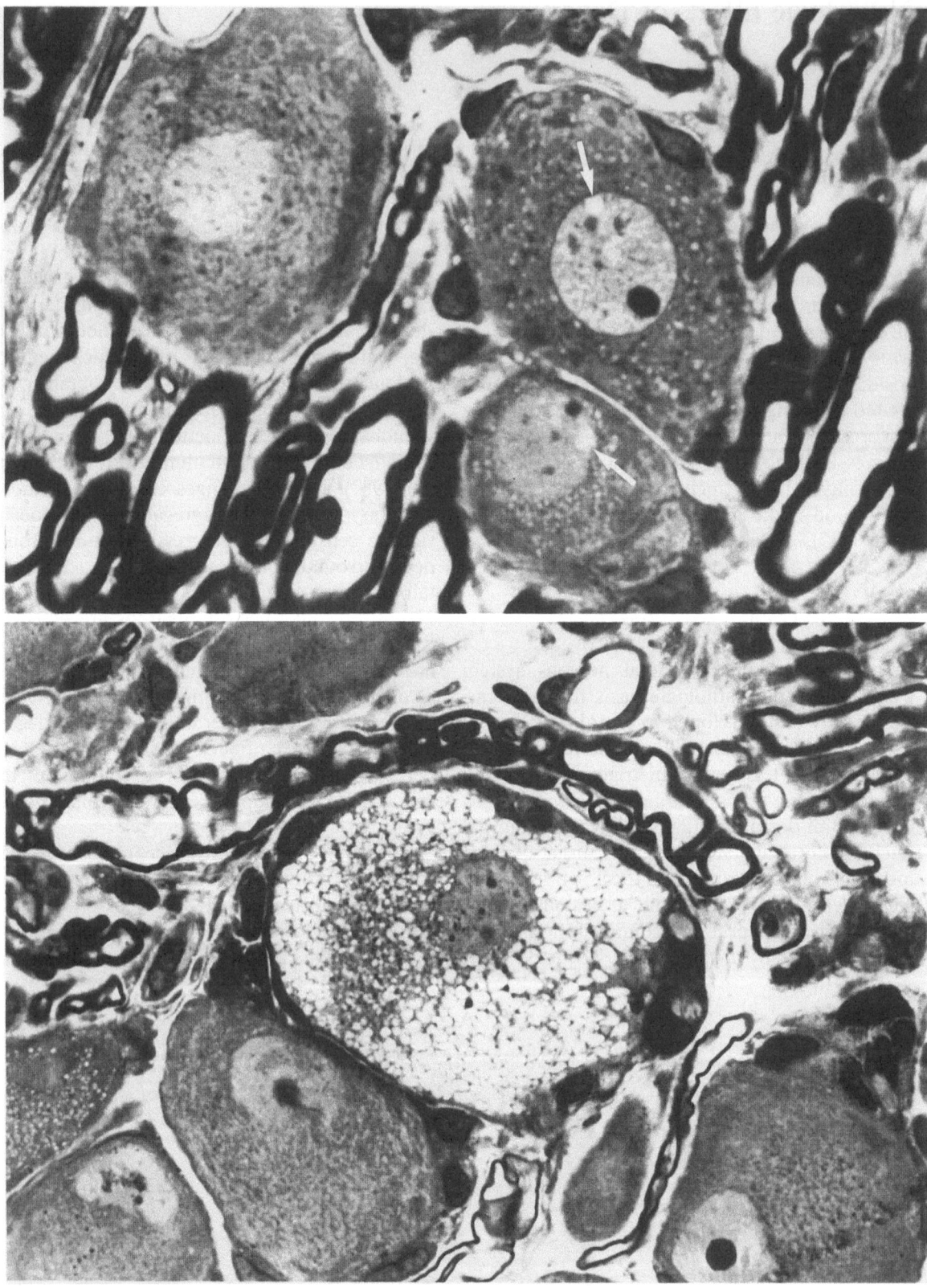

Fig. 22 *(above)*. Discrete regions of nuclear (chromatin) clearing *(arrows)* in neurons of dorsal root ganglion following doxorubicin administration. Toluidine blue – safranin stain, × 1450

Fig. 23 *(below)*. Marked cytoplasmic vacuolization of a neuron in a dorsal root ganglion in doxorubicin-induced neurotoxicity. Toluidine blue – safranin stain, × 1500

within 10 days (Eddy 1983). Quelamycin, an iron-containing (triferric) derivative of doxorubicin elicits a greatly diminished neurotoxic effect (Jortner and Cho 1981).

Differential Diagnosis

Differentiation of doxorubicin neurotoxicity is not a major consideration. In rats it is an experimental disease with lesions quite distinctive in distribution and nature.

Biologic Features

Doxorubicin has proved to be an effective antineoplastic agent, useful against a variety of malignancies including a number of solid tumors (Calabresi and Parks 1985). Several cellular actions of the anthracyclines (daunomycin is the other clinically important anthracycline antibiotic) are thought to give rise to this chemotherapeutic effect (Gianni et al. 1983). These compounds bind to deoxyribonuclei acid (DNA), by intercalation between base pairs resulting in stiffening, elongation, and conformational changes in the double helix, uncoiling of supercoiled DNA, and strand breaks. These changes are associated with inhibition of DNA and in particular preribosomal ribonucleic acid (RNA) synthesis, both important factors in anthracycline-induced antitumor activity. The anthracyclines have also been demonstrated to bind to membrane phospholipids such as cardiolipin and phosphatidylserine, causing a significant change in membrane structure and function. Upon reduction, these drugs form toxic free radicals such as semiquinone, oxygen, and alkylating drug radicals. The DNA injury (such as strand scission) may relate in part to free radical-induced effects.

Several toxic effects of the anthracyclines restrict the extent of their therapeutic use. As might be expected, rapidly dividing cell populations, such as the gastrointestinal epithelium and hematopoietic system, are potential targets. In addition, a major limiting factor is the dose-related cardiomyopathy seen with these compounds. This myocardial lesion has been related to free radical injury or direct membranotoxic events (Gianni et al. 1983).

The basis for the striking distribution of neuronal lesion in rats, primarily affecting peripheral ganglia, is thought to reside in the inability of doxorubicin to cross intact blood-brain or blood-nerve barriers. Thus, its neurotoxic action is restricted to regions where such barriers are normally absent, such as peripheral sensory and autonomic ganglia (Cho et al. 1980a, b). In these areas blood-borne doxorubicin can enter the tissue and gain access to neuronal and glial cells. Regions of central nervous system lying outside the blood-brain barrier, such as the area postrema, median eminence, and neurohypophysis, are also injured following intravenous administration of doxorubicin (Bigotte and Olsson 1983a). Altering the blood-brain barrier with intravenous mannitol will also permit injury due to blood-borne doxorubicin although this produces hemorrhagic infarcts in affected brain tissue (Neuwelt et al. 1981). Infusion of the compound into the cerebrospinal fluid leads to subpial necrotizing angiopathy (Merker et al. 1978). Evidence for retrograde axonal transport of locally administered doxorubicin, with subsequent nerve cell body injury, has been demonstrated (Bigotte and Olsson 1983b). This does not appear to be a factor in its systemic neurotoxicity.

Nuclear lesions appear to be primary in the pathogenesis of the doxorubicin-induced neuronal injury in peripheral ganglia. As noted above, doxorubicin has a deleterious effect on DNA in other cell populations and may similarly affect these neurons. The neuronal nuclear changes of clearing and diminished staining may be the morphologic substrate of this drug-induced nucleoprotein damage (Cho et al. 1980a, b). The basis of the particular susceptibility of neurons among the ganglionic components remains speculative. Differences in genomic packaging between neurons and other cells have been noted and may play a role (Brown 1978). The drug-induced genomic defects may diminish neuronal DNA or DNA-dependent RNA synthesis normally required for cellular repair (McIlwain and Bachelard 1985; Parhad et al. 1984). In addition, a diminished ability to carry out DNA excision repair has been observed in developing neural (retinal) cell populations (Karran et al. 1977). It has, therefore, been suggested that doxorubicin-induced DNA damage may lead to gradual depletion of material necessary for neuronal integrity (Cho et al. 1980b). This may lead to metabolic defects in affected neurons. As an example, delay in neuronal cellular processing of amino acids for axonal transport has been demonstrated in this toxicity (Sahenk and Mendell 1979). In another study, transient retinal ganglion cell axonal neurofilamentous swelling preceded wallerian degeneration after intravitreous injection of doxorubicin (Parhad et al. 1984). This suggested a defect in slow transport of cytoskeletal elements. Whatever the definitive mechanism, the slower pace of neuropathy in rats given smaller doses of doxorubicin suggests that the rate of this depletion of "vital" material is determined by the degree of nucleic acid injury (Jortner and Cho 1980).

Comparison with Other Species

Neurotoxicity is not a feature of doxorubicin chemotherapy in man. Multiple small, divided intravenous doses of doxorubicin elicit a ganglioneuropathy in rabbits which is qualitatively similar to that in rats when cumulative doses exceeded 16 mg/kg (Bronson et al. 1982). A rhesus monkey under a similar experimental regimen had severe ganglioneuropathy after receiving a total of 20 mg/kg doxorubicin over a 10-month period (Bronson et al. 1982) indicating that primates are susceptible to this neuropathy.

References

Bigotte L, Olsson Y (1983a) Toxic effects of adriamycin on the central nervous system. Ultrastructural changes in some circumventricular organs of the mouse after intravenous administration of the drug. Acta Neuropathol (Berl) 61: 291-299

Bigotte L, Olsson Y (1983b) Cytotoxic effects of adriamycin on the mouse hypoglossal neurons following retrograde axonal transport from the tongue. Acta Neuropathol (Berl) 61: 161-168

Bronson RT, Henderson IC, Fixler H (1982) Ganglioneuropathy in rabbits and a rhesus monkey due to high cumulative doses of doxorubicin. Cancer Treat Rep 66: 1349-1355

Brown IR (1978) Analysis of gene activity in the mammalian brain. In: Roberts S, Lajtha A, Gispen WH (eds) Mechanisms, regulation and special functions of protein synthesis in the brain. Elsevier North Holland, Amsterdam, pp 29-46

Calabresi P, Parks PE jr (1985) Chemotherapy of neoplastic diseases. In: Gilman AG, Goodman LS, Rail TW, Murad F (eds) Goodman and Gilman's The pharmacological basis of therapeutics, 7th edn. Macmillan, New York, pp 1240-1306

Cho E-S (1977) Toxic effects of adriamycin on the ganglia of the peripheral nervous system: a neuropathological study. J Neuropathol Exp Neurol 36: 907-915

Cho E-S, Spencer PS, Jortner BS, Schaumberg HH (1980a) A single intravenous injection of doxorubicin (Adriamycin[R]) induces sensory neuronopathy in rats. Neurotoxicology 1: 583-591

Cho E-S, Spencer PS, Jortner BS (1980b) Doxorubicin. In: Spencer PS, Schaumberg HH (eds) Experimental and clinical neurotoxicology. Williams and Wilkins, Baltimore, pp 430-439

Eddy EL (1983) Neuronal loss from cervical dorsal root ganglia in adriamycin induced peripheral neuropathy - a quantitative study. Anat Anz (Jena) 153: 83-90

Eddy EL, Nathaniel EJH (1982) An ultrastructural study of the effects of adriamycin on the dorsal root ganglia of young and adult rats. Exp Neurol 77: 275-285

Gianni L, Corden BJ, Myers CE (1983) The biochemical basis of anthracycline toxicity and antitumor activity. Rev Biochem Toxicol 5: 1-82

Jortner BS, Cho E-S (1980) Neurotoxicity of adriamycin in rats: a low-dose effect. Cancer Treat Rep 64: 257-261

Jortner BS, Cho E-S (1981) Neurotoxicity of quelamycin in the rat. Neurotoxicology 2: 789-792

Karran P, Moscona A, Strauss B (1977) Developmental decline in DNA repair in neural retina cells of chick embryos. Persistent deficiency of repair competence in a cell line derived from late embryos. J Cell Biol 74: 274-286

McIlwain H, Bachelard HS (1985) Nucleic acids and proteins. In: McIlwain H, Bachelard HS (eds) Biochemistry and the central nervous system, 5th edn. Churchill Livingston, Edinburgh, pp 202-243

Merker PC, Lewis MR, Walker MD, Richardson EP jr (1978) Neurotoxicity of adriamycin (doxorubicin) perfused through the cerebrospinal fluid spaces of the rhesus monkey. Toxicol Appl Pharmacol 44: 191-205

Neuwelt EA, Pagel M, Barnett P, Glassberg M, Frenkel EP (1981) Pharmacology and toxicity of intracarotid adriamycin administration following osmotic blood-brain barrier modification. Cancer Res 41: 4466-4470

Parhad IM, Griffin JW, Clark AW, Koves JF (1984) Doxorubicin intoxication: neurofilamentous axonal changes with subacute neuronal death. J Neuropathol Exp Neurol 43: 188-200

Sahenk Z, Mendell JR (1979) Analysis of fast axoplasmic transport in nerve ligation and adriamycin-induced neuronal perikaryon lesions. Brain Res 171: 41-53

Neurotoxic Effects of Clinoquinol, Mouse

Makoto Koga, Jun Tateishi, Yuji Sato, and K. Matsuki

Synonyms. Hippocampal sclerosis, toxic encephalopathy associated with convulsion, subacute myelo-optic neuropathy (in man, dog and cat).

Gross Appearance

Clioquinol (synonyms: 5-chloro-7-iodo-8-hydroxyquinoline, iodochlorhydroxyquinoline, chinoform, Enterovioform, Vioform) was admixed by 0.2%–2.0% with a powder diet and given to mice. They lost weight and some had abrupt generalized convulsions without preceeding loss of consciousness. In these animals the brain seemed to be small.

After the application of 10% clioquinol ointment to the shaved back skin of mice, regrowth of the hair was impaired and the treated skin showed evidence of erosion, while the hair regrew in the control mice treated with Tween 80 or Vaseline alone.

Microscopic Features

Moderate loss of nerve cells in the hippocampus, especially in CA1 and CA3, was seen in a mouse which died on the 62nd day after oral clioquinol administration. Astroglial proliferation of moderate degree and mild spongiosis or small cavity formation were evident in these areas. Degradation products were minimal and no vascular abnormality was observed. Atrophic nerve cells with darkly stained cytoplasm and nuclei were scattered in surrounding hippocampal areas. Almost total loss of hippocampal neurons, except for few remaining ones in CA2 and CA4, was evident in all of four mice sacrificed on the 191st day. A dense network of gliosis, a few destruction products, and no vascular change was observed in these areas (Figs. 24, 25). The rest of the nervous system, including spinal cord and peripheral nerves, remained intact.

Püschner and Fankhauser (1969) reported repeated convulsions in mice after the administration of clioquinol for 2 weeks. Similar but milder changes were found in the hippocampus. Hippocampal lesions in mice chronically intoxicated with clioquinol successively expand, but remain circumscribed and corresponded well to the clas-

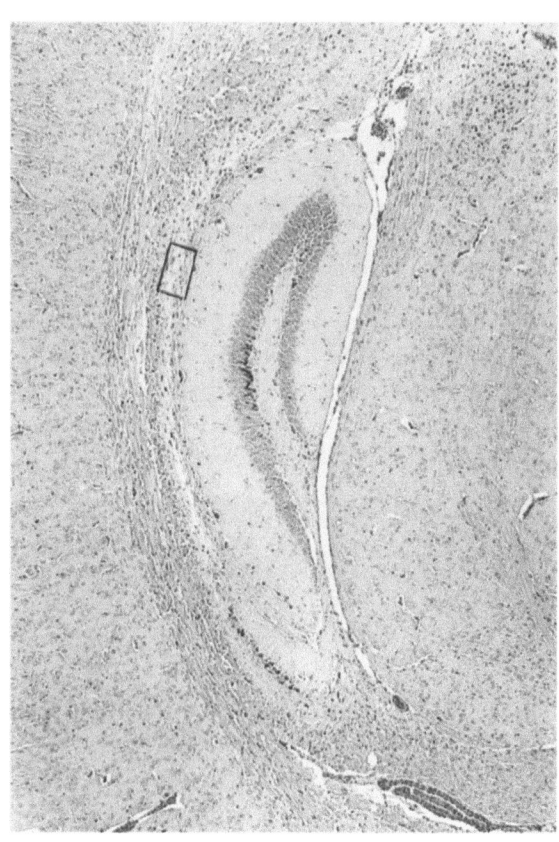

Fig. 24. Hippocampus, mouse, following oral administration of clioquinol. Note loss of neurons and gliosis, especially in CA1 and CA3. *Outlined area* enlarged in Fig. 25. H and E, × 47

sical concept of hippocampal sclerosis due to repeated convulsions (Scholz 1951). Krinke et al. (1978) also reported similar hippocampal lesions in mice after a few oral doses of clioquinol and compared them with lesions induced by amphetamine. They attributed the lesion to toxic encephalopathy produced by the convulsive treatments. Epileptogenic effect of clioquinol has been reported in other animal species and humans and will be discussed later. The skin of the mice to which clioquinol had been applied underwent severe inflammation with necrosis of the hair follicle.

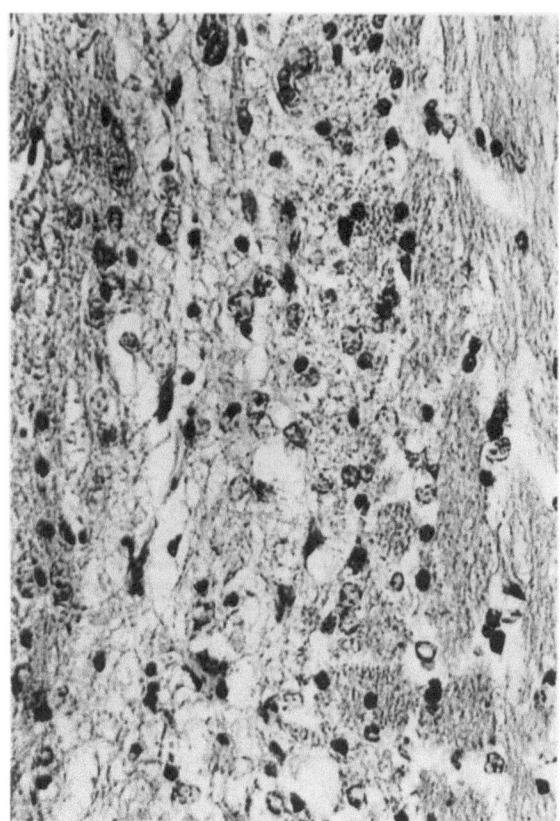

Fig. 25. Higher magnification of CA1 (in Fig. 24) showing complete neuronal loss and astroglial proliferation. H and E, × 400

Biologic Features

Toxic doses of clioquinol differ greatly in different species as well as strains of animals. Tamura (1975) reported that the onset of neurologic symptoms was more dependent on the concentration of unconjugated clioquinol in the circulation than on the daily or total dosage.

Absorption and accumulation of clioquinol given orally to mice has been studied and reported (Tateishi et al. 1975). Clioquinol concentration reached up to 17.3 µg/g plasma in an average of 15 mice after the administration of clioquinol (about 22.5 mg/kg daily) through a gavage tube. Percutaneous absorption was measured in mice applied with 10% clioquinol ointment to the shaved back skin, after the installation of body corsets to prevent the mice from licking the drug. The concentration reached 3.42 ± 2.69 µg/ml plasma after 12 hours, and about 50% of it was unconjugated clioquinol (Table 4).

Yamanaka et al. (1973) indicated that clioquinol induced uncoupling of oxidative phosphorylation in the mitochondria. Our in vitro study revealed that the exposure of clioquinol to explanted dorsal root ganglia from mice resulted in marked mitochondrial swelling in the neurons.

Comparison with Other Species

The neurotoxic effects of clioquinol are of particular interest because of the widespread use of this drug in humans as an intestinal amebicide. The Japanese episode of "subacute myelo-optic-neuropathy" (SMON) gave a warning that an old drug such as clioquinol is not safe, particularly when the method of administration changes in some way during the passage of time (Kono 1975). It has been well demonstrated in epidemiologic studies that long-term administration of clioquinol to Japanese patients with digestive disorders caused SMON.

The main pathologic features of this human toxicity are distal dominant axonopathy in the optic tracts, posterior funicles of the spinal cord, less severe changes in the corticospinal tract and peripheral nerves (Shiraki 1971). These lesions can be totally or partially reproduced by chronic oral administration of clioquinol to dogs, cats, monkeys (Tateishi et al. 1973, 1977; Egashira and Matsuyama 1982) and rabbits (Sakurama 1973).

Table 4. Clioquinol concentration in mice plasma after application of 10% clioquinol ointment on shaved back skin

Form of clioquinol	Un-conjugated (µg/ml)	Glucuronate-conjugated (µg/ml)	Sulfate-conjugated (µg/ml)	Total concentration (µg/ml)
6 h (n=6)	0.17 ± 0.09	0.06 ± 0.05	0.08 ± 0.05	0.31 ± 0.18
12 h (n=6)	1.70 ± 1.35	0.69 ± 0.58	1.02 ± 0.76	3.42 ± 2.69

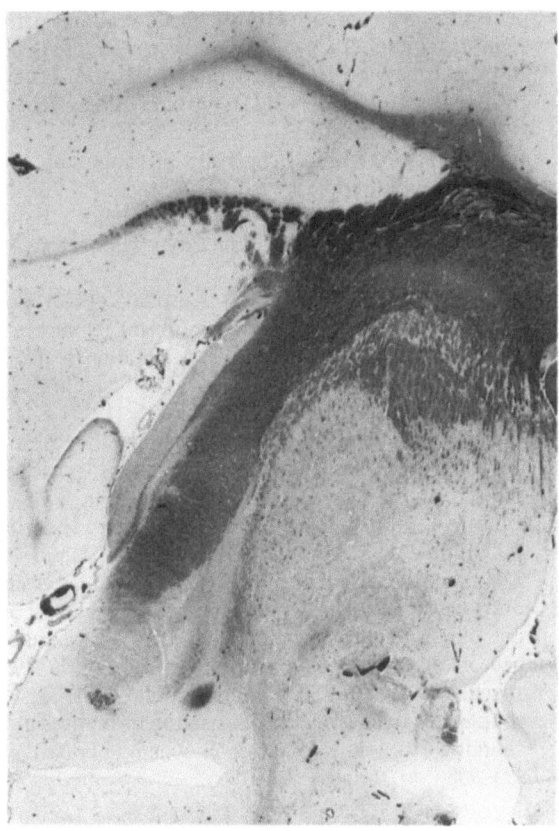

Fig. 26. Degeneration in the optic tract of a mongrel dog following oral doses up to 90 mg/kg daily for 185 days. Klüver-Barrera stain. ×9

In dogs given clioquinol, there was severe degeneration in the distal portion of the optic tracts (Fig. 26) and posterior funicles of the spinal cord, less severely in the corticospinal tract. Involvement of the peripheral nerves was not a common finding (Tateishi et al. 1977; Krinke et al. 1979). Clioquinol, therefore, produced central distal-dominant axonopathy in the primary sensory neurons in dogs (Spencer and Schaumburg 1976; Thomas et al. 1984).

Average daily doses of clioquinol administered to many affected patients were 20–40 mg/kg, while doses given to mongrel dogs were 60–144 mg/kg and higher in other species.

Rats fed a maize diet and given clioquinol for 146 days lost body weight, and half of them died. The peripheral nerve terminals in the foot muscle were decreased in number, associated with loss of nerve endings in the muscle spindles. However, we could not reproduce degeneration of Goll's tract in the spinal cord of rats, as reported by Jones et al. (1973).

Intraperitoneal injection of the drug (200–400 mg/kg daily) caused generalized convulsions in a few rats, and many animals died within 3 weeks. At autopsy, there were marked peritoneal adhesions and retention of clioquinol, which resulted from a difficulty in absorption of the drug and permitted long survival in some rats. Intraperitoneal injections into our rats produced no lesions in the nervous system, yet other authors did find lesions in the peripheral nerves (Kotaki et al. 1983) and in the optic nerves and small neurons of the dorsal root ganglia in similar experiments (Ozawa et al. 1986).

In addition to the chronic neurotoxicity of the drug there have been reports of acute toxicity. Shortly after the ingestion of a large amount of clioquinol, a young adult patient went into an acute state of mental confusion, presumably due to direct toxic effects of the drug (Kaeser and Scollo-Lavizzari 1970). Many dogs and cats showed convulsions shortly after a single or a few oral administrations of clioquinol and died in convulsive state (Tateishi et al. 1973). Hangartner (1965) reported that a cat died after repeated convulsions within a few days after skin application of clioquinol powder. It was not known whether oral ingestion or cutaneous absorption occurred in this case. Our experiments of cutaneous application in mice indicated distinct absorption through the skin.

Acknowledgements. K. Hatanaka and K. Beppu provided technical and secretarial assistance, and M. Ohara kindly commented on the manuscript. This work was supported in part by a grant from the Japanese Ministry of Health and Welfare.

References

Egashira Y, Matsuyama H (1982) Subacute myelo-optico-neuropathy (SMON) in Japan, with special reference to the autopsy cases. Acta Pathol Jpn (Suppl 1) 32: 101–116

Hangartner D (1965) Troubles nerveux observés chez le chien après absorption d'Entero-Vioforme Ciba. Schweiz Arch Tierheilkd 107: 43–47

Jones EL, Searle CE, Smith WT (1973) Peripheral neuropathy in ageing rats fed clioquinol and a maize diet. Acta Neuropathol (Berl) 24: 256–262

Kaeser HE, Scollo-Lavizzari G (1970) Akute zerebrale Störungen nach hohen Dosen eines Oxychinolinderivates. Dtsch Med Wochenschr 95: 394–397

Kono R (1975) Introductory review of subacute myelo-optico-neuropathy (SMON) and its studies done by the SMON research commission. Jpn J Med Sci Biol (Suppl) 28: 1–21

Kotaki H, Nakajima K, Tanimura Y, Saitoh Y, Nakagawa F, Tamura Z, Nagashima K (1983) Appearance of intoxication in rats by intraperitoneal administration of clioquinol. J Pharmacobiodyn 6: 773–783

Krinke G, Pericin C, Thomann P, Hess R (1978) Toxic encephalopathy with hippocampal lesions. Zentralbl Veterinarmed [A] 25: 277–296

Krinke G, Schaumburg HH, Spencer PS, Thomann P, Hess R (1979) Clioquinol and 2,5-hexanedione induced different types of distal axonopathy in the dog. Acta Neuropathol (Berl) 47: 213–221

Ozawa K, Saida K, Saida T (1986) Experimental clioquinol intoxication in rats: abnormalities in optic nerves and small nerve cells of dorsal root ganglia. Acta Neuropathol (Berl) 69: 272–277

Püschner H, Fankhauser R (1969) Neuropathologische Befunde bei experimenteller Vioform-Vergiftung der weißen Maus. Schweiz Arch Tierheilkd 3: 371

Sakurama N (1973) An experimental study on pathological changes induced by iodochlorhydroxyquinoline (chinoform) in rabbits. Kumamoto Med J 47: 234–252

Scholz W (1951) Die Krampfschädigungen des Gehirns. Springer, Berlin Heidelberg New York (Monographien aus dem Gesamtgebiete der Neurologie und Psychiatrie, vol 75)

Shiraki H (1971) Neuropathology of subacute myelo-optico-neuropathy, "SMON". Jpn J Med Sci Biol 24: 217–242

Spencer PS, Schaumburg HH (1976) Central and peripheral distal axonopathy – the pathology of dying-back polyneuropathies. In: Zimmermann HH (ed) Progress in neuropathology, vol III. Grune and Stratton, New York, pp 253–295

Tamura Z (1975) Clinical chemistry of clioquinol. Jpn J Med Sci Biol (Suppl) 28: 69–77

Tateishi J, Kuroda S, Saito A, Otsuki S (1973) Experimental myeloneuropathy induced by clioquinol. Acta Neuropathol (Berl) 24: 304–320

Tateishi J, Ogata M, Watanabe S, Kuroda S (1975) Blood concentration of clioquinol (chinoform) in mice after repeated oral administrations. Jpn J Public Health 22: 231–233

Tateishi J, Kuroda S, Ikeda H, Otsuki S (1977) Experimental subacute myeloopticoneuropathy. In: Roizin L, Shiraki H, Grcevic N (eds) Neurotoxicology. Raven, New York, pp 345–351

Thomas PK, Bradley DJ, Bradley WA, Degen PH, Krinke G, Muddle J, Schaumburg HH, Skelton-Stroud PN, Thomann P, Tzebelikos E (1984) Correlated nerve conduction, somatosensory evoked potential and neuropathological studies in clioquinol and 2,5-hexanidione neurotoxicity in the baboon. J Neurol Sci 64: 277–295

Yamanaka N, Imanari T, Tamura Z, Yagi K (1973) Uncoupling of oxidative phosphorylation of rat liver mitochondria by chinoform. J Biochem (Tokyo) 73: 993–998

Neurotoxic Effects of Hexacarbons (*n*-Hexane, Methyl-*n*-Butylketones; 2,5-Hexane-Dione; 1,4-Diketones)

Gisela Stoltenburg-Didinger and Holger Altenkirch

Synonyms. *n*-Hexane (CH_3-CH_2-CH_2-CH_2-CH_2-CH_3); 2-hexanone (methyl-*n*-butylketone, MBK) (CH_3-CO-CH_2-CH_2-CH_2-CH_3); 2,5-hexanedione (2,5-HD) (CH_3-CO-CH_2-CH_2-CO-CH_3); butanone (methylethyl ketone, MEK), (CH_3-CO-CH_2-CH_3).

Gross Appearance

Lesions in the peripheral and central nervous system are not seen grossly.

Microscopic Features

Light-microscopic examination of peripheral nerves reveals the characteristic pattern of scattered multifocal giant axonal swellings (Figs. 27–29). In the beginning these alterations

Fig. 27 *(upper left).* Hexacarbon neuropathy, early stage, ▶ rat. Multifocal giant axonal swellings in longitudinal sections of rat tibial nerve. Enlargement of axonal diameters in the paranodal region *(black arrow)* precedes thinning of myelin sheaths *(open arrow).* Toluidine blue, × 600

Fig. 28 *(lower left).* Hexacarbon neuropathy, early stage, rat. Two large axonal swellings, note thinning of myelin sheath and increased axoplasmic density. Swellings are located proximal as well as distal to node of Ranvier. Toluidine blue, × 600

Fig. 29 *(upper right).* Hexacarbon neuropathy, early stage, rat. Cross section of tibial nerve, several demyelinated giant axonal swellings. Toluidine blue, × 800

Fig. 30 *(lower right).* Hexacarbon neuropathy, early stage, rat. Caudal portion of the ventrolateral tract in lumbar spinal cord with several axonal swellings, one already demyelinated *(arrow).* Toluidine blue, × 800

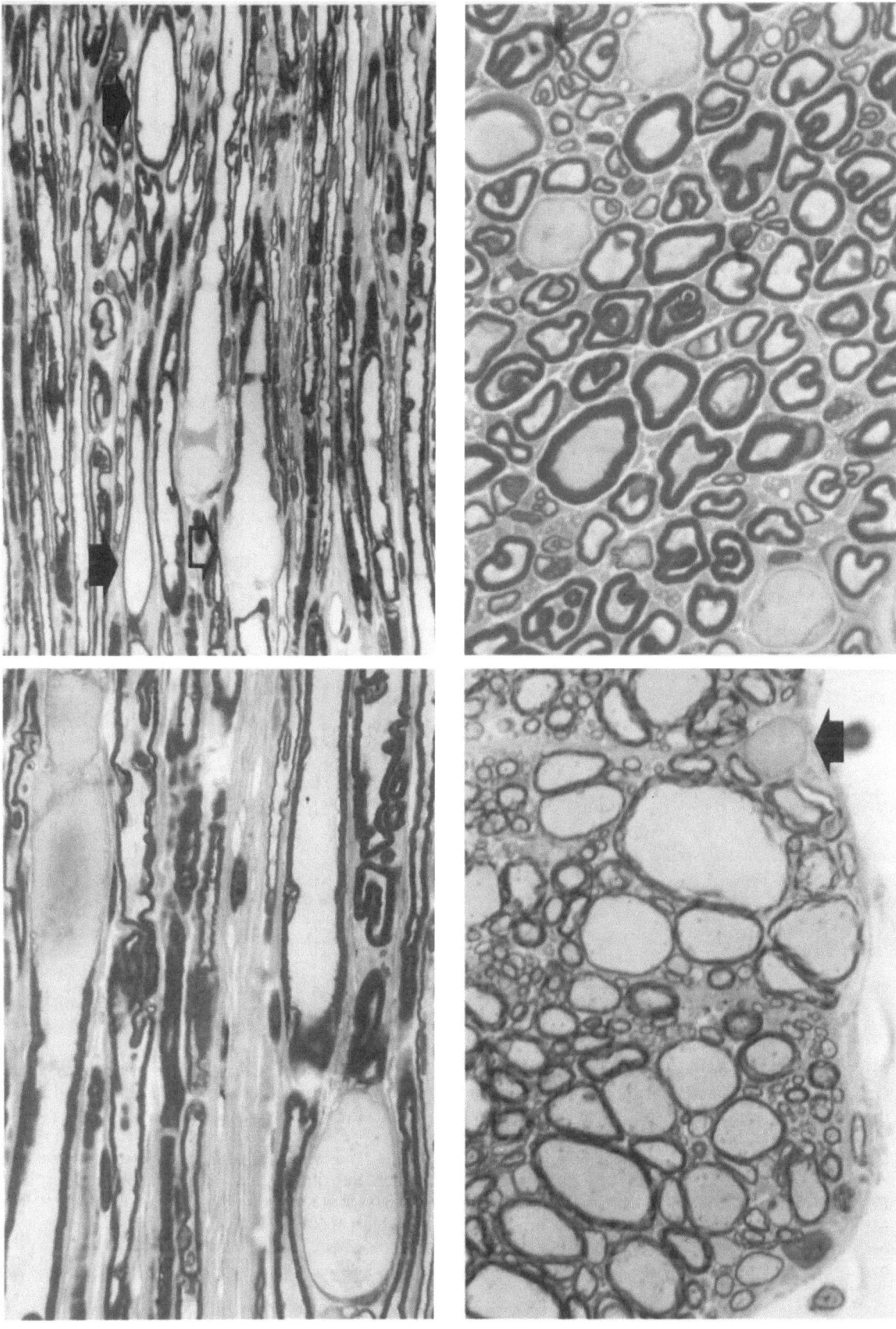

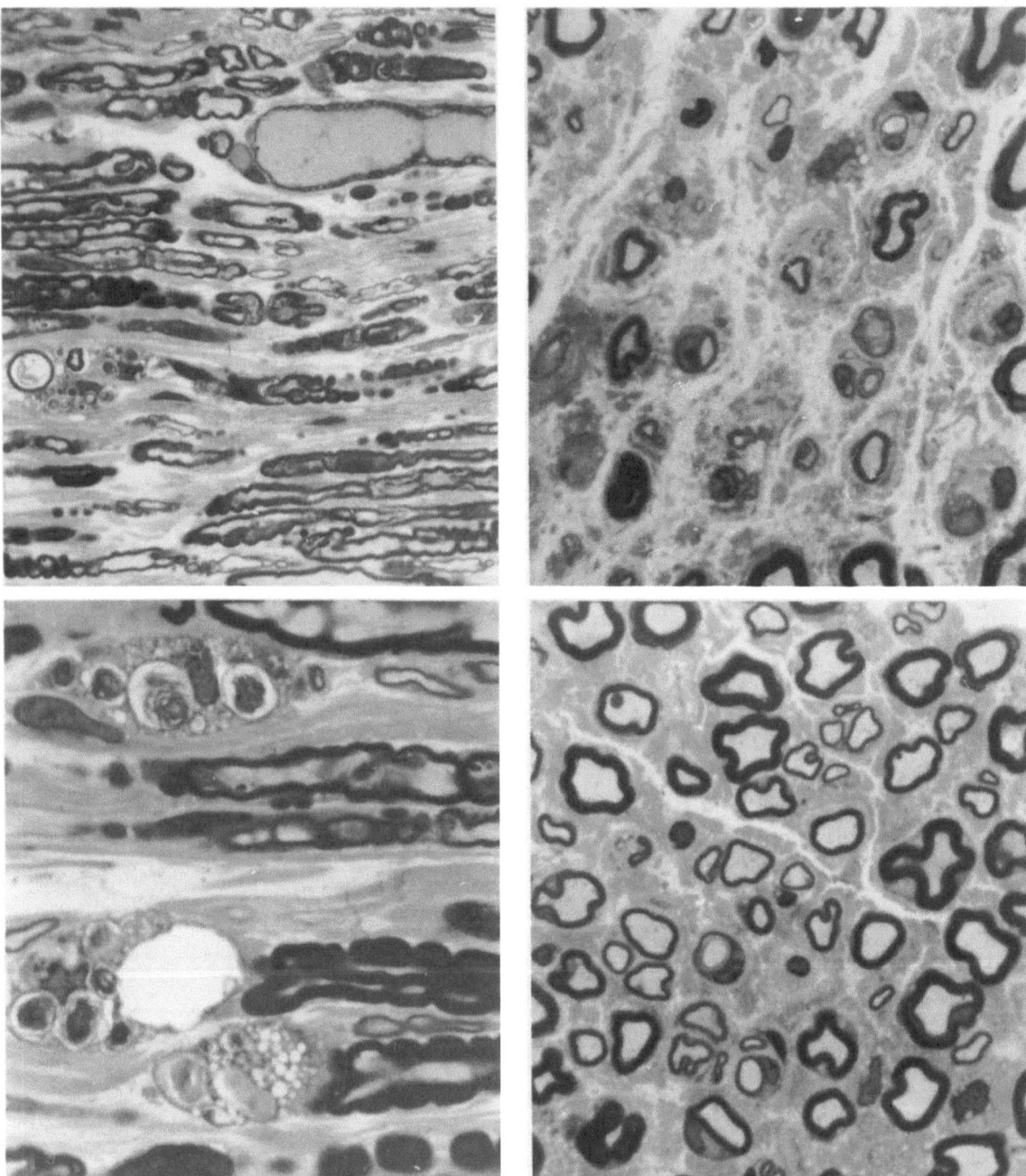

Fig. 31 *(upper left).* Late stage of hexacarbon intoxication. Only axons of small diameter are preserved, in the rest of the section acute and progressive lesions may be seen at the same time: axonal swelling and ovoid formation of former large diameter fibers. Toluidine blue, × 600

Fig. 32 *(lower left).* Late stage of hexacarbon intoxication. Myelin is corrugated in the proximal part of the nerve fiber, the distal part is degenerated to a row of myelin ovoids indicating wallerian degeneration. Toluidine blue, × 1100

Fig. 33 *(upper right).* Cross sections of tibial nerve, hexacarbon intoxication, rat. Early regeneration and remyelination. Toluidine blue, × 600

Fig. 34 *(lower right).* Cross sections of tibial nerve, hexacarbon intoxication, rat. Regeneration in later stages. Axon/myelin ratio still differs from normal fibers. Toluidine blue, × 600

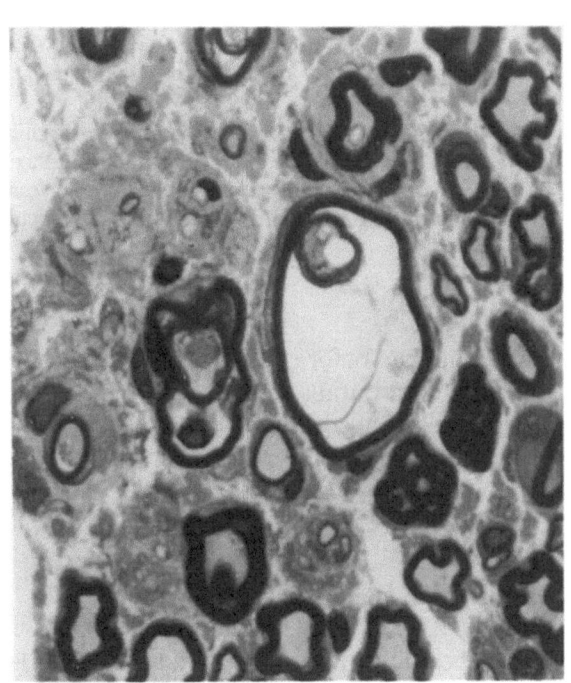

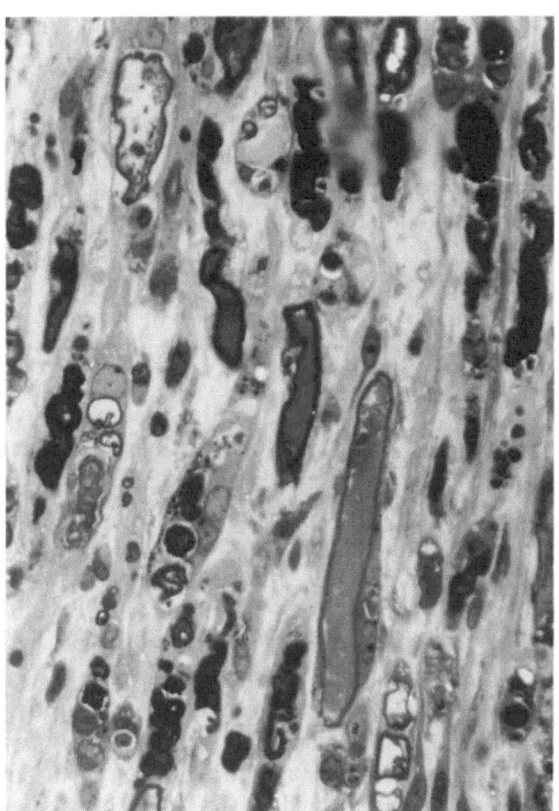

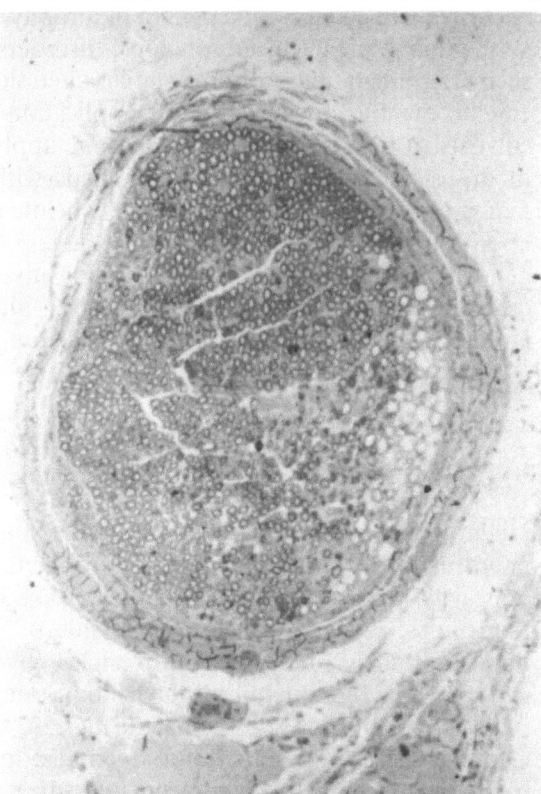

Fig. 35 *(upper left).* Cross sections of tibial nerve, hexacarbon intoxication, rat. Persisting splitting of myelin 6 months after last exposure. Toluidine blue, ×600

Fig. 36 *(upper right).* Tibial nerve, rat, following local application of *n*-hexane. Longitudinal section, most of the fibers have undergone breakdown or swellings. Toluidine blue, ×600

Fig. 37 *(lower right).* Tibial nerve, rat, following local application of MEK. Intact perineurium covers spreading of axonal swellings below application site. H and E, ×25

are mainly localized to the branches of the tibial nerve supplying the calf muscles, but are also seen in other portions of the sciatic nerve, other peripheral nerves, and the spinal cord (Fig. 30). Giant axonal swellings appear in the immediate proximity of the nodes of Ranvier (Figs. 27, 28). In these regions there is a secondary attenuation and retraction of the myelin sheath. Areas of swollen axons display increased axoplasmic density (Figs. 28, 29).

In the course of the intoxication the acute axonal lesions appear concomitantly with distal fiber breakdown (Fig. 31). While the initial axonal swelling undergoes local shrinkage and remyelination, the distal part of the fiber degenerates into a chain of myelin ovoids (Fig. 32).

During and after exposure, signs of regeneration in the form of axonal sprouting with subsequent remyelination are visible (Figs. 33, 34). Even in periods of regeneration, certain myelin alterations are persistent, i.e., corrugation and splitting of the myelin lamellae (Fig. 35). In acute stages of intoxication, skeletal muscles undergo single fiber necrosis indicating a primarily myotoxic action of hexacarbons, whereas in later stages the muscle will reflect the nerve damage exclusively in a neurogenic pattern of atrophy.

While this sequence of morphologic disorders is seen after inhalation exposure, similar alterations can be demonstrated by topical application of solvents to rat nerves in vivo. n-Hexane applied in drops to the living tibial nerve leads within 4 days to axonal swellings immediately below the application site. The fibers are subsequently degenerated in the typical pattern forming myelin ovoids (Fig. 36). Strikingly similar local alterations are evident after topical application of MEK (Fig. 37).

Ultrastructure

Giant axonal swellings contain masses of 10-nm neurofilaments. The condensed neurofilaments appear to be normal in shape and size (Fig. 38). Sometimes, especially on the distal side of the node of Ranvier, mitochondria, vesicles, glycogen granules, neurotubules, and smooth endoplasmic reticulum are accumulated (Figs. 39, 40). Glycogen granules can be found free in the axoplasm in myelinated or unmyelinated fibers or delimited by a single membrane. Regeneration occurs in the form of sprouting of axons. Some of the newly formed axons contain neurofilaments and glycogen exclusively (Fig. 41).

Fig. 38 *(above)*. Cross section of paranodal region of ▶ myelinated nerve fibers, rat. Normal axoplasm with neurotubules, neurofilaments and vesicles, myelin sheath is constructed of several lamellae. TEM, × 31 700

Fig. 39 *(middle)*. Cross section of paranodal region of myelinated nerve fibers, rat. Swollen part of axon, axoplasm contains masses of neurofilaments, myelin sheath *(left)* is reduced to a few lamellae. TEM, × 22 000

Fig. 40 *(below)*. Cross section of paranodal region of myelinated nerve fibers, rat. Part of axon distal to axonal swelling, axoplasm is packed with mitochondria, vesicles, neurotubules, and cisternae of endoplasmic reticulum. TEM, × 20 000

As mentioned before, splitting of myelin lamellae persists even during regeneration periods. Ultrastructurally phagocytic cells are found between the axon and the myelin sheath which is transformed into myelin bubbles.

Differential Diagnosis

The specific morphologic alteration, i.e., large swellings of the axon with intraaxonal accumulation of 10-nm neurofilaments, occurs in several conditions:

- Canine hereditary spinal muscular atrophy
- Amyotrophic lateral sclerosis (ALS)
- Giant axonal neuropathy ("kinky hair disease")
- Intoxications induced by acrylamide, carbon disulfide (CS$_2$),

iminodipropionitrile (IDPN), aluminium, and maytansine (Goldman and Yen 1986).

In all cases the accumulated neurofilaments appear to be normal in shape and structure. The site of the initial cytoskeletal disturbance is, however, different – the filamentous accumulation starts in the proximal portion of the axon in ALS and IDPN intoxication, whereas hexacarbon, CS$_2$, and acrylamide neuropathies begin in the distal portion of the axon.

Biologic Features

Certain aliphatic hydrocarbons are designated as hexacarbons because of their configuration with six C atoms. Normal hexane (n-hexane) and MBK are considered together in this chapter because they are metabolically linked by 2,5-hexan-

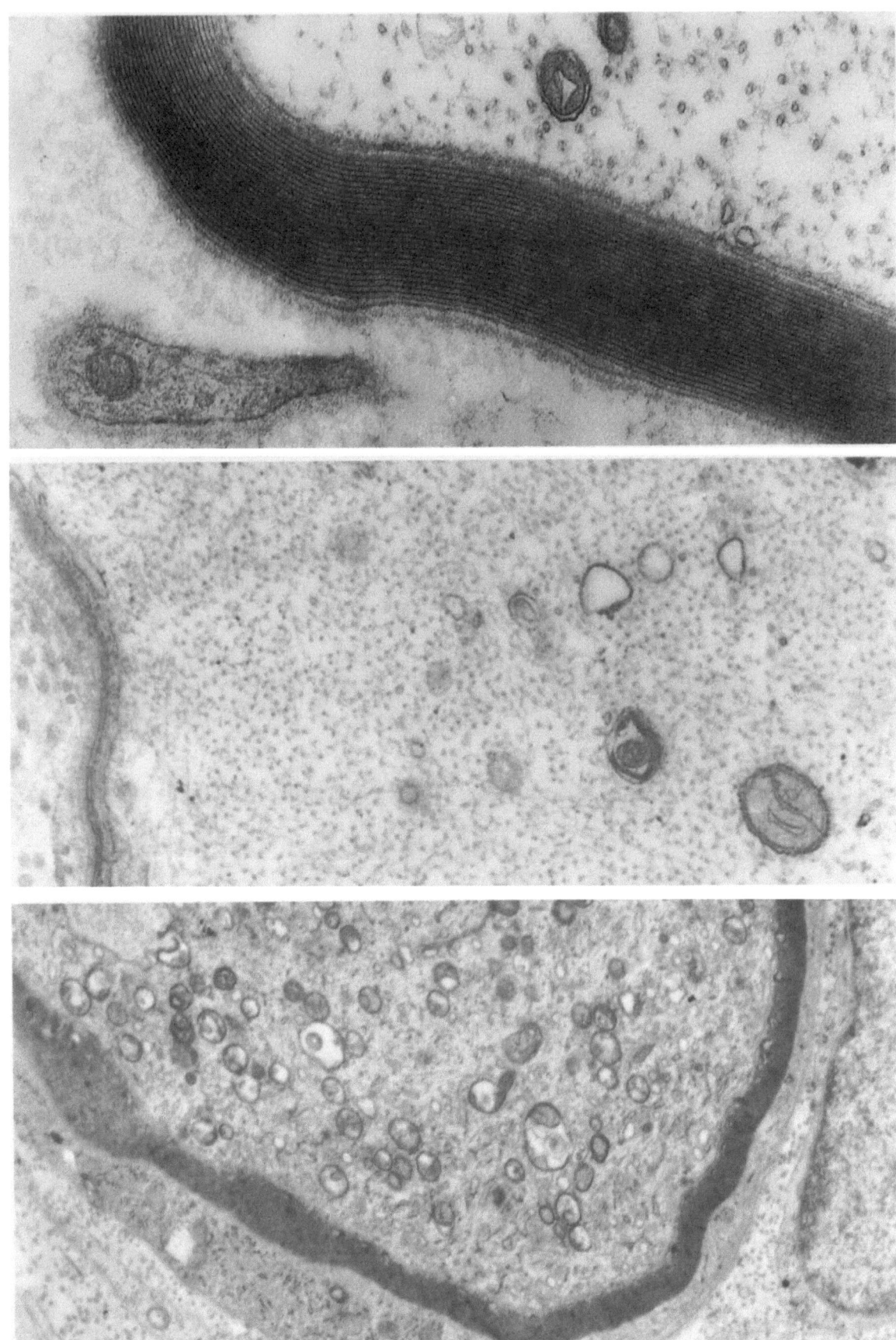

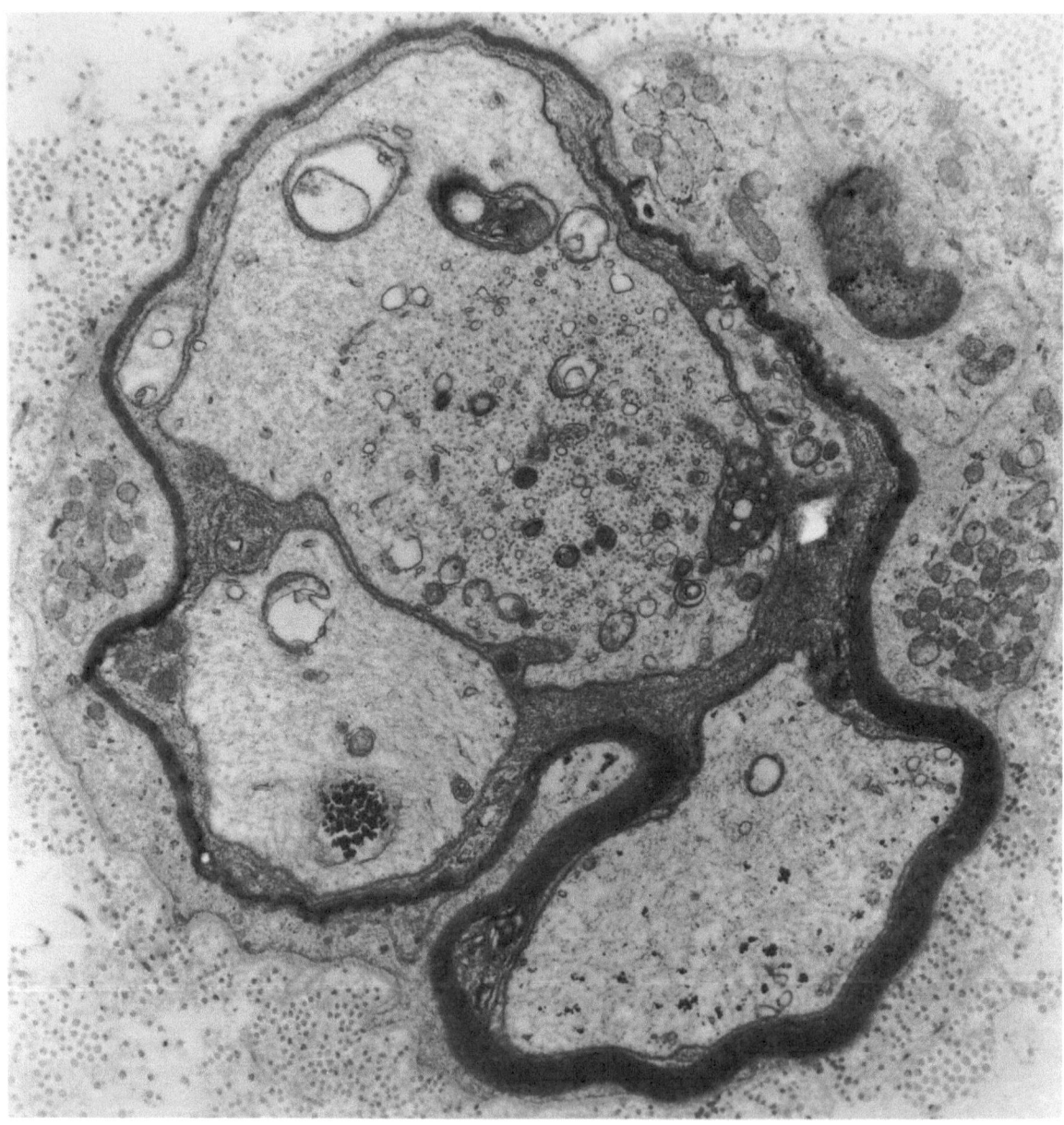

Fig. 41. Regenerating sprouts within one myelin sheath, two of them containing neurofilaments and glycogen. The larger one contains clusters of vesicles and neurotubules. TEM, × 10000

edione, a diketone which is thought to be the decisive neurotoxic metabolite in hexacarbon neurotoxicity. Other gamma-diketones, such as 2,5-heptane-dione and 3,6-octane-dione also cause neuropathy (Spencer et al. 1980a). The widely used industrial solvent MEK, although not a hexacarbon, will be included in this chapter because of its potentiating effects on hexacarbon neurotoxicity (Altenkirch et al. 1982a).

Naturally occurring animal disease secondary to hexacarbons has not been reported. In experimental animal studies, all species tested (chicken,

mouse, rat, dog, cat, monkey) developed a peripheral neuropathy following subacute or subchronic exposure to neurotoxic hexacarbons (Spencer et al. 1980b). Although most experiments use the inhalation exposure, other routes of application such as respiratory, dermal subcutaneous, intraperitoneal and oral have also induced peripheral neuropathies.

Rats exposed continuously by inhalation to 500 ppm of n-hexane display signs of a motor neuropathy after 9 weeks. A mixture of 500 ppm of n-hexane and 200 ppm MEK induces neuro-

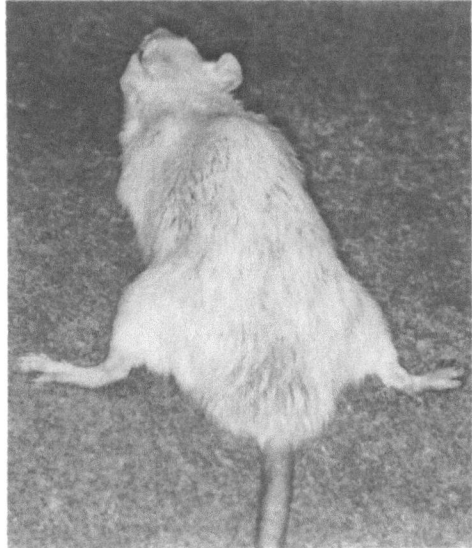

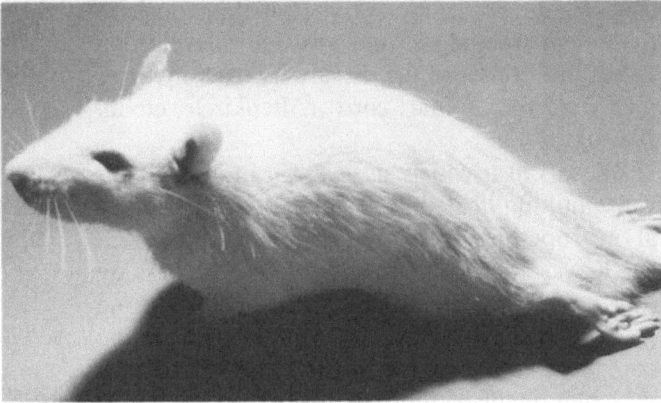

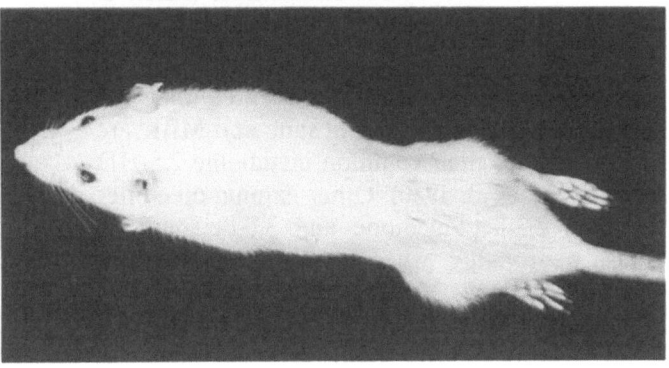

Fig. 42 *(left).* Rat with functional impairment in hexacarbon neuropathy. Slight paresis as earliest clinical sign of peripheral neuropathy. Eversion of the hindlimbs and waddling gait

Fig. 43 *(upper right).* Rat with functional impairment in hexacarbon neuropathy. Severe paraparesis of the hindlimbs, crawling gait

Fig. 44 *(lower right).* Rat with functional impairment in hexacarbon neuropathy. Paralysis manifested by severe tetraparesis and atrophy of hindlimbs and lower trunk

pathy within 4 weeks, i.e., the development of neurotoxic signs can be enhanced by MEK (Altenkirch et al. 1982a).

Clinical Signs. Intoxicated animals develop a motor deficit which evolves as follows:

- Slight paresis manifested by an eversion of the hindlimbs with a waddling gait due to proximal weakness of the hindlimbs (Fig. 42).
- Severe paresis – in this stage rats show a crawling gait moving mainly by means of the forelimbs and are unable to drag the hindlimbs under the trunk (Fig. 43).
- Paralysis – most severely affected animals are unable to move at all. Severe paresis is generally accompanied by atrophy of the hindlimb muscles (Fig. 44).

Human Disease. n-Hexane is widely used as a component of organic solvent mixtures in indus-

try and households. In industrial workers exposed to hexane-containing solvent mixtures endemic outbreaks of neuropathies have occurred in Japan, the United States, Italy, Austria, France, and other European countries. n-Hexane, although a neurotoxin with a specific mechanism of action, has a low neurotoxic effect which can be potentiated by MEK, another industrial solvent of widespread use (Altenkirch et al. 1982a). Mixtures of MEK and n-hexane have been frequently implicated in outbreaks of neuropathy associated with occupational exposures or following deliberate solvent abuse (sniffing). Neuromyelopathies with a particularly severe clinical course have been reported in juveniles who chronically inhaled n-hexane/MEK mixtures. The neurologic picture consists of considerable weight loss, flaccid tetraparesis, muscular atrophy, glove- and stocking-type sensory deficits, and characteristic autonomous disorders in the form of an excessive hyperhidrosis and rubeosis of the extremities. Hyperreflexia, positive pyramidal tract signs, and spasticity developing 1 year after onset of the disease indicate involvement of the spinal cord (Altenkirch et al. 1982 b).

MBK was also widely used as an industrial solvent until implicated in an outbreak of peripheral neuropathies in a factory in Ohio in 1973. MBK was substituted in the printing process by (the non-neurotoxic) methylisobutyl ketone (MIBK) in an attempt to reduce atmospheric contamination. Again MEK acted as a potentiating component of the solvent mixture (Allen et al. 1975).

Pathogenesis. It is generally accepted that the neurotoxic properties of *n*-hexane and MBK are attributable to their common metabolite 2,5-HD (Krasavage et al. 1980). Other gamma-diketones such as 2,5-heptanedione and 3,6-octanedione cause neuropathy, whereas related compounds (2,4-hexanedione, 2,3-hexanedione and 2,6-heptanedione), which lack the 1,4 spacing of the carbonyl groups, fail to produce experimental neuropathy. Presumably, circulating 2,5-HD disrupts neuronal axonal function and results in massive, focal accumulations of neurofilaments in distal regions of certain axons (Spencer et al. 1980 b). The following hypotheses have been suggested for the mechanism of toxic action:

- A defect in energy metabolism has been proposed as the key mechanism of toxic action. Spencer et al. (1979) suggested that neurotoxic hexacarbons bind to glycolytic enzymes in the nerve fibers causing a dose-dependent inhibition of enzyme activity along the entire length of the axon. Under these circumstances, the neuronal perikaryon would be unable to supply the elevated demand for glycolytic enzyme so that the distal regions would become enzyme deficient. This would result in a diminished energy supply with subsequent axonal transport malfunction and nerve fiber degeneration.
- Another hypothesis states that the toxic metabolite (2,5-HD) results in covalent cross-linking of neurofilaments during the progression of slow axonal transport. The reduction in axonal diameter at the nodes of Ranvier presents obstructions to the proxio-distal flow of the growing mass of neurofilaments, and, when the aggregate of neurofilaments is too large to pass through the nodes of Ranvier, the subsequent obstruction of axonal transport leads to

a proximal axonal enlargement and degenerative changes in the axon distal to this point (Graham 1980).
- Another mechanism was proposed by DeCaprio et al. (1982) who demonstrated in experimental studies that pyrrole adduct formation is the precipitating factor in diketone neuropathies.

Comparison with Other Species

Most experimental studies concerning the morphologic alterations of hexacarbons were performed on rats. In our own experience the morphology and topography of hexacarbon-induced lesions within the peripheral nervous system are comparable in human biopsies and animal experimental studies. In animals, central nervous system damage is located in the long ascending and descending spinal cord tracts, cerebellar white matter, optic nerve, and mamillary bodies. In humans no such data on central nervous system damage induced by *n*-hexane are available. Spastic gait and impaired vision and memory are believed to represent the human correlates of this pathologic substrate found in animals (Spencer et al. 1980 b).

References

Allen N, Mendell JR, Billmaier DJ, Fontaine RE, O'Neill J (1975) Toxic polyneuropathy due to methyl-*n*-butyl-ketone. Arch Neurol 32: 209–218

Altenkirch H, Wagner HM, Stoltenburg-Didinger G, Steppat R (1982a) Potentiation of hexacarbon-neurotoxicity by methyl-ethyl-ketone (MEK) and other substances: clinical and experimental aspects. Neurobehav Toxicol Teratol 4: 623–627

Altenkirch H, Wagner HM, Stoltenburg-Didinger G, Spencer PS (1982b) Nervous system responses of rats to subchronic inhalation of *n*-hexane and *n*-hexane + methyl-ethyl-ketone mixtures. J Neurol Sci 57: 209–219

DeCaprio AP, Olavos EJ, Weber P (1982) Covalent binding of a neurotoxic *n*-hexane metabolite. Conversion of primary amines to substituted pyrrole adducts by 2,5-hexanedione. Toxicol Appl Pharmacol 65: 440–450

Goldman JE, Yen SH (1986) Cytoskeletal protein abnormalities in neurodegenerative diseases. Ann Neurol 19: 209–223

Graham DG (1980) Hexane neuropathy: a proposal for pathogenesis of a hazard of occupational exposure and inhalant abuse. Chem Biol Interact 32: 339–345

Krasavage WJ, O'Donoghue JL, DiVincenco GD, Terhaar CJ (1980) The relative neurotoxicity of methyl-*n*-butyl-ketone, *n*-hexane and their metabolites. Toxicol Appl Pharmacol 52: 433–441

Spencer PS, Sabri MI, Schaumburg HH, Moore CL (1979) Does a defect of energy metabolism in the nerve fiber underlie axonal degeneration in polyneuropathies? Ann Neurol 5: 501–507

Spencer PS, Couri D, Schaumburg HH (1980a) n-Hexane and methyl-n-butylketone. In: Spencer PS, Schaumburg HH (eds) Experimental and clinical neurotoxicology. Williams and Wilkins, Baltimore, pp 456–475

Spencer PS, Schaumburg HH, Sabri MI, Veronesi B (1980b) The enlarging view of hexacarbon neurotoxicity. CRC Crit Rev Toxicol 7: 279–356

Organophosphorus Ester-Induced Delayed Neuropathy, Rat

Bernard S. Jortner

Synonyms. Organophosphorus ester-induced delayed neurotoxicity, distal symmetrical neuropathy, distal progressive axonopathy, polyneuropathy, dying-back neuropathy.

Gross Appearance

No gross lesion is evident in the nervous system.

Microscopic Features

The pathologic features of organophosphorus ester-induced delayed neurotoxicity have been determined from studies in species other than the rat, mainly the cat and chicken. These need to be summarized prior to consideration of the rodent model of this condition. This delayed neuropathy differs from acute cholinergic effects elicited by many organophosphates (see Biologic Features) and occurs following a latent period of about 1–2 weeks after dosing with appropriate compounds. Neurons are the target cell with progressive bilateral lesions elicited in distal regions of longer, larger myelinated fibers in both central and peripheral nervous system. In the latter, these changes are thus best seen in distal regions of sciatic nerve branches such as the plantar and common peroneal nerves (Cavanagh 1954, 1964; Prineas 1969) and the recurrent laryngeal nerve (Bouldin and Cavanagh 1979a, b). Lesions in the central nervous system are most evident in the rostral cervical spinal cord and brain stem levels of ascending pathways such as the spinocerebellar and gracilis tracts, and lumbosacral regions of descending fibers as in the reticulospinal and corticospinal tracts (Beresford and Glees 1963; Cavanagh 1954; Cavanagh and Patangia 1965; Jortner 1982, 1984; Jortner et al. 1983). The cerebellar white matter may also have distal fiber tract lesions (Cavanagh 1954; Cavanagh and Patangia 1965).

Initial morphologic effects are seen in axons. At the light-microscopic level these consist of distal, nonterminal swelling, axoplasmic densities, and increased argyrophilia which are followed by wallerian degeneration of the fiber (Fig. 45) (Beresford and Glees 1963; Bouldin and Cavanagh 1979a; Cavanagh 1954; Jortner and Ehrich 1987; Jortner et al. 1983; Preissig and Abou-Donia 1978). There is a phagocytic and glial reaction to these in the central or peripheral nervous system, with a potential for regeneration in the latter region.

Ultrastructure

Ultrastructural changes in affected axons prior to breakdown of the fiber include accumulation of branching cisternal structures resembling agranular endoplasmic reticulum, swelling and rarefaction of axoplasm, granular degeneration of neurofilaments, mitochondrial degeneration, and the presence of dense and membranous bodies (Bischoff 1967, 1970; Bouldin and Cavanagh 1979b; Jortner and Ehrich 1987; Le Vay et al. 1971; Prineas 1969) (Figs. 46, 47, 48). Transmission electron microscopy of teased fibers of the feline recurrent laryngeal nerve have revealed that diisopropylfluorophosphate (DFP), a direct-acting neurotoxin, elicits early, focal, distal but not terminal varicosities due to the presence of intramyelinic or intra-axonal vacuoles (Bouldin and Cavanagh 1979a, b).

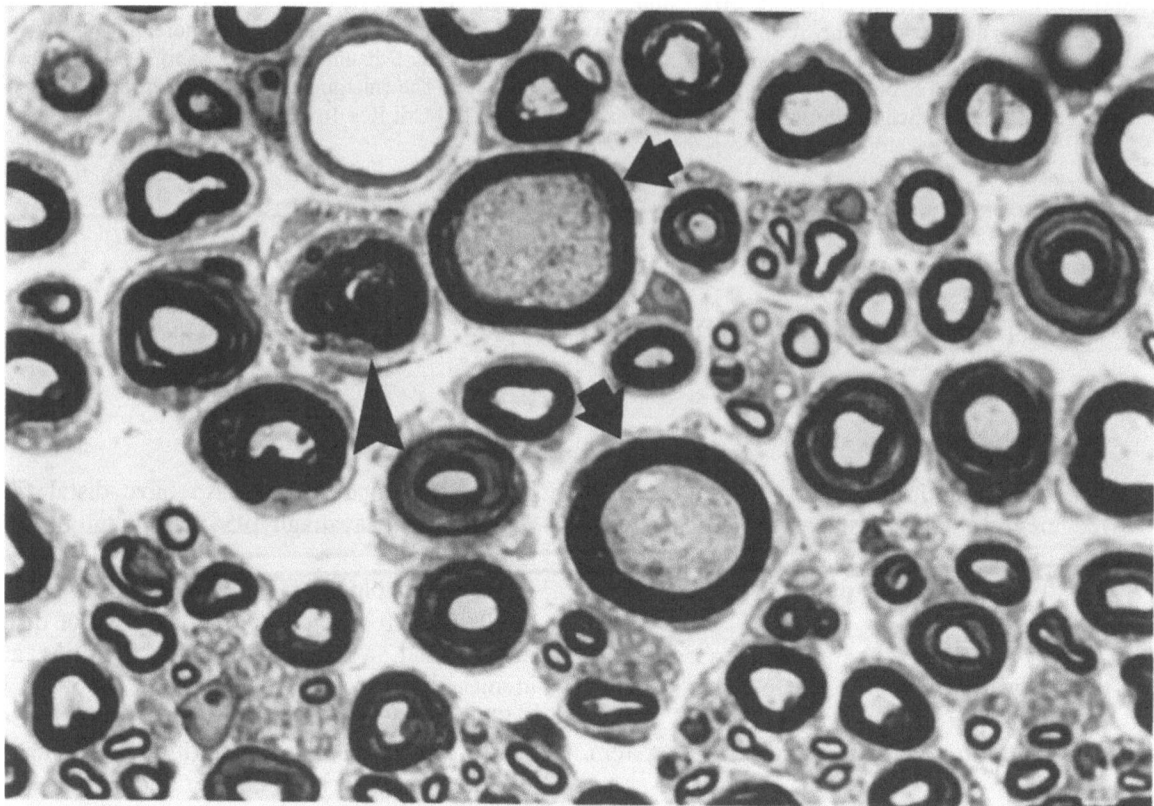

Fig. 45. Cross section of dorsal metatarsal nerve of chicken with delayed neuropathy due to organophosphorus ester. Note swollen, dark-staining, debris-laden myelinated axons *(arrows)* and another fiber undergoing wallerian degeneration *(arrowhead).* Toluidine blue-safranin, × 1700

Differential Diagnosis

The presence of bilateral, distal, centripetal neuropathy, with lesions of axonopathy and subsequent wallerian degeneration in myelinated fibers of peripheral nerves and long pathways of the spinal cord, is suggestive of delayed neuropathy induced by organophosphates. Definitive diagnosis requires additional historical or biochemical data. A history of exposure to an organophosphorus-delayed neurotoxin weeks prior to onset of clinical disease is of considerable significance. Chemical detection of the compound in body tissues is not possible at the time clinical evidence of the neuropathy exists. The toxins elicit their effects and are metabolized in the interval between exposure and clinical onset (Davis and Richardson 1980). Similarly, known biochemical effects of these toxins must be detected shortly after exposure. As discussed below, the depression of neurotoxic esterase activity is manifest within 40 h of dosing and returns to normal by the time nerve fibers are undergoing degradative changes (Johnson 1975, 1982; Ehrich

Fig. 46 *(above).* Dorsal metatarsal nerve of a chicken ▶ 14–24 days following administration of 360 mg/kg triorthotoyl phosphate. Note increased intra-axonal agranular endoplasmic reticulum cisternae *(arrows)* and a dense body *(arrowhead).* TEM, × 21 666

Fig. 47 *(below).* Dorsal metatarsal nerve of a chicken 14–24 days following administration of 360 mg/kg triorthotoyl phosphate. Note local intra-axonal increase in mitochondria and dense bodies. TEM, × 21 945

et al. 1986; Jortner and Ehrich 1987). Other esterases inhibited by organophosphorus compounds (e.g., cholinesterase and carboxylesterases) also tend to recover in days to weeks following toxin adminstration (Ehrich et al. 1986).

A range of other toxin elicit a similar pattern of lesions of the nervous system, the "dying-back" central and peripheral neuropathy (Cavanagh 1979). Some of these, such as acrylamide, carbon disulfide, and the hexacarbons, tend to elicit axonal swelling due to often massive accumulation of 10-nm neurofilaments. This is a rather distinctive lesion and can be detected by electron mi-

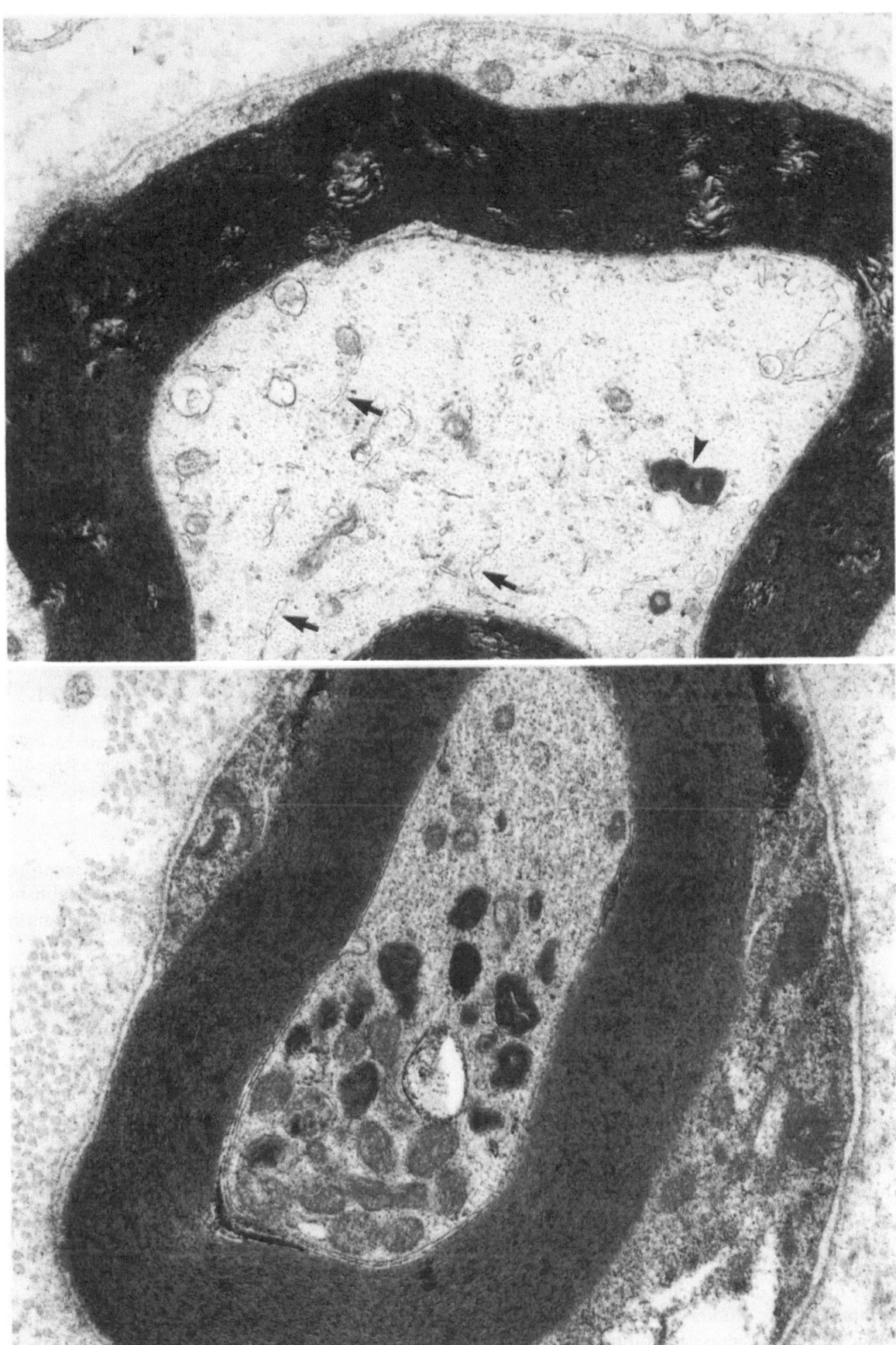

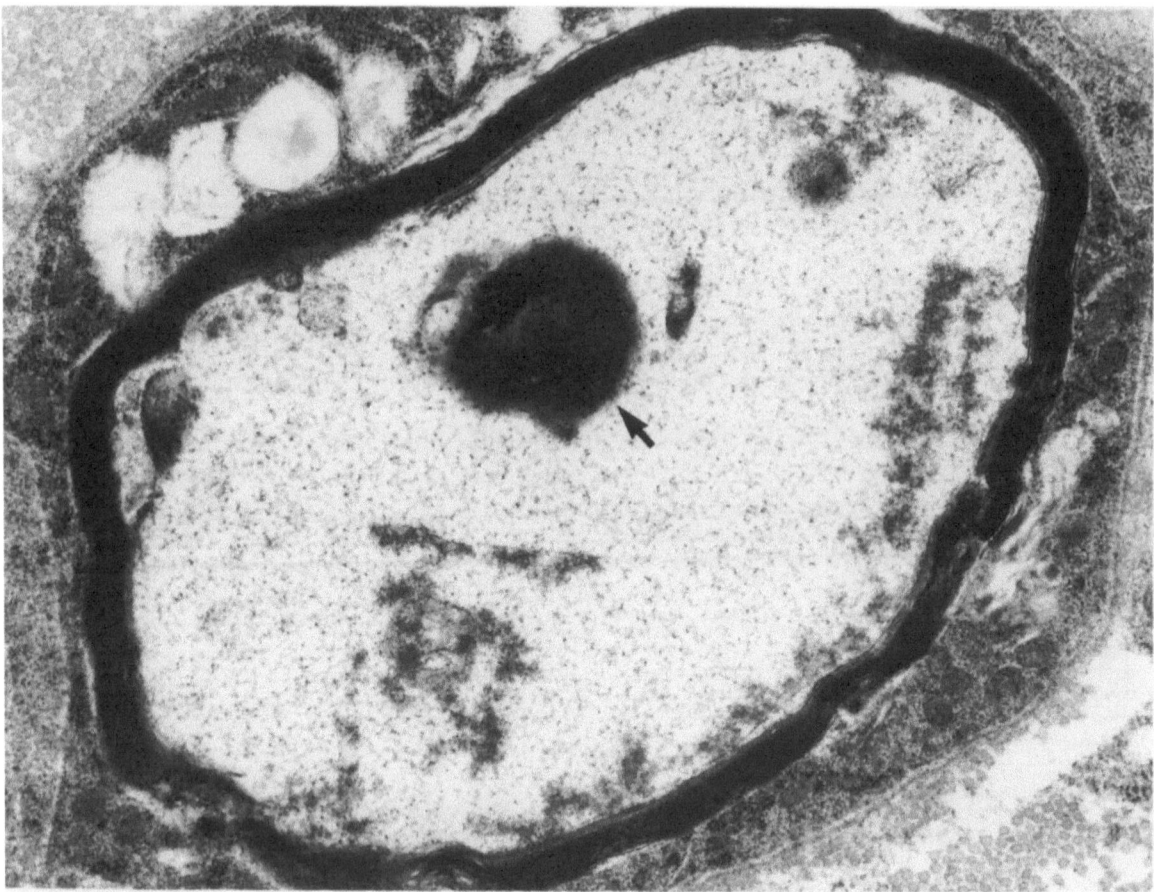

Fig. 48. Dorsal metatarsal nerve of a chicken 14–24 days following administration of 360 mg/kg triorthotoyl phosphate. Note swollen axon with granular debris (most likely representing neurofilament degeneration) and a large dense body *(arrow).* TEM, ×21259

croscopy. Organophosphorus compounds do not have this ability, but they do tend to elicit intra-axonal membranous accumulations and, in some studies, fiber vacuoles (Bouldin and Cavanagh 1979b; Jortner and Ehrich 1987; Veronesi 1984). As stated above, definitive diagnosis must be supported by historical and biochemical data.

Biologic Features

The precise mechanisms by which an appropriate dose of an organophosphate delayed neurotoxin produces distal axonopathy and subsequent wallerian degeneration some days to weeks later is not known. Some correlates of in vivo biochemical effects such compounds and development of the neuropathy have been attempted. Early studies relating the acute effects such as cholinesterase inhibition and associated cholinergic clinical signs to the delayed neuropa-

thy have been discarded (Davis and Richardson 1980). A clear relationship has been established between the nature of the reaction of certain organophosphorus compounds (delayed neurotoxins) with neurotoxic esterase, an enzyme found in the nervous system (and other tissues), and the development of delayed neuropathy (Johnson 1975, 1982). A wide variety of protoxicants (including triorthocresyl phosphate) and direct-acting compounds (including mipafox, phenyl saligenin phosphate, DFP) have the ability to inhibit transiently some 75% or more of the activity of brain or spinal cord neurotoxic esterase following a single oral or parenteral neurotoxic dose. To be neurotoxic, this process undergoes certain necessary steps. Initially there is phosphorylation (or phosphonylation, etc.), followed by "aging." The latter is a rapid cleavage process yielding an ionized acidic group on the phosphorus atom of the neurotoxic esterase-organophosphorus complex (Johnson 1982). It has been suggested that the charged group on the aged neurotoxic esterase (or on the portion cleaved from it) upset the normal milieu of the neuron and leads to the axonopathy (Johnson 1982). This must be a brief interaction since neurotoxic esterase activity returns to normal by the time neuropathy occurs. Multiple smaller doses of these delayed neurotoxins can elicit the neuropathy if a plateau of some 50%–65% neurotoxic esterase inhibition is maintained.

The Long-Evans hooded rat model has been evaluated in part as to its toxic metabolic similarity to more traditional experimental forms. The relationship of significant delayed neuropathy to the degree of acute inhibition of neurotoxic esterase activty has been established as in other species. Direct-acting (mipafox) and metabolically activated (triorthocresyl phosphate) delayed neurotoxins elicited prominent axonal injury following inhibition of $\geq 66\%$ brain and $\geq 72\%$ spinal cord neurotoxic esterase activity (Padilla and Veronesi 1985; Veronesi et al. 1986). As in other species, the ability of a nonaging inhibitor of neurotoxic esterase (phenylmethylsulfonyl fluoride) to protect against organophosphorus-delayed neurotoxins has also been established in rats (Veronesi and Padilla 1985). This confirms the significance of the aging reaction of neurotoxic esterase in the evolution of lesions in this species.

What happens to the neuron following these episodes, leading to the neuropathy, is not understood. A number of hypotheses have been put forth. The predilection for lesions to develop distally in the longest, largest nerve fibers has led to suggestion that the high level of synthesis, transport, or utilization of essential materials needed by such cells might be particularly prone to interference by the neurotoxic organophosphorus compound (Cavanagh 1973). Glazer et al. (1978) have suggested that a trophic substance necessary for neuronal preservation might be changed.

Alteration of some aspect of axonal transport may well be a factor in the evolution of this neuropathy, although a definite pattern of dysfunction has yet to emerge (Bradley and Williams 1973; James and Austin 1970; Moretto et al. 1986; Pleasure et al. 1969; Reichert and Abou-Donia 1980). An effect on neuronal membranes as a major event has been supported by the ultrastructural prominence of early membranous changes in affected axons and by the work of Bouldin and Cavanagh (1979a, b). The latter suggest that an early breakdown of membrane control of intra-extracellular ionic gradients leads to early influx of water and to subsequent wallerian degeneration.

Comparison with Other Species

As early experimental approaches were made to this delayed neuropathy, it was believed that rodents (rats and mice) were not suitable laboratory animals. Although these species were susceptible to the acute (cholinergic) effects of organophosphorus compounds, the delayed neuropathy was inconsistently produced, even using multiple doses of documented neurotoxins (Abou-Donia 1981; Barnes and Denz 1953; Johnson 1975, 1982). A basis for this refractoriness was thought to lie in more rapid metabolism and excretion of such compounds by these animals compared to susceptible species (Abou-Donia 1981). Other considerations have included inhibitor specificity of neurotoxic esterase (also known as "neuropathy target esterase"; see Biologic Features) forms in brains of different species, or the inability of active metabolites of neurotoxic compounds to reach the site of action in sufficient concentration (Soliman et al. 1982).

Continuing interest in developing a small mammalian experimental model has led to reevaluation of the laboratory rat for this purpose. Although clinical signs of this neuropathy in the rat are often subtle and difficult to evaluate, neuropathologic changes are present and can be quantitated (Veronesi 1984). A model using Long-Evans hooded male rats of about 90 days of age has been developed (Padilla and Veronesi 1985; Veronesi 1984; Veronesi et al. 1986). Rats require larger doses of the organophosphate than chickens to elicit lesions.

Single-dose gavage studies indicate 834–3480 mg/kg of the protoxicant triorthotoyl phosphate is needed to produce this delayed neuropathy in $\geq 90\%$ of rats, but only 360 mg/kg is required in chickens (Ehrich et al. 1986; Jortner and Ehrich 1987; Padilla and Veronesi 1985). Following these large doses, cholinergic complications are not uncommon in rats. Clinical signs of delayed neurotoxicity, such as walking on hocks or crossing of rear legs when the animal is lifted by the tail, have been observed in the above-noted rat model.

However, evaluation of the severity of toxic effects rests with semiquantitative light-microscopic assessment of lesions involving the fasciculus gracilis ascending tract at the C-2 levels of the spinal cord (Padilla and Veronesi 1985; Veronesi 1984; Veronesi et al. 1986).

In spite of the larger doses required, lesions elicited by organophosphorus delayed neurotoxins in the rat are not dissimilar from those in chickens and other experimental animals. A progressive, centripetal distal axonopathy is produced affecting longer, larger diameter myelinated fibers most severely and leading to fiber degeneration. As noted above, lesions can be best evaluated in the rostral cervical (distal) levels of the fasciculus gracilis. The extent of swollen axons, intra-axonal hyaline bodies and myelin vacuoles are used to score the severity of pathologic lesions (Veronesi 1984). Electron-microscopic study of the swollen axons at a relatively early time point (2 weeks) reveals intra-axonal accumulation of tubulovesicular profiles derived from smooth endoplasmic reticulum or large intramyelinic or intra-axonal vacuoles. Later (6 weeks) swollen axons are packed with massive quantities of mitochondria, dense bodies, and vesicular profiles in granular cytoplasm making up the hyaline bodies. Lesions in peripheral nerves appear similar and lead to distal, centripetal wallerian degeneration (Itoh et al. 1985; Veronesi 1984). Attempts to quantify profiles of the latter (myelin ellipsoids) in nerve cross sections are confounded in early stages (2 or 6 weeks in a multidose study) by the presence of regenerating axons, a feature less obvious at 12 weeks (Veronesi 1984).

Other attempts to produce a rat model of the delayed neuropathy caused by organophosphorus have met with varying degrees of success. Itoh et al. (1985) have produced this syndrome by using relatively young animals, 7-week-old Sprague-Dawley rats, and 12 semiweekly subcutaneous doses of 600 mg/kg triorthotoyl phosphate. Acute cholinergic effects, often transiently delayed rear leg weakness, and consistent lesions in peripheral nerves and fasciculus gracilis in spinal cord and brain stem were seen. Other attempts to elicit this syndrome in rats have been less successful (Sprague et al. 1985). The use of mice has similarly given mixed results (Lapadula et al. 1985; Soliman et al. 1982).

The Long-Evans hooded rat model appears most reliable (Padilla and Veronesi 1985; Veronesi 1984; Veronesi et al. 1986). Lesions and their distribution and mechanisms of the neuropathy appear generally similar to those of experimental models such as chickens and cats. The rat appears less sensitive than chickens as doses required for its elucidation are much higher. The rat is also better able to clinically mask the effects of the neuropathy.

Human cases of delayed neuropathy due to organophosphorus ester have a similar delayed onset of clinical signs which take the form of a distal sensorimotor neuropathy (Cavanagh 1979). Mild cases may undergo clinical recovery, but more severe ones retain evidence of an upper motor neuron lesion.

Acknowledgement. I wish to acknowledge my collaborative association with Dr. M. Ehrich and the support provided by the National Institutes of Environmental Health Sciences, grant 03384.

References

Abou-Donia MB (1981) Organophosphorus ester-induced delayed neurotoxicity. Annu Rev Pharmacol Toxicol 21: 511–548

Barnes JM, Denz FA (1953) Experimental demyelination with organophosphorus compounds. J Pathol Bacteriol 65: 597–606

Beresford WA, Glees P (1963) Degeneration in the long tracts of the cords of the chicken and cat after triortho-cresylphosphate poisoning. Acta Neuropathol (Berl) 3: 108–118

Bischoff A (1967) The ultrastructure of tri-ortho-cresyl phosphate poisoning. I. Studies on myelin and axonal alterations in the sciatic nerve. Acta Neuropathol (Berl) 9: 158–174

Bischoff A (1970) Ultrastructure of tri-ortho-cresyl phosphate poisoning in the chicken. II. Studies on spinal cord alterations. Acta Neuropathol (Berl) 15: 142–155

Bouldin TW, Cavanagh JB (1979a) Organophosphorus neuropathy. I. A teased-fiber study of the spatio-temporal spread of axonal degeneration. Am J Pathol 94: 241–252

Bouldin TW, Cavanagh JB (1979b) Organophosphorus neuropathy. II. A fine-structural study of the early stages of axonal degeneration. Am J Pathol 94: 253–270

Bradley WG, Williams MH (1973) Axoplasmic flow in axonal neuropathies. I. Axoplasmic flow in cats with toxic neuropathies. Brain 96: 235–246

Cavanagh JB (1954) The toxic effects of tri-ortho-cresyl phosphate on the nervous system. An experimental study in hens. J Neurol Neurosurg Psychiatry 17: 163–172

Cavanagh JB (1964) Peripheral nerve changes in ortho-cresyl phosphate poisoning in the cat. J Pathol Bacteriol 87: 365–383

Cavanagh JB (1973) Peripheral neuropathy caused by chemical agents. CRC Crit Rev Toxicol 2: 365–417

Cavanagh JB (1979) The 'dying back' process. A common denominator in many naturally occurring and toxic neuropathies. Arch Pathol Lab Med 103: 659–664

Cavanagh JB, Patangia GN (1965) Changes in the central nervous system in the cat as a result of tri-*o*-cresyl phosphate poisoning. Brain 88: 165–180

Davis CS, Richardson RJ (1980) Organophosphorus compounds. In: Spencer PS, Schaumberg HH (eds) Experimental and clinical neurotoxicology. Williams and Wilkins, Baltimore, pp 527-544

Ehrich M, Jortner BS, Gross WB (1986) Dose-related beneficial and adverse effects of dietary corticosterone on organophosphorus-induced delayed neuropathy in chickens. Toxicol Appl Pharmacol 83: 250-260

Glazer EJ, Baker T, Riker WF (1978) The neuropathology of DFP at cat soleus neuromuscular junction. J Neurocytol 7: 741-758

Itoh H, Kishida H, Takeuchi E, Tadokoro M, Uchikoshi T, Oikawa K (1985) Studies on the delayed neurotoxicity of organophosphorus compounds - (III). J Toxicol Sci 10: 67-82

James KAC, Austin L (1970) The effect of DFP on axonal transport of protein in chicken sciatic nerve. Brain Res 18: 192-194

Johnson MK (1975) Organophosphorus esters causing delyed neurotoxic effects: mechanisms of action and structure activity studies. Arch Toxicol 34: 259-288

Johnson MK (1982) The target for initiation of delayed neurotoxicity by organophosphorus esters: biochemical studies and toxicological applications. Rev Biochem Toxicol 4: 141-212

Jortner BS (1982) Selected aspects of the anatomy and response to injury of the chicken (Gallus domesticus) nervous system. Neurotoxicology 3: 299-310

Jortner BS (1984) Pathology of organophosphorus-induced delayed neurotoxicity. In: MacEwen JD, Vernot EH (eds) Proceedings, 14th annual conference of environmental toxicology. National Technical Information Service, Springfield, VA, pp 106-117

Jortner BS, Ehrich M (1987) Neuropathological effects of phenyl saligenin phosphate in chickens. Neurotoxicology 8: 97-108

Jortner BS, Pope AM, Heavner JE (1983) Haloxon-induced delayed neurotoxicity: effect of plasma A (aryl) esterase activity on severity of lesions in sheep. Neurotoxicology 4: 241-246

Lapadula DM, Patton SE, Campbell GA, Abou-Donia MB (1985) Characterization of delayed neurotoxicity in the mouse following chronic oral administration of tri-o-cresyl phosphate. Toxicol Appl Pharmacol 79: 83-90

Le Vay S, Meier C, Glees P (1971) Effects of tri-ortho-cresyl-phosphate on spinal ganglia and peripheral nerves of chicken. Acta Neuropathol (Berl) 17: 103-113

Moretto A, Lotti M, Sabri MI, Spencer PS (1986) Reduced retrograde transport heralds OP axonopathy. Trans Am Soc Neurochem 17: 162

Padilla S, Veronesi B (1985) The relationship between neurological damage and neurotoxic esterase inhibition in rats acutely exposed to tri-ortho-cresyl phosphate. Toxicol Appl Pharmacol 78: 78-87

Pleasure DE, Mishler KC, Engel WK (1969) Axonal transport of proteins in experimental neuropathies. Science 166: 524-525

Preissig SH, Abou-Donia MB (1978) The neuropathology of leptophos in the hen: a chronologic study. Environ Res 17: 242-250

Prineas J (1969) The pathogenesis of dying-back polyneuropathies. I. An ultrastructural study of experimental tri-ortho-cresyl phosphate intoxication in the cat. J Neuropathol Exp Neurol 28: 571-597

Reichert BL, Abou-Donia MB (1980) Inhibition of fast axoplasmic transport by delayed neurotoxic organophosphorus esters: a possible model of action. Mol Pharmacol 17: 56-60

Soliman SA, Linder R, Farmer J, Curley A (1982) Species susceptibility to delayed toxic neuropathy in relation to in vivo inhibition of neurotoxic esterase by neurotoxic organophosphorus esters. J Toxicol Environ Health 9: 189-197

Sprague GL, Fordan BL, Bickford AA, Castles TR (1985) Failure of piperonyl butoxide to alter TOCP lethality or delayed neurotoxicity in rats. Toxicologist 5: 194

Veronesi B (1984) A rodent model of organophosphorus-induced delayed neuropathy: distribution of central (spinal cord) and peripheral nerve damage. Neuropathol Appl Neurobiol 10: 357-368

Veronesi B, Padilla S (1985) Phenylmethylsulfonyl fluoride protects rats from mipafox-induced delayed neuropathy. Toxicol Appl Pharmacol 81: 258-264

Veronesi B, Padilla S, Lyerly D (1986) The correlation between neurotoxic esterase inhibition and mipafox-induced neuropathic damage in rats. Neurotoxicology 7: 207-216

Neurotoxic Effects of Ethidium Bromide, Rat

Kinuko Suzuki

Gross Appearance

Pathologic lesions are produced by a direct exposure of the central and peripheral nervous tissues to ethidium bromide which is a red dye. Therefore the lesion appears red or reddish-orange and softer than the surrounding tissue.

Microscopic Features

Central Nervous System. Within 24 h of exposure to ethidium bromide, well-defined, rod-shaped structures appear in the swollen cytoplasm of oligodendrocytes. They are usually found in the perikaryal region, but often appear to extend to

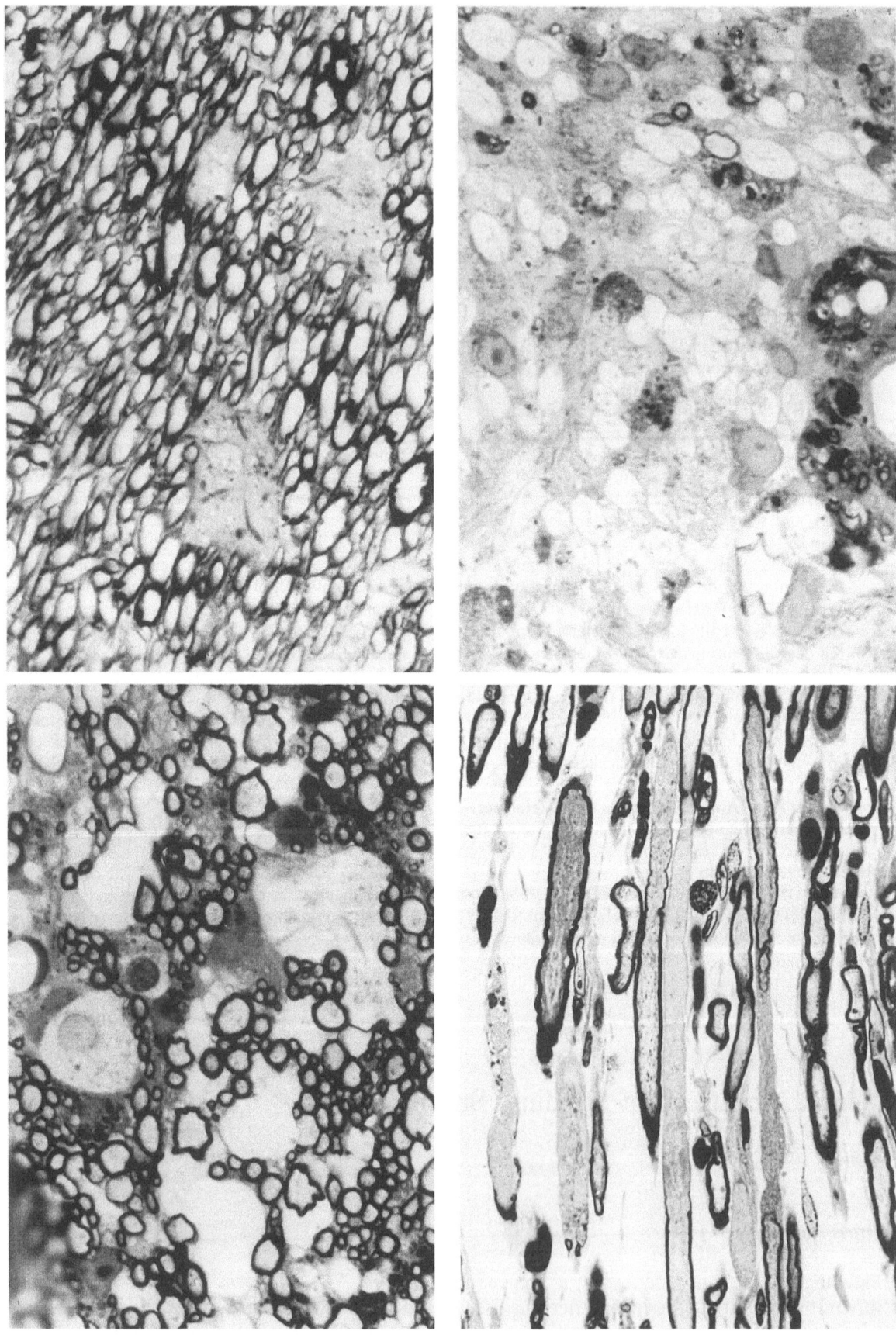

the exterior of the cell body of oligodendrocytes (Fig. 49). These rod-shaped structures stain deeply basophilic in toluidine blue-stained sections. Deeply basophilic granules, which most likely represent cross-sectional profiles of these structures, are also identified in the cytoplasm of oligodendrocytes (Fig. 49). Nuclear chromatin of these oligodendrocytes is dispersed to the peripheral border of the nuclei. Diffuse status spongiosus due to vacuolation of myelin, associated with degeneration of oligodendrocytes, gradually develops (Fig. 50). Macrophages appear within a few days, and by the 6th day total demyelination has occurred (Fig. 51). Some axonal degeneration is also observed. The demyelinated axons are remyelinated spontaneously after the 9th–12th days by oligodendrocytes as well as by Schwann's cells.

Peripheral Nervous System. Schwann's cells at the exposed site undergo similar dispersion of nuclear chromatin. Their cytoplasm is swollen and often vesiculated, but rod-shaped structures as observed in oligodendrocytes are not found. Gradual degeneration of Schwann's cells and demyelination develop (Fig. 52) and are followed by spontaneous remyelination.

Ultrastructure

The cytoplasm of oligodendrocytes undergoes various degrees of degenerative change. Proliferation of microtubules and cisternae of endoplasmic reticulum, which often fuse to form linear structures, is very conspicuous. Dense bodies, myelin figures, and clear vacuoles of various size are numerous. The rod-shaped structures are very similar to the cytoplasmic "scrolls" described in the oligodendrocytes in young rats treated with the hypocholesterolemic drugs (Suzuki and Zagoren 1974). The cross-sectional profile of the scrolls is that of compactly or loosely packed concentric lamellae. Sheets of parallel lamellae connecting to the endoplasmic reticulum are seen in profile in longitudinal sections (Fig. 53). Normal cytoplasmic constituents such as ribosomes, microtubules, the cisternae of the endoplasmic reticulum, and mitochondria can be identified between these sheets of lamellae.

Clear vacuoles in the myelin sheaths are formed by the separation of myelin lamellae at the intraperiod lines and occasional dilatation of periaxonal space. The pattern of demyelination is very similar to that caused by various demyelinating agents. Myelin lamellae disintegrate to form numerous honeycomb structures (Fig. 54). Compacted myelin lamellae are removed by infiltrating macrophages. Many axons are completely demyelinated by the 6th day (Fig. 54). In remyelinating axons after the 9th–12th days, thin myelin sheaths are formed by oligodendrocytes as well as by Schwann's cells.

In the peripheral nerve, ultrastructural changes in Schwann's cells are essentially identical to those of oligodendrocytes. Although rod-shaped structures are not found at light-microscopic level, alteration of the endoplasmic reticulum to form small scrolls is frequently found in the cytoplasm of Schwann's cells. Schwann's cells of unmyelinated fibers appear more susceptible than those of myelinated fibers. In an advanced stage of degeneration, the cytoplasm of the Schwann's cell of unmyelinated fibers is fragmented, and eventually only clusters of unmyelinated axons surrounded by the basal laminae remain (Fig. 55). An axon surrounded by a redundant basal lamina in an empty space bordered by an irregular basal lamina may be found on some occasions. Demyelination and spontaneous remyelination as noted in the central nervous system occur in the peripheral nerve as well (Fig. 56). In comparison with the central nervous system, however, axonal damage appears to be more frequent in the peripheral nerve.

◀ **Fig. 49** *(upper left).* Brain stem, rat. Rod-shaped structures in the perikarya of oligodendrocytes in a nerve fiber tract. Granules seen in the perikarya probably represent cross-sectional profiles of rod-like structures. No degenerative changes are seen in the myelinated fibers. Glutaraldehyde, postosmicated, Epon-embedded, toluidine blue, × 1000

Fig. 50 *(lower left).* Brain stem, rat. Status spongiosus of the nerve fiber tract formed by many vacuoles within the myelin sheaths. Rod-shaped structures and granules are seen in the perikarya of two degenerating oligodendrocytes. Glutaraldehyde, postosmicated, Epon-embedded, toluidine blue, × 1000

Fig. 51 *(upper right).* Brain stem, rat. Totally demyelinated axons in a nerve fiber tract. Macrophages contain myelin debris. Glutaraldehyde, postosmicated, Epon-embedded, toluidine blue, × 1000

Fig. 52 *(lower right).* Peripheral nerve fibers with segmental demyelination. Axonal degeneration is indicated by numerous fine granules and loss of myelin sheaths. Glutaraldehyde, postosmicated, Epon-embedded, toluidine blue, × 500

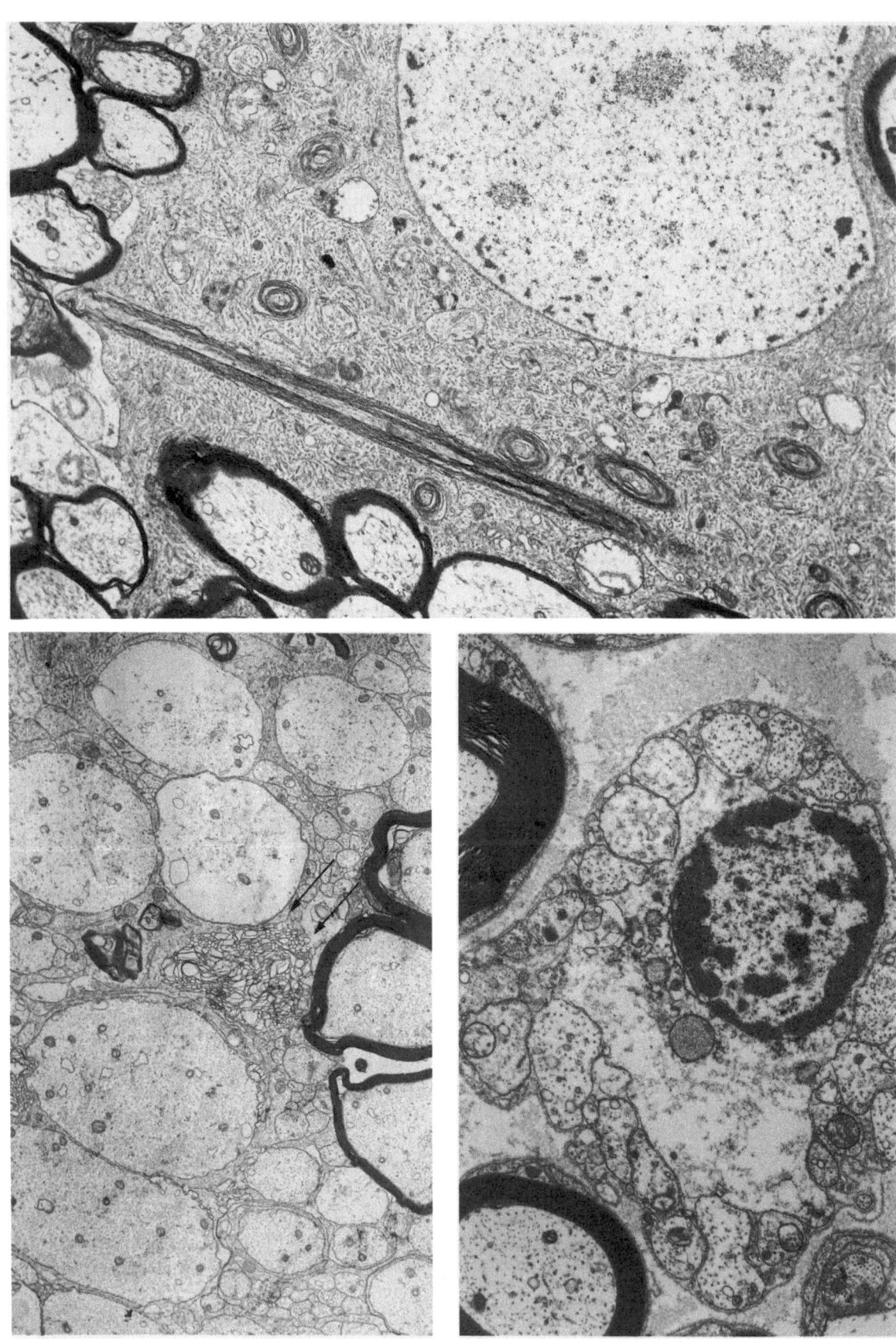

Differential Diagnosis

Rod-shaped structures in oligodendrocytes are also noted in the young rats which receive intraperitoneal injections of hypocholesterolemic drugs (Suzuki and Zagoren 1974). In addition, an ultrastructural feature of "scrolls" is found in the neurologic mutant mouse, "jimpy," which has severe hypomyelination of the central nervous system (Meier and Bischoff 1974). Spongy changes due to formation of intramyelinic vacuoles are common neuropathologic features and are caused by a variety of neurotoxic substances such as cuprizone (Suzuki and Kikkawa 1969), triethyltin (Aleu et al. 1963), isoniazid (Blakemore et al. 1972), and hexachlorophene (Lampert et al. 1973). The pattern of demyelination is similar to that seen in many demyelinating conditions including immune-mediated, viral, toxic, and traumatic demyelination (Ludwin 1981).

Biologic Features

Ethidium bromide is a phenylphenanthridine compound and has been used for the treatment of trypanosomiasis (Browlee et al. 1950; Woolfe 1952). It is a DNA-intercalating drug and is known to inhibit or suppress mitochondrial DNA, RNA, and protein synthesis in mammalian cells (Zylber et al. 1969; Leibowitz 1971). Since it emits a bright red fluorescent light, it is used as a fluorescent stain for quantitative and qualitative observations of the DNA contents of cells (Plumbridge and Brown 1977; Bengtsson et al. 1977). Cultured mammalian cells consistently undergo alterations of mitochondrial structures and function (Soslau and Nass 1971; McGill et al. 1973). With a single intraperitoneal injection of ethidium bromide in weanling male mice, matrix-enriched megamitochondria, structurally identical to those produced by a copper-chelating agent, cuprizone (Suzuki 1969), are produced in the hepatocytes (Albring et al. 1973).

An intracysternal injection of ethidium bromide (Sigma Chemical Co., St. Louis, MO) 2.5 μg in physiologic saline to weanling male Sprague-Dawley strain of rats produced alterations of oligodendrocytes and demyelination, followed by remyelination by both oligodendrocytes and Schwann's cells in the subpial fiber tracts of the brain stem (Yajima and Suzuki 1979 a, b). In the peripheral nerve, demyelination can be produced by intraneural injection of the same amounts of ethidium bromide with a glass micropipette

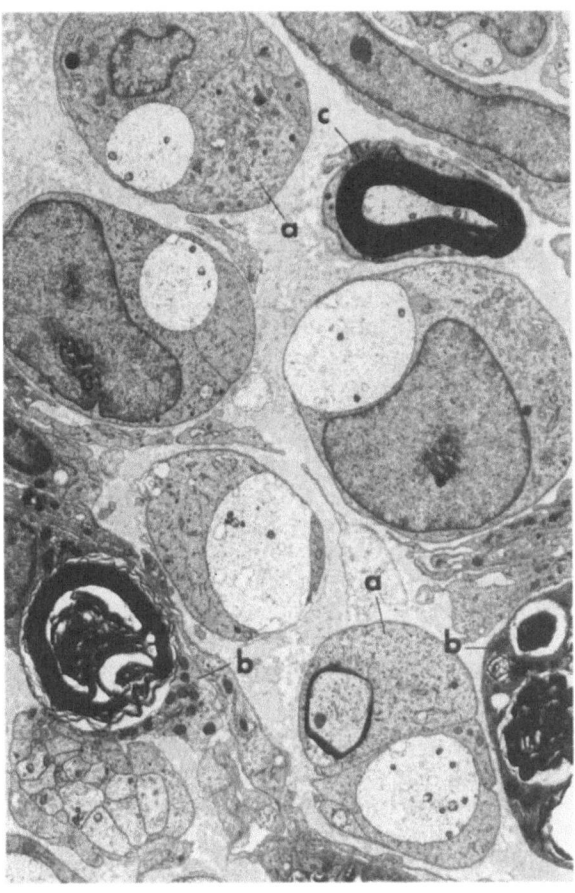

Fig. 56. Demyelinated peripheral nerve fibers, brain, rat, surrounded by Schwann's cells *(a)*. Macrophages *(b)* containing myelin debris are also noted. A single intact myelinated fiber *(c)* is seen in this field. TEM, × 5400

◀ **Fig. 53** *(above)*. Oligodendrocyte, brain, rat, contains many myelin scrolls. The cytoplasm is packed with numerous smooth cisternae and microtubules. The nuclear chromatin is dispersed. Adjacent myelinated fibers have a normal appearance. TEM, × 10 000

Fig. 54 *(lower left)*. Demyelinated axons, brain, rat. Three normally myelinated fibers are seen *(right)*. *Arrows* indicate honeycomb structures of degenerated myelin. Scattered myelin debris is seen within the processes of macrophages. TEM, × 8100

Fig. 55 *(lower right)*. A degenerating Schwann's cell of unmyelinated fiber. The perikarya is electronlucent, and clusters of dilated cisternae of rough endoplasmic reticulum are adjacent to the nucleus. Unmyelinated axons are well preserved. Myelin sheaths and Schwann's cells of myelinated fibers have a normal appearance. TEM, × 12600

(50-100 μm tip) connected by fine vinyl tubing to the syringe. Intravenous administration of the same amounts into weanling male rats is toxic enough to kill the animals. However, adult male albino mice can tolerate an intravenous injection of 1.0 ml 0.1%, 0.5%, and 1% solution. Under the fluorescence mircoscope, bright red fluorescence of ethidium bromide can be detected in the areas lacking blood-brain barrier such as choroid plexus, area postrema, and circumventricular organs of the brain (neurohypophysis, organum vasculosum laminae terminalis, and median eminence). Fluorescence disappears after 24 h and so far no lesion has been reported in these regions (Cesarini et al. 1985).

Etiology and Frequency. Neurotoxic effects have been reported only under experimental conditions in rat, cat, and cockroach (Yajima and Suzuki 1979 a, b; Blakemore 1982; Smith et al. 1984). Blakemore injected a small volume of ethidium bromide into the dorsal column of the spinal cord of cats and found morphologic alterations in oligodendrocytes and astrocytes 2 days after the injection. Demyelination occurred 8-14 days after the injection and was followed by remyelination by oligodendrocytes and Schwann's cells (Blakemore 1982). In vivo application of ethidium bromide to the cockroach central nervous system is reported to cause extensive destruction of the neurologia within 24 h (Smith et al. 1984).

Comparison with Other Species

As described above, the cat is the only other mammal in which neuropathologic changes have been demonstrated. The pathologic changes are essentially the same as those seen in the rat (Yajima and Suzuki 1979 a, b), but rod-shaped cytoplasmic structures in oligodendrocytes are not observed in the cat (Blakemore 1982).

References

Albring M, Radsak K, Thoenes W (1973) Giant mitochondria. II. Induction of matrix enriched megamitochondria in mouse liver parenchymal cells by ethidium bromide. Virchows Arch [B] 14: 373-377

Aleu FP, Katzman R, Terry RD (1963) Fine structure and electrolyte analyses of cerebral edema induced by alkyl tin intoxication. J Neuropathol Exp Neurol 22: 403-413

Bengtsson A, Grimelius L, Johansson H, Ponten J (1977) Nuclear DNA-content of parathyroid cells in adenomas, hyperplastic and normal glands. Acta Pathol Microbiol Scand [A] 85: 455-460

Blakemore WF (1982) Ethidium bromide induced demyelination in the spinal cord of the cat. Neuropathol Appl Neurobiol 8: 365-375

Blakemore WF, Palmer AC, Noel PRB (1972) Ultrastructural changes in isoniazid-induced brain edema in the dog. J Neurocytol 1: 263-278

Browlee G, Gross MD, Goodwin LG, Woodbine M, Wall LP (1950) The chemotherapeutic action of phenanthridine compounds. Br J Pharmacol 5: 261-275

Cesarini K, Atillo A, Brigotte L, Hussain ST, Olsson Y (1985) Cytofluorescence localization of ethidium bromide in the nervous system of the mouse. I. Ethidium bromide: its distribution in regions within and without the blood-brain barrier after intravenous injection. Acta Neuropathol (Berl) 68: 273-278

Lampert PW, O'Brien J, Garrett R (1973) Hexachlorophene encephalopathy. Acta Neuropathol (Berl) 23: 326-333

Leibowitz RD (1971) The effect of ethidium bromide on mitochondrial DNA synthesis and mitochondrial DNA structure in HeLa cells. J Cell Biol 51: 116-122

Ludwin SK (1981) Pathology of demyelination and remyelination. In: Waxman SG, Ritchie JM (eds) Demyelinating disease: basic and clinical electrophysiology. Raven, New York, pp 123-168

McGill M, Hsu TC, Brinkley BR (1973) Electron-dense structures in mitochondria induced by short-term ethidium bromide treatment. J Cell Biol 59: 260-265

Meier C, Bischoff A (1974) Dysmyelination in "jimpy" mouse. Electron microscopic study. J Neuropathol Exp Neurol 33: 343-353

Plumbridge TW, Brown JF (1977) Spectrophotometric and fluorescence polarization studies of the binding of ethidium, daunomycin and mepacrine to DNA and to poly(IC). Biochim Biophys Acta 479: 441-449

Smith PJS, Leech CA, Treherne JE (1984) Glial repair in an insect central nervous system: effects of selective glial disruption. J Neurosci 4: 2698-2711

Soslau G, Nass MMK (1971) Effects of ethidium bromide on the cytochrome content and ultrastructure of L-cell mitochondria. J Cell Biol 51: 514-524

Suzuki K (1969) Giant hepatic mitochondria: production in mice fed with cuprizone. Science 163: 81-82

Suzuki K, Kikkawa Y (1969) Status spongiosus of CNS and hepatic changes induced by cuprizone (biscyclohexanone oxalyldihydrazone). Am J Pathol 54: 307-325

Suzuki K, Zagoren JC (1974) Degeneration of oligodendroglia in the central nervous system of rats treated with AY9944 or triparanol. Lab Invest 31: 503-515

Woolfe G (1952) The trypanocidal action of phenanthridine compounds. Ann Trop Med Parasitol 46: 285-296

Yajima K, Suzuki K (1979a) Ultrastructural changes of oligodendroglia and myelin sheaths induced by ethidium bromide. Neuropathol Appl Neurobiol 5: 49-62

Yajima K, Suzuki K (1979b) Demyelination and remyelination in the rat central nervous system following ethidium bromide injection. Lab Invest 41: 385-392

Zylber E, Vesco C, Penman S (1969) Selective inhibition of the synthesis of mitochondria-associated RNA by ethidium bromide. J Mol Biol 44: 195-204

Neurotoxic Effects of 6-Aminonicotinamide, Mouse

Hisashi Aikawa and Kinuko Suzuki

Gross Appearance

Suckling mice injected intraperitoneally with 6-aminonicotinamide (6-AN) in one dose of 25 mg/kg body weight consistently develop enlargement of the head 7-9 days after injection (Aikawa and Suzuki 1985a, 1986). In coronal sections of the cerebrum, marked hydrocephalus is evident due to dilatation of the lateral ventricles (Fig. 57). The fourth ventricle is not dilated and the aqueduct is always narrowed and obliterated (Aikawa et al. 1984). No hydrocephalus is seen in adult mice treated with 6-AN.

Microscopic Features

Spongy degeneration in the subcortical gray matter, especially in the brain stem, cerebellum, and spinal cord, is the most striking feature in 6-AN-treated mice (Fig. 58). These spongy changes are due to intracytoplasmic vacuolation of astrocytes and oligodendrocytes. Neurons and blood vessels appear to be intact at the light-microscopic level. Ependymal and subependymal cells in the entire ventricular system, even in the central canal of the spinal cord, also undergo cytoplasmic vacuolation (Figs. 59, 60). The lumen of the aqueduct is obliterated by these edematous ependymal and glial cells, resulting in aqueductal stenosis. These intracytoplasmic hydropic changes of ependymal and glial cells gradually disappear 20 days after injection, and by the 30th day the aqueduct is totally obliterated with loss of the aqueductal lumen and ependymal cells. Only a cluster of ependymal cells remain at the dorsal and ventral portions of the aqueduct (Aikawa and Suzuki 1985b; Aikawa et al. 1986). In the white matter, especially in the corpus callosum, swollen oligodendrocytes and macrophages are frequently noted. Spongy change of enteric glial cells in the myenteric plexus is also conspicuous in the 6-AN-treated suckling mice (Aikawa and Suzuki 1985a; 1986). Spongy changes of ependymal cells are rarely seen in adult animals.

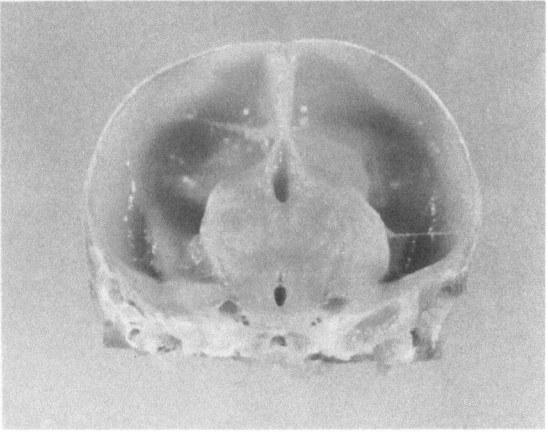

Fig. 57. Coronal section of the cerebrum of a mouse 9 days after injection with 6-AN. Note marked dilatation of the lateral and third ventricles. × 5

Ultrastructure

In the acute stage of 6-AN neurotoxicity, ultrastructural features of the edematous ependymal and glial cells are characterized by half-moon-shaped nuclei and dilatation of the perinuclear cisterns and cisterns of the rough endoplasmic reticulum (RER) (Figs. 61, 62). Nuclear blebs, composed of aggregated actin filaments are frequently observed in the dilated perinuclear cisterns (Aikawa et al. 1986). In neurons in the anterior horn of the spinal cord, nuclei are invaginated and the endoplasmic cisterae are dilated. In the rER of the neurons, cisterns are reduced in numbers and ribosomes are dissociated or dispersed. Neurofilaments and microtubules are increased in number. Ultrastructural features of neurons in mice treated with 6-AN are compatible to those of so-called "chromatolytic" changes (Aikawa and Suzuki 1986). On the 30th day following injection, surviving ependymal cells in the obliterated aqueduct contain abundant intermediate filaments and lipid droplets in the cytoplasm. They are similar to those reported in the astrocytes of rats treated with 6-AN in the chronic stage (Chui and Garcia 1979). Electron-microscopic features of the swollen enteric glial cells in the myenteric plexus are essentially identical to those lesions of the central nervous system in the 6-AN-treated mice (Aikawa and Suzuki 1986).

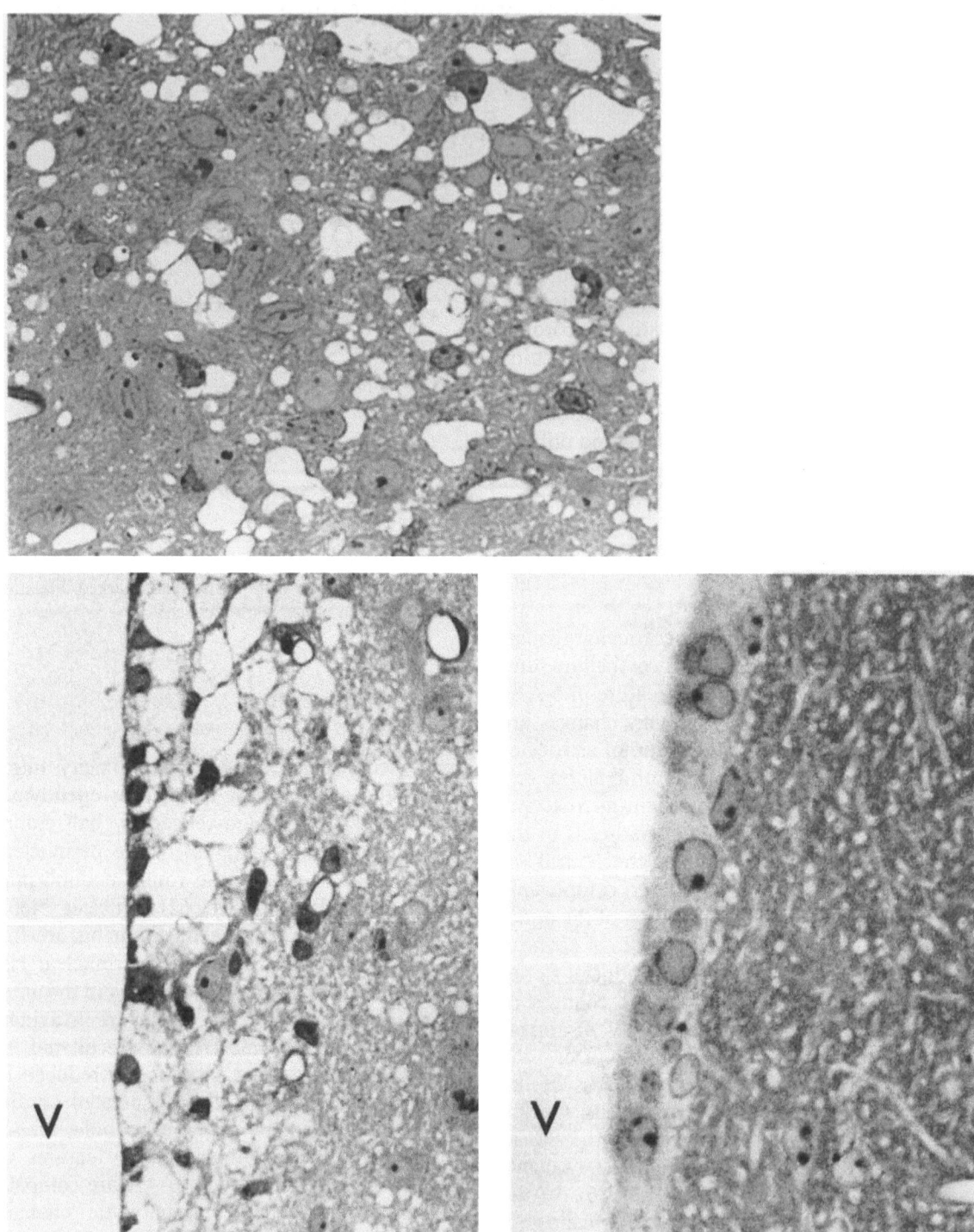

Fig. 58 *(above)*. Anterior horn of the lumbar spinal cord of a mouse 5 days after injection with 6-AN. Note that glial cells contain intracytoplasmic vacuoles (spongy changes), but neurons appear to be intact. 1-μm Epon section, toluidine blue, × 170

Fig. 59 *(lower left)*. Degeneration of ependymal cells, mouse, 5 days after injection with 6-AN. Almost all ependymal cells and subependymal glial cells are vacuolated. *V,* Ventricle. 1-μm Epon section, toluidine blue, × 1000

Fig. 60 *(lower right)*. Ependymal cells of normal control for Fig. 59. Toluidine. blue, × 1000

Fig. 61 *(above)*. Vacuolated ependymal cells in the lateral ▶ ventricle of a treated mouse 5 days following injection with 6-AN. Perinuclear cisterns *(P)* and the endoplasmic reticulum *(E)* are dilated. *V,* Ventricle. TEM, × 9000

Fig. 62 *(below)*. A normal ependymal cell of the littermate control for Fig. 61. TEM, × 9000

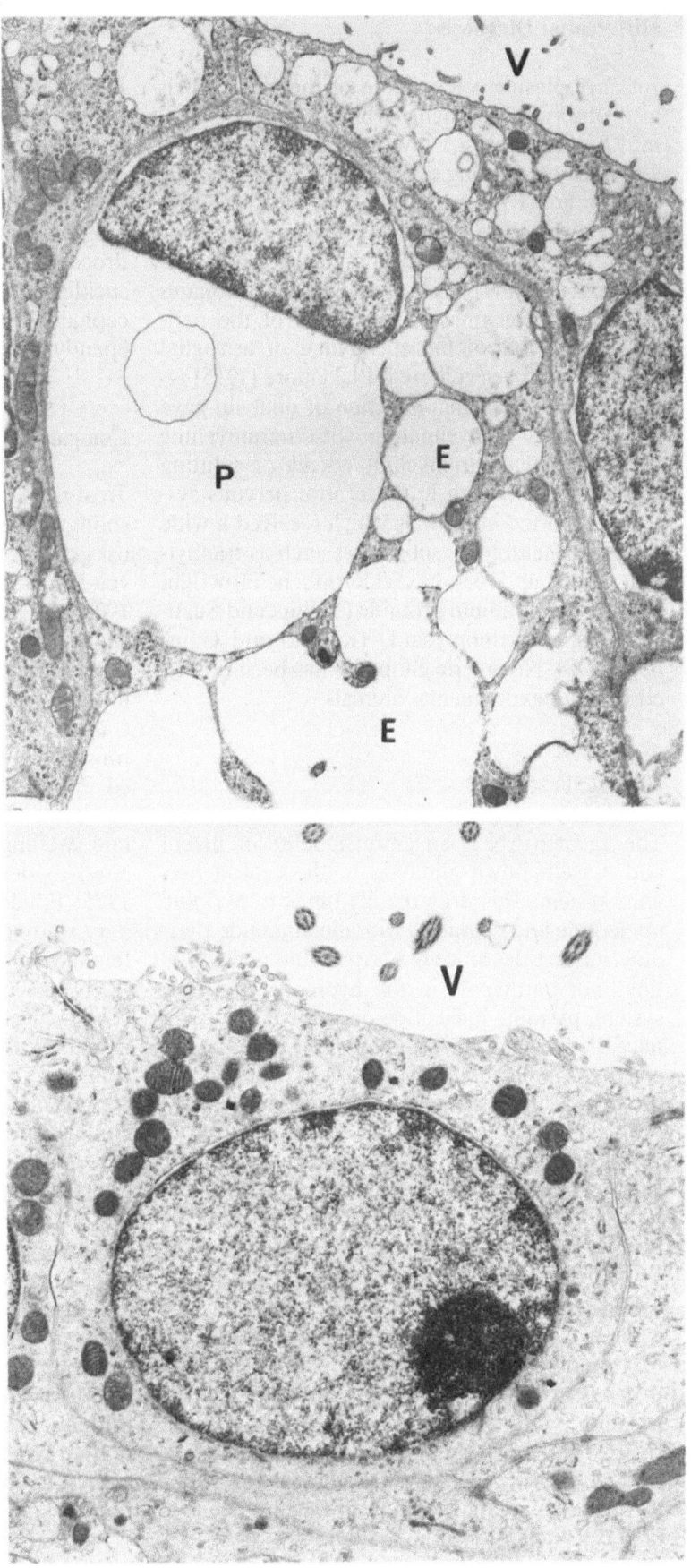

Differential Diagnosis

Intracytoplasmic vacuolation of the glial cells is also observed in rodents which received a vitamin B_1 antagonist, pyrithiamine (Watanabe 1978), or a chelating agent of copper, cuprizone (Suzuki and Kikkawa 1969). Ouabain, which interferes with the energy-dependent transport system, also produces astrocytic edema when it is injected into the brain (Towfighi and Gonates 1973). However, marked dilatation of the perinuclear cisterns of the ependymal or astroglial cells has not been reported. Blakemore (1975) reported that intraspinal injection of ouabain gave rise to local demyelination with intramyelinic edema. Similar intramyelinic edema or splitting of the myelin sheath in the central nervous system is reported in animals which received a wide variety of neurotoxic substances such as triethyltin (Aleu et al. 1963), hexachlorophene (Towfighi et al. 1974), ethidium bromide (Yajima and Suzuki 1979), or actinomycin D (Rizzuto and Gambetti 1978). No enteric gliopathy has been reported in other experimental animals.

Biologic Features

The agent 6-AN is an antimetabolite of niacin and a well-known gliotoxin to the central nervous system. This drug readily binds to pyridine nucleotide and competes with nicotinamide pyridine nucleotide. Since 6-AN-pyridine nucleotide does not participate in the hydrogen transport system, pyridine nucleotide-dependent oxidation may be disturbed. 6-AN is reported to block the activity of 6-phosphogluconate dehydrogenase in the pentose phosphate pathway and subsequently to impair glycolysis of the cell (Herken et al. 1974; Griffiths et al. 1981). In our experiments, suckling mice received a single intraperitoneal injection of 6-AN at the dose of 25 mg/kg of body weight on various postnatal days.

Etiology. 6-AN-induced hydrocephalus may be caused by the stenosis of the aqueduct which may result from the combination of ependymal degeneration and dysfunction, brain stem compression by the dilated lateral ventricles, and periaqueductal edema. Glial cells are most sensitive to 6-AN toxicity. The mice treated with 6-AN develop status spongiosus due to degeneration of glial cells regardless of age. Etiology of 6-AN-induced gliopathy is considered to be due to the inhibition of nicotinamide-adenine-dinucleotide phosphate (NADP)-dependent dehydrogenases which are exclusively localized in glial cells. However, there are some age differences in the development of the lesions. In adult mice, ependymal degeneration is rarely seen and no hydrocephalus is noted. In suckling mice, in addition to glial vulnerability, the ependymal cell is the most susceptible to the toxic action of 6-AN. Hydrocephalus is consistently observed only in suckling mice. Therefore, 6-AN-induced hydrocephalus may depend on the maturation of the ependymal cells.

Comparison with Other Species

Treatment with 6-AN consistently results in spongy degeneration of glial cells in the subcortical gray matter in adult rats (Schneider and Cervos-Navarro 1974; Blakemore 1975; Horita et al. 1978; Sasaki 1982) and pigs (O'Sullivan and Blakemore 1980). Ultrastructural features of these lesions in rats and pigs are identical. Ocular lesions are described in rabbits (Render and Carlton 1985). Chromatolytic changes of the neurons at the electron-microscopic level are reported in rats (Horita et al. 1978). In the peripheral nervous system, the inner Schwann-cell cytoplasmic swelling is reported when 6-AN is administered to developing rats (Brzoska and Adhami 1975; Friede and Bischhausen 1978). A preliminary study on 6-AN susceptibility in several different animals suggests that species difference of 6-AN toxicity depends on the maturation of the central nervous system because newborn cats treated with 6-AN do not develop ependymal lesions and hydrocephalus (unpublished data). Teratogenic effects of this agent are reported in chick (Landauer 1957), mice (Pinsky and Fraser 1959), rats (Chamberlain 1970), and rabbits (Schardein et al. 1967). In these studies, cleft palate, hydrocephalus, and skeletal anomalies are frequently reported. In vitro study of 6-AN reveals that vacuolar alteration of the satellite cells and myelinated fibers occurs in ganglion culture (Kim and Wenger 1973; Yonezawa et al. 1980).

Acknowledgements. This investigation was supported in part by grant No. 86-5-41 from NCNP of the Ministry of Health and Welfare, Japan, and grants NS-24453 and ES-01104 from the National Institutes of Health, USA.

References

Aikawa H, Suzuki K (1985a) Enteric gliopathy in niacin-deficiency induced by CNS glio-toxin. Brain Res 334: 354-356

Aikawa H, Suzuki K (1985b) Aqueduct stenosis induced by a single injection of antivitamin. Dev Brain Res 22: 284-287

Aikawa H, Suzuki K (1986) Lesions in the skin, intestine, and central nervous system induced by an antimetabolite of niacin. Am J Pathol 122: 335-342

Aikawa H, Suzuki K, Ito N, Iwasaki Y, Nonaka I (1984) 6-aminonicotinamide-induced hydrocephalus in suckling mice. J Neuropathol Exp Neurol 43: 511-521

Aikawa H, Kobayashi S, Suzuki K (1986) Aqueductal lesions in 6-aminonicotinamide-treated suckling mice. Acta Neuropathol (Berl) 71: 243-250

Aleu FP, Katzman R, Terry RD (1963) Fine structure and electrolyte analyses of cerebral edema induced by alkyl tin intoxication. J Neuropathol Exp Neurol 22: 403-413

Blakemore WF (1975) Remyelination by Schwann cells of axons demyelinated by intraspinal injection of 6-aminonicotinamide in the rat. J Neurocytol 4: 745-757

Brzoska HR, Adhami H (1975) Electronmicroscopic study of the effect of 6-AN on the sciatic nerve in newborn rats. Acta Neuropathol (Berl) 33: 59-66

Chamberlain JG (1970) Early neurovascular abnormalities underlying 6-aminonicotinamide (6-AN)-induced congenital hydrocephalus in rats. Teratology 3: 377-385

Chui E, Garcia JH (1979) Pathogenesis of 6-aminonicotinamide neurotoxicity: new structural analysis. In: Zimmermann HM (ed) Progress in neuropathology, vol 4. Raven, New York, pp 341-359

Friede RL, Bischhausen R (1978) How do axons control myelin formation? The model of 6-aminonicotinamide neuropathy. J Neurol Sci 35: 341-353

Griffiths IR, Kelly PAT, Grome JJ (1981) Glucose utilization in the central nervous system in the acute gliopathy due to 6-aminonicotinamide. Lab Invest 44: 547-552

Herken H, Lange K, Kolbe H, Keller K (1974) Antimetabolic action on the pentose phosphate pathway in the central nervous system induced by 6-aminonicotinamide. In: Genazzani E, Herken H (eds) Central nervous system. Studies on metabolic regulation and function. Springer, Berlin Heidelberg New York, pp 41-54

Horita N, Oyanagi S, Ishii T, Izumiyama Y (1978) Ultrastructure of 6-aminonicotinamide (6-AN)-induced lesions in the central nervous system of rats. I. Chromat-olysis and other lesions in the cervical cord. Acta Neuropathol (Berl) 44: 111-119

Kim SU, Wenger BS (1973) Neurotoxic effects of 6-aminonicotinamide on cultures of central nervous tissue. Acta Neuropathol (Berl) 26: 259-264

Landauer W (1957) Niacin antagonist and chick development. J Exp Zool 136: 509-529

O'Sullivan BM, Blakemore WF (1980) Acute nicotinamide deficiency in the pig induced by 6-aminonicotinamide. Vet Pathol 17: 748-758

Pinsky L, Fraser FC (1959) Production of skeletal malformations in the offspring of pregnant mice treated with 6-aminonicotinamide. Biol Neonate 1: 106-112

Render JA, Carlton WW (1985) Ocular lesions of 6-aminonicotinamide toxicosis in rabbits. Vet Pathol 22: 72-77

Rizzuto N, Gambetti PL (1978) Status spongiosus of rat central nervous system induced by actinomycin D. Acta Neuropathol (Berl) 36: 21-30

Sasaki S (1982) Brain edema and gliopathy induced by 6-aminonicotinamide intoxication in the central nervous system of rats. Am J Vet Res 43: 1691-1695

Schardein JL, Wooley ET, Peltzer MA, Kaump DH (1967) Congenital malformations induced by 6-aminonicotinamide in rabbit kits. Exp Mol Pathol 6: 335-346

Schneider H, Cervos-Navarro J (1974) Acute gliopathy in spinal cord and brain stem induced by 6-aminonicotinamide. Acta Neuropathol (Berl) 27: 11-23

Suzuki K, Kikkawa Y (1969) Status spongiosus of CNS and hepatic changes induced by cuprizon (biscyclohexanon oxalyldihydrazone). Am J Pathol 54: 307-325

Towfighi J, Gonatas NK (1973) Effect of intracerebral injection of ouabain in adult and developing rats. An ultrastructural and auto-radiographic study. Lab Invest 28: 170-180

Towfighi J, Gonatas NK, McCree L (1974) Hexachlorophene-induced changes in central and peripheral myelinated axons of developing and adult rats. Lab Invest 31: 712-721

Watanabe I (1978) Pyrithiamine-induced acute thiamine-deficient encephalopathy in the mouse. Exp Mol Pathol 28: 381-394

Yajima K, Suzuki K (1979) Demyelination and remyelination in the rat central nervous system following ethidium bromide injection. Lab Invest 41: 385-392

Yonezawa T, Bornstein MB, Peterson ER (1980) Organotypic cultures of nerve tissue as a model system for neurotoxicity investigation and screening. In: Spencer PS, Schaumburg HH (eds) Experimental and clinical neurotoxicology. William and Wilkins, Baltimore, pp 788-802

Neurotoxic Effects of Trimethyltin

Georg J. Krinke

Synonym. Trimethyltin neuronal toxicity (neuron-opathy).

Gross Appearance

A bilateral reduction in the size of the hippocampal formation, mainly in the area of the fascia dentata, may be seen after slicing the fixed brains of affected animals (Brown et al. 1979; Dyer et al. 1982).

Microscopic Features

In most species, the predominant pathologic changes are present in the hippocampal formation and the basal (piriform/entorhinal) cortex of the brain. Other areas of the nervous system may be affected as well, such as the neocortex, basal ganglia, cerebellum, brain stem, spinal cord, dorsal root ganglia, olfactory cortex, retina, and the inner ear (Brown et al. 1979; Bouldin et al. 1981; Chang and Dyer 1983; Brown et al. 1984a).

The major pathologic finding is neuronal necrosis. The neurons are shrunken, their cytoplasm appears pale with the Nissl stain and eosinophilic with hematoxylin and eosin, and their nuclei are pyknotic. The early change is characterized by a loss of Nissl substance (Fig. 63), which is followed by condensation and clumping of the cytoplasm and subsequent shrinkage and fragmentation of the nucleus (Brown et al. 1979). Advanced neuronal necrosis, with proliferation of glial cells and neuronophagia, results in a loss of neurons and astrocytic gliosis. Less susceptible neurons may appear morphologically intact at the light-microscopic level despite the presence of ultrastructural alterations (Chang and Dyer 1983).

Ultrastructure

During the first 24 h following the intoxication, small (approximately 100-200 nm) vesicular or tubular, electron-dense particles occur within the cytoplasm (Fig. 64). They are formed at the expense of the rough endoplasmic reticulum and appear to arise either from the rough endoplas-

mic reticulum devoid of ribosomes or, more probably, from the smooth endoplasmic reticulum (Brown et al. 1984a). In some neurons, dilation of the cisternae of the endoplasmic reticulum and of the Golgi complex is apparent (Fig. 65). At a more advanced stage, the cytoplasm contains larger, electron-dense bodies (approximately 300-400 nm) intermingled with well-preserved mitochondria (Fig. 66). These bodies have occasional lamellar arrays and resemble autophagic vacuoles; the high activity of acid phosphatase confirms their lysosomal character (Bouldin et al. 1981).

The loss of the rough endoplasmic reticulum together with the relative concentration of the mitochondria may account for the cytoplasmic eosinophilia of these neurons seen under the light microscope.

Differential Diagnosis

Histologic features similar to those of trimethyltin-induced neuronal necrosis, such as the cytoplasmic eosinophilia and nuclear pyknosis with hematoxylin and eosin staining have been observed in experimental intoxication with benzoic acid (Kreis et al. 1967) and trialkyllead (Seawright et al. 1980). Since this type of neurotoxic lesion closely resembles the nonspecific necrosis caused by disturbances in energy metabolism in nervous tissue ("ischemic nerve cell change"), attempts should be made to discriminate between these two conditions.

Electron microscopy is helpful in this respect by showing the microvacuolization of neuronal cytoplasm due to mitochondrial swelling in anoxic ischemia (Brown and Brierley 1973) but not in trimethyltin toxicity. The formation of cytoplasmic, electron-dense particles characteristic of the trimethyltin effect is not a feature of the ischemic nerve cell change, although small clusters of dense material may occur in the latter condition as well (Kirino and Sano 1984). Distention of the endoplasmic reticulum and the Golgi complex is not confined to the effect of trimethyltin since it has been observed in conditions such as status epilepticus (Evans et al. 1983) and hypoglycemic brain damage (Auer et al. 1985).

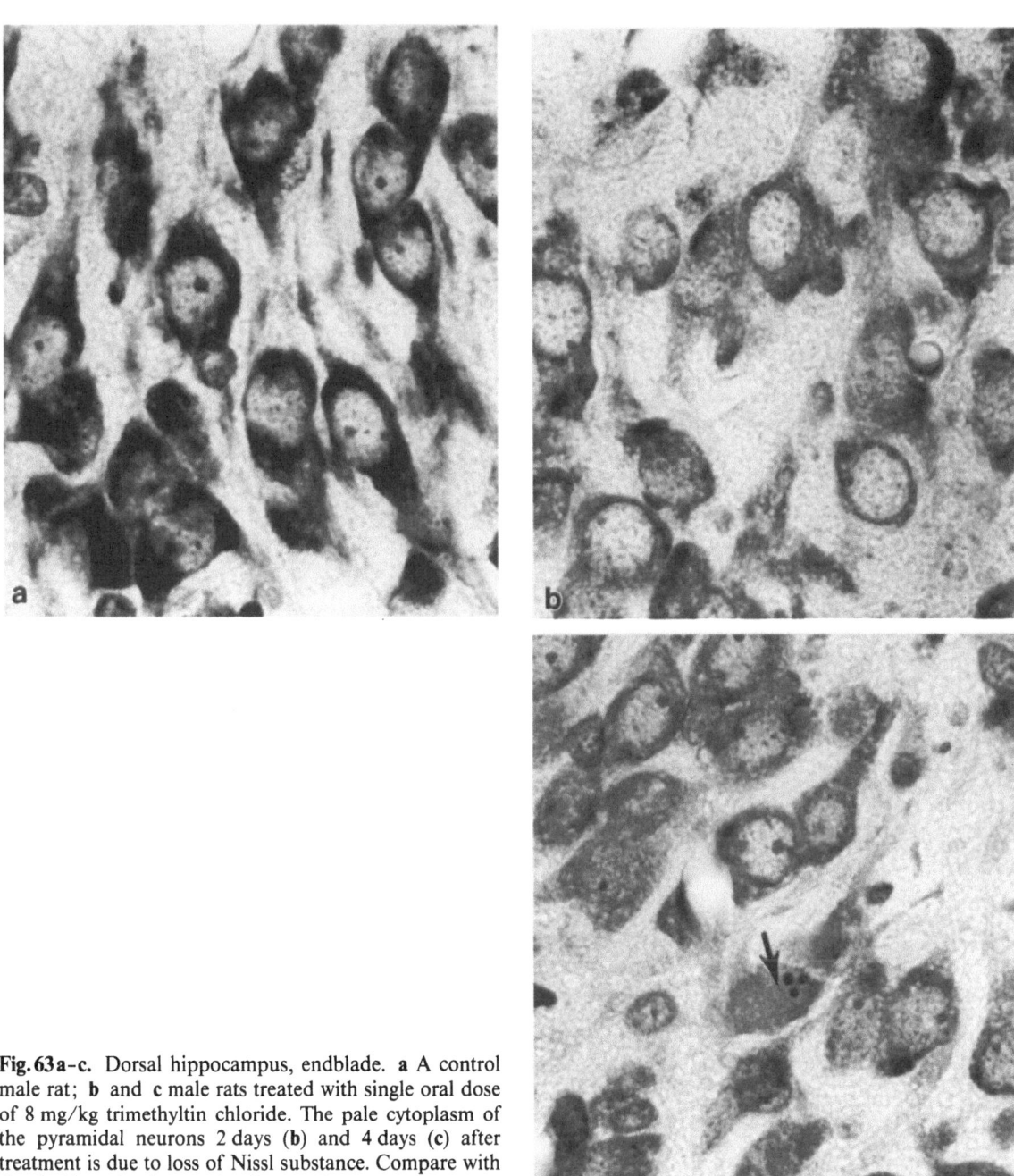

Fig. 63 a–c. Dorsal hippocampus, endblade. **a** A control male rat; **b** and **c** male rats treated with single oral dose of 8 mg/kg trimethyltin chloride. The pale cytoplasm of the pyramidal neurons 2 days (**b**) and 4 days (**c**) after treatment is due to loss of Nissl substance. Compare with the darkly stained control cells (**a**). Note necrotic neuron *(arrow)* with fragmented nucleus in the center of **c**. Perfusion fixation with glutaraldehyde, paraffin section, cresyl violet, × 1000

Another feature of the trimethyltin lesion to be considered in differential diagnosis is the susceptibility of the hippocampus to neuronal damage. Since the hippocampus is very vulnerable to indirect (secondary) effects, especially seizures accompanied by respiratory, circulatory, and thermoregulatory deficiency, the interpretation of hippocampal lesions is frequently a matter of controversy. The predilection site in the hippo-campus for secondary lesions of the anoxic ischemic kind is the "Sommer's sector," while another area, the so-called endblade (Fig. 67), has a tendency to manifest the primary toxic effects of certain compounds (Krinke et al. 1978). In trimethyltin toxicity the damage is more prominent in the endblade, although both portions of the hippocampus may be affected (Brown et al. 1979; Dyer et al. 1982; Krinke and Hess 1983).

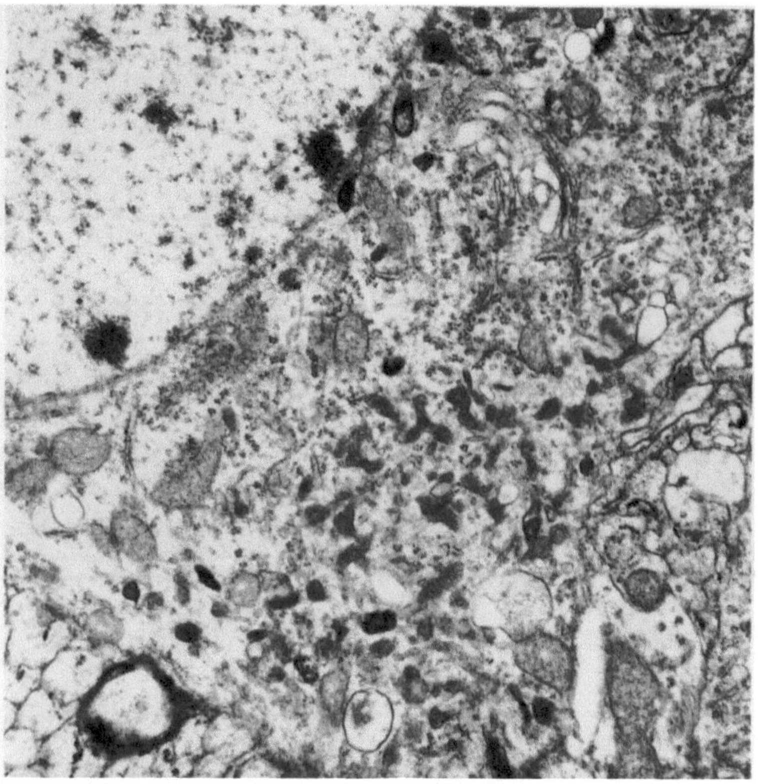

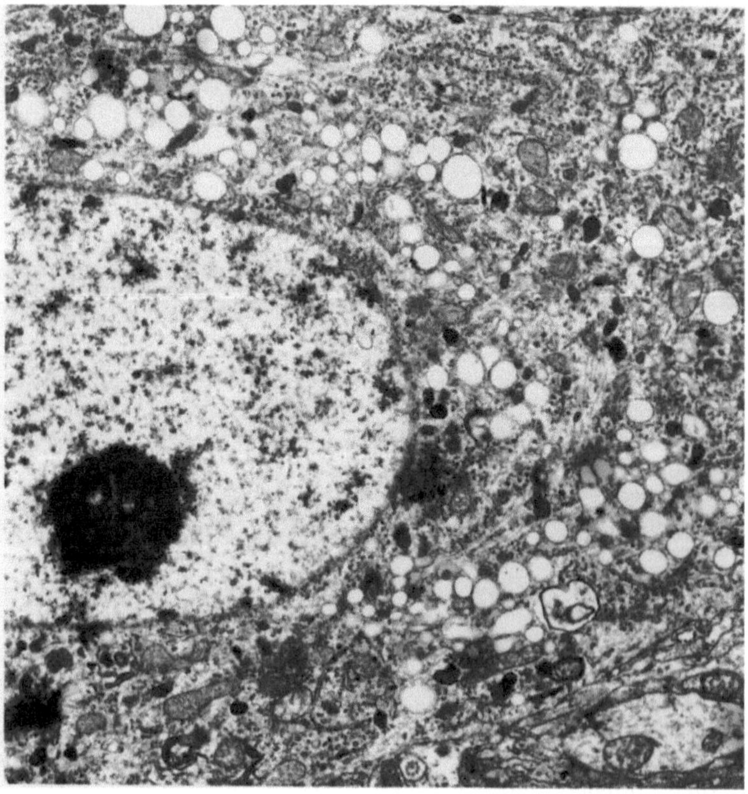

60   Georg J. Krinke

Fig. 64 *(above).* Pyramidal neuron, 1 day after administration of trimethyltin chloride. Initial formation of vesicular and tubular electron-dense particles within the cytoplasm. Same area and treatment as in Fig. 63 b, c. Uranyl acetate and lead citrate, × 20300

Fig. 65 *(below).* A pyramidal neuron 2 days after treatment. Distended cisternae of endoplasmic reticulum and Golgi complex together with the presence of electron-dense particles. Same area and treatment as in Fig. 63 b, c. Uranyl acetate and lead citrate, × 9900

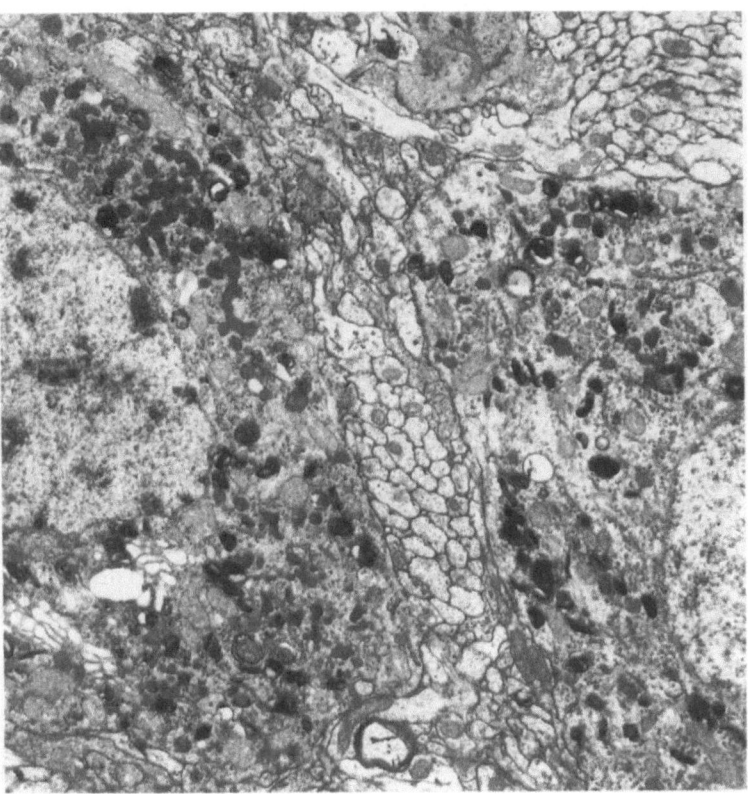

Fig. 66. The cytoplasm of pyramidal neurons contains numerous electron-dense bodies, well-preserved mitochondria, and a reduced amount of rough endoplasmic reticulum. Seven days following treatment, same area as in Fig. 63b, c. Uranyl acetate and lead citrate, ×9100

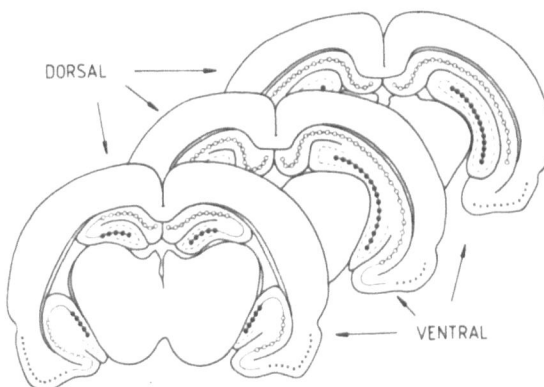

Fig. 67. Topography of hippocampal formation and basal cortex in rat brain. *White circles,* Sommer's sector; *black circles,* endblade; *broken line,* fascia dentata; *crosses,* basal (entorhinal and piriform) cortex

Biologic Features

Natural History. Metallic tin has a low degree of toxicity. The organic alkyltin derivatives are, however, highly toxic; this was dramatically illustrated when about 100 persons died of brain edema following ingestion of a drug containing triethyltin (Fortemps et al. 1978).

Trimethyltins, which are not sold commercially, are generated as byproducts during the manufacture of dimethyltin dichloride, a substance used as a plastic stabilizer. Accidental exposure of humans to trimethyltin chloride has demonstrated its potent neurotoxic effect (Fortemps et al. 1978; Rey et al. 1983). Owing to its propensity for damaging the brain and inducing behavioral changes, trimethyltin has recently become a standard model substance widely used for the validation of behavioral tests in experimental animals.

Etiology and Pathogenesis. There is a striking difference in the toxicity of the two closely related chemical agents trimethyltin and triethyltin. Swelling of the brain white matter occurs in triethyltin toxicity, and this effect may be due to a strong inhibition of oxidative phosphorylation by this compound; trimethyltin, which does not damage the brain white matter, is 30–40 times less active as an inhibitor of oxidative phosphorylation (Aldridge and Rose 1969).

The exact mechanism of trimethyltin toxicity remains uncertain. According to Bouldin et al. (1981), the subcellular target structure may be a specialized (Golgi-associated) region of the neuronal endoplasmic reticulum in which lysosomes are formed. Although the loss of Nissl substance is indicative of a (direct or indirect) disturbance in protein synthesis (Brown et al. 1979; Chang and Dyer 1983), specific experiments have demonstrated only a slight inhibition of protein synthetic process by trimethyltin. Possibly, the changes in the Golgi complex disturb subsequent processing of synthesized protein (Brown et al. 1984a).

In animal experiments, trimethyltin is usually administered as a chloride. It is very likely, in the animal body, that some of the chloride ions are substituted by hydroxide ions so that both hydroxides and chlorides are present; since both forms are soluble in water and in lipids, the rapid passage of trimethyltin through the cellular membranes is possible. The presence of significant amounts of trimethyltin in the nervous system is compatible with the occurrence of pathologic changes; however, there is no evidence that the selective damage of certain neurons is associated with focal concentrations of trimethyltin (Brown et al. 1984b). Additional factors, such as the functional state of neurons with hyperactivation of selected systems, may account for their particular vulnerability (Chang and Dyer 1985).

Behavioral Observations. In animals, the signs of poisoning include tremors, hyperexcitability, aggressive behavior, spontaneous seizures, sensory system disturbances, learning and memory impairment, and self-mutilation of the tail (Brown et al. 1984b). Subjective and psychic disturbances have been observed in humans including headache, loss of vigilance, insomnia, anorexia, disorientation, sensation of pain, tinnitus, cophosis, and a semiconscious state; one severely intoxicated individual developed a persistent hypotonic hyperkinetic syndrome (Fortemps et al. 1978; Rey et al. 1983).

Comparison with Other Species

Both species- and strain-related differences in the susceptibility to trimethyltin toxicity may occur. A single dose of approximately 3 mg/kg trimethyltin chloride is lethal for Syrian hamsters, gerbils, marmosets, and probably humans, while the LD_{50} for the rat is much higher: 12.6 mg/kg; this reduced toxicity for the rat may be related to a partial inactivation of trimethyltin by its binding to hemoglobin, which does not occur in other species (except the cat) (Brown et al. 1984b). Mice (BALB/c and C57BL/6) treated with 3 mg/kg trimethyltin chloride p. o. show a greater toxicity than rats treated with 7.5 mg. Long-Evans rats are more sensitive than the Sprague-Dawley strain (Chang et al. 1983).

The distribution of lesions within the nervous system, which indicates the hierarchy of neuronal susceptibility, may vary from species to species, and even within one species depending on the age and dosing regimen. For instance, adult mice show the greatest damage in the hippocampal fascia dentata, while in rats and the young mice it occurs in the hippocampal pyramidal cells and the olfactory cortex (Dyer et al. 1982; Chang et al. 1983; Reuhl et al. 1983). In the hamster, the neurons in the neocortex and basal cortex are more affected than in the hippocampus (Brown et al. 1984b).

Minor differences in clinical signs also exist, such as the absence of aggression in gerbils and hamsters and of seizures in hamsters; there is no record of tremors in humans (Brown et al. 1984b).

Light-microscopic examination of the brain from a man who died 12 days after accidental exposure to trimethyltin chloride revealed loss of Nissl substance with shrinkage and eosinophilia of cytoplasm (Rey et al. 1983), pathologic alterations known to occur in animal studies.

References

Aldridge WN, Rose MS (1969) The mechanism of oxidative phosphorylation, a hypothesis derived from studies of trimethyltin and triethyltin compounds. FEBS Lett 4: 61–68

Auer RN, Kalimo H, Olsson Y, Siesjö BK (1985) The temporal evolution of hypoglycemic brain damage. II. Light- and electron-microscopic findings in the hippocampal gyrus and subiculum of the rat. Acta Neuropathol (Berl) 67: 25–36

Bouldin TW, Goines ND, Bagnell CR, Krigman MR (1981) Pathogenesis of trimethyltin neuronal toxicity. Am J Pathol 104: 237–249

Brown AW, Brierley JB (1973) The earliest alterations in rat neurones and astrocytes after anoxia-ischaemia. Acta Neuropathol (Berl) 23: 9-22

Brown AW, Aldridge WN, Street BW, Verschoyle RD (1979) The behavioral and neuropathologic sequelae of intoxication by trimethyltin compounds in the rat. Am J Pathol 97: 59-82

Brown AW, Cavanagh JB, Verschoyle RD, Gysbers MF, Jones HB, Aldridge WN (1984a) Evolution in the intracellular changes in neurons caused by trimethyltin. Neuropathol Appl Neurobiol 10: 267-283

Brown AW, Verschoyle RD, Street BW, Aldridge WN (1984b) The neurotoxicity of trimethyltin chloride in hamsters, gerbils and marmosets. J Appl Toxicol 4: 12-21

Chang LW, Dyer RS (1983) Trimethyltin induced pathology in sensory neurons. Neurobehav Toxicol Teratol 5: 673-696

Chang LW, Dyer RS (1985) Septotemporal gradients of trimethyltin-induced hippocampal lesions. Neurobehav Toxicol Teratol 7: 43-49

Chang LW, Wenger GR, McMillan DE, Dyer RS (1983) Species and strain comparison of acute neurotoxic effects of trimethyltin in mice and rats. Neurobehav Toxicol Teratol 5: 337-350

Dyer RS, Deshields TL, Wonderlin WF (1982) Trimethyltin-induced changes in gross morphology of the hippocampus. Neurobehav Toxicol Teratol 4: 141-147

Evans M, Griffiths T, Meldrum B (1983) Early changes in the rat hippocampus following seizures induced by bicuculline or L-allylglycine: a light and electron microscope study. Neuropathol Appl Neurobiol 9: 39-52

Fortemps E, Amand G, Bomboir A, Lauwerys R, Laterre EC (1978) Trimethyltin poisoning. Report of two cases. Int Arch Occup Environ Health 41: 1-6

Kirino T, Sano K (1984) Fine structural nature of delayed neuronal death following ischemia in the gerbil hippocampus. Acta Neuropathol (Berl) 62: 209-218

Kreis H, Frese K, Wilmes G (1967) Physiologische und morphologische Veränderungen an Ratten nach peroraler Verabreichung von Benzoesäure. Fd Cosmet Toxicol 5: 505-511

Krinke G, Hess R (1983) Trimethylzinn-induzierte Läsion im Hippocampus als Beispiel für selektive Vulnerabilität. Schweiz Med Wochenschr 113: 799

Krinke G, Pericin C, Thomann P, Hess R (1978) Toxic encephalopathy with hippocampal lesions. Zentralbl Veterinarmed [A] 25: 277-296

Reuhl KR, Smallridge EA, Chang LW, Mackenzie BA (1983) Developmental effects of trimethyltin intoxication in the neonatal mouse. I. Light microscopic studies. Neurotoxicology 4: 19-28

Rey CH, Weilemann LS, Besser R, Limbourg P, Majdandzic J (1983) Akzidentelle gewerbliche Di- und Trimethylzinnchlorid-Vergiftung. Erfahrungen an sechs Patienten. Schweiz Med Wochenschr 113: 1172

Seawright AA, Brown AW, Aldridge WN, Verschoyle RD, Street BW (1980) Neuropathological changes caused by trialkyllead compounds in the rat. In: Holmstedt B, Lauwerys R, Mercier M, Roberfroid M (eds) Mechanisms of toxicity and hazard evaluation. Proceedings of the 2nd international congress on toxicology. Elsevier North Holland, Amsterdam, pp 71-74

Neurotoxic Effects of Lysolecithin, Mouse, Rat

Susan M. Hall

Synonyms. Lysolecithin; lysophosphatidyl choline (LPC).

Gross Appearance

Experimental lesions are produced by the injection of varying amounts of lysolecithin directly into the central nervous system or peripheral nerves. The sites and techniques of injection will be described in following sections of this report. Gross lesions are not usually observed.

Microscopic Features

Lesions are small and focal: their spatial extent and overall shape reflect not only the volume and concentration of lysolecithin solution injected, but also the fascicular geometry of the peripheral nerve fiber or central tract under study since this determines the spread of the injected bolus. In both peripheral and central nervous system, demyelination is initiated rapidly. The first signs of myelin loss occur within 1 h post injection.

Peripheral Nervous System. In resin-embedded toluidine blue-stained 1 μm sections, the lesion most often appears as a crescent-shaped area beneath the perineurium. In transverse sections, many myelin sheaths appear to have split into two or three concentric rings separated by pale regions. With time all recognizable compact myelin disappears and is replaced by masses of foamy material. In longitudinal sections and in teased fiber preparations, these changes can be seen to begin most often at Schmidt-Lanterman incisures and paranodes (Fig. 68 a, b) and to spread 3–4 days after injection to involve whole internodes. Demyelinated axons are initially associated with debris-containing cells (Figs. 69, 70), but within 2 weeks most are seen to be pro-myelinated, i.e., ensheathed by debris-free Schwann's cells. Remyelination is established for

50%–60% of affected axons by 3 weeks after injection (Fig. 71), and for 95 + % axons by 6 weeks. In teased preparations, remyelinating axons may be recognized because they are surrounded by myelin sheaths that are inappropriately thin (for the caliber of the fiber proximal and distal to the zone of remyelination) and internodal lengths that are uniformly short (ca. 400 µm). It is not unusual to see very short intercalated internodes (10–50 µm in length) (Fig. 72). There is an obvious increase in the number of intratubal nuclei with time (intratubal cells are those cells lying within the Schwann-cell basal lamina tubes). In part, this increase is attributable to a Schwann-cell gliosis that accompanies repair and, in part, it reflects an influx of macrophages. Mononuclear cells enter the endoneurium via endoneurial blood vessels from the 3rd day after inoculation. Lipid-laden macrophages constitute a prominent component of the cellular population of the nerve during the acute debris-clearing phase of repair. Some accumulate in a subperineurial position where they can be seen to undergo degeneration with liberation of lipid droplets. Debris-containing phagocytes rarely persist within a remyelinated lesion after 1 month.

Central Nervous System. Injection of lysolecithin into the corpus callosum of the rabbit produces both degeneration an demyelination. The site of the lesion appears as a light zone in which myelin loss can be demonstrated by an absence of Luxol fast blue staining, and the maintenance of axonal continuity within fiber fascicles by

Fig. 68 a, b. Sciatic nerve, adult mouse, 1 h after injection of lysolecithin. Teased, osmicated single fibers. Loss of osmiophilia at Schmidt-Lanterman incisures (**a**) and paranodes (**b**) indicates onset of demyelination. × 500

Fig. 69 *(upper left).* Sciatic nerve, adult mouse, 6 days after ▶ injection. Demyelinating axons are surrounded by debris-laden intratubal cells and/or by decompacting myelin. Toluidine blue-stained resin section, × 1200

Fig. 70 *(upper right).* Sciatic nerve, adult mouse, 6 days after injection. Teased, osmicated single fiber. Junction between normally myelinated internode and demyelinated, debris-containing segment. × 500

Fig. 71 *(lower left).* Sciatic nerve, adult mouse, 3 weeks after injection. Remyelinating axons and occasional pro-myelinated axons lie in the endoneurium. Many axons are surrounded by processes of supernumerary Schwann's cells *(arrows).* Toluidine blue-stained resin section, × 700

Fig. 72 *(lower right).* Sciatic nerve, adult mouse, 3 weeks after injection. Teased, osmicated single fiber. Short intercalated remyelinating internode. × 300

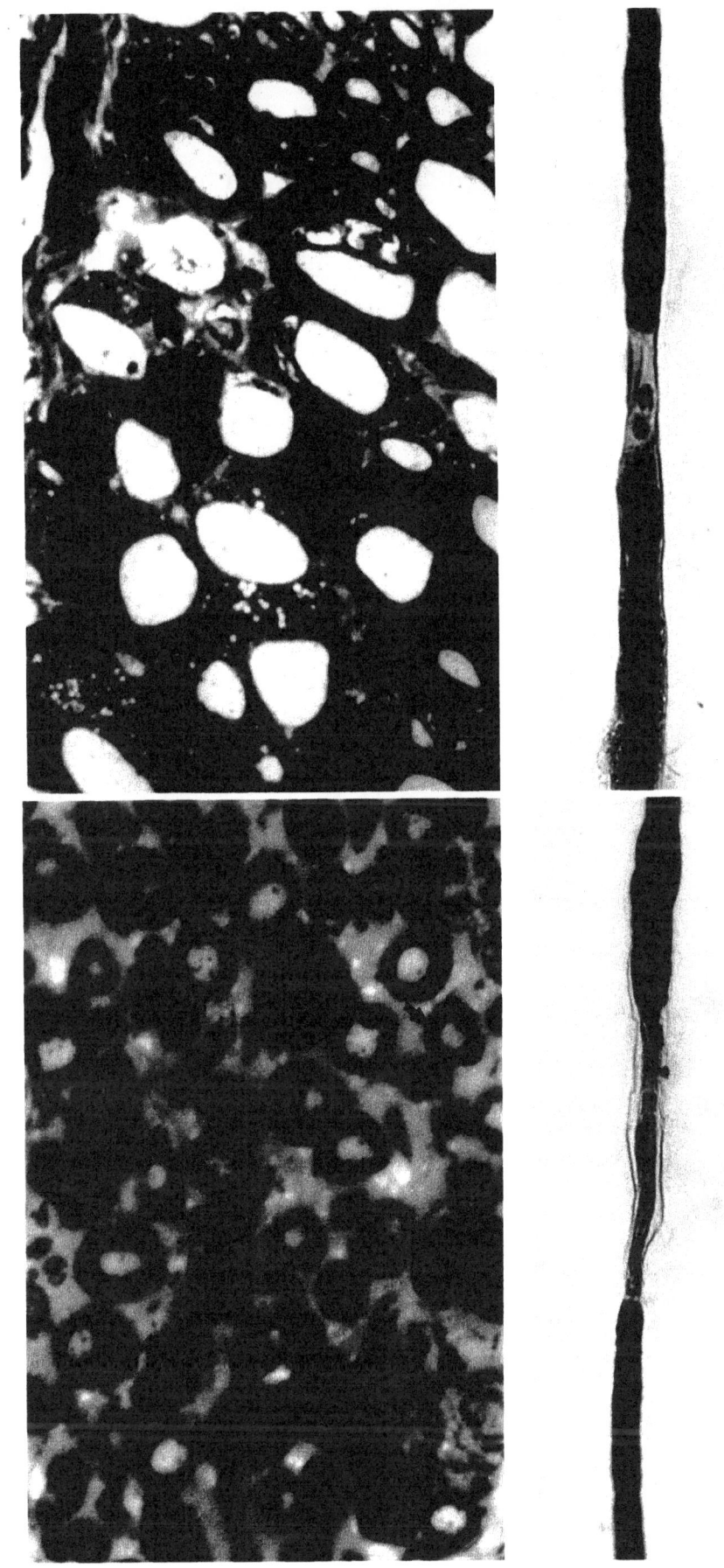

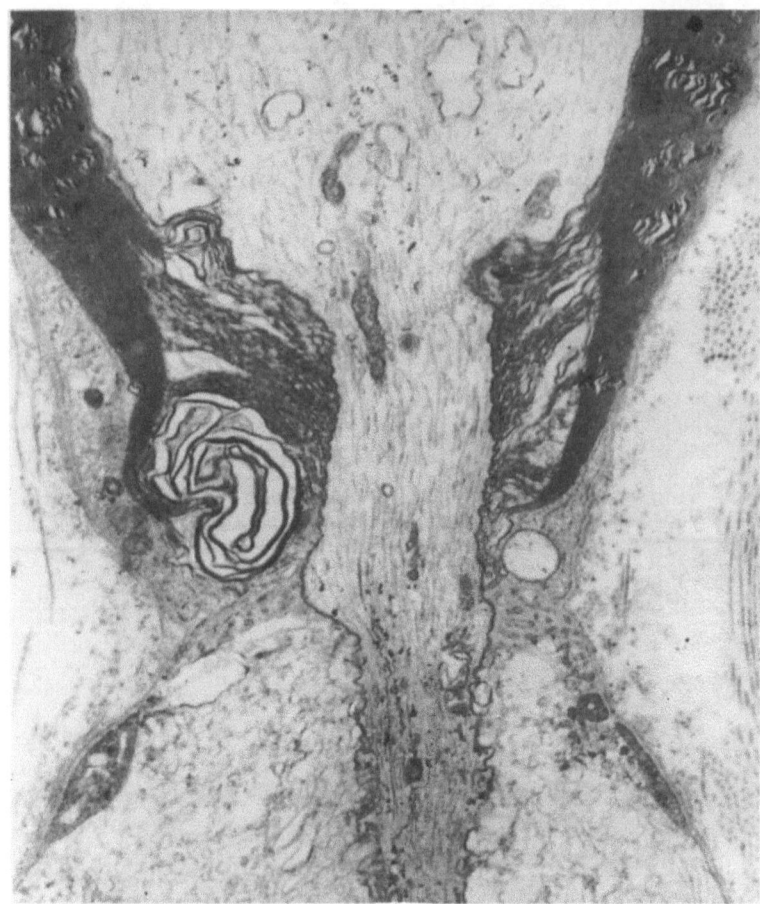

Fig. 73. Sciatic nerve, adult mouse, 1 h after injection. Node of Ranvier. Myelin of one paranode has already undergone vesicular breakdown. TEM, × 24 000

Holmes silver nitrate staining (Waxman et al. 1979). Intraspinal injection typically produces a single demyelination lesion extending 5-10 mm along the length of the cord and approximately 1 mm² in transverse section (mouse, Hall 1972; rat, Blakemore 1976; cat, Blakemore et al. 1977; rabbit, Blakemore 1978). Axonal degeneration and glial cell necrosis is always present in the center of the lesion around the site of injection and may be more extensive, particularly in the rabbit where lesions are cystic and accompanied by wallerian degeneration cranial and caudal to the zone of demyelination (Blakemore 1978). At the edges of the lesion axonal continuity is maintained and most axons undergo demyelination. Within 1 h after injection, myelinated fibers are seen to be dispersed within an edematous extracellular space. Myelin disorganization begins during the first 12 h and many axons are completely demyelinated by 24 h. Astrocytes at the edge of the lesions frequently exhibit signs of hypertrophy. In both spinal cord and corpus callosum, lesion sites are extensively infiltrated by macrophages. Remyelination by both Schwann's

Fig. 74 *(above)*. Sciatic nerve, adult mouse, 1 h after injection. Varying degrees of vesicular change have occurred in the myelin sheaths. Axons appear normal. TEM, × 8300 ▶

Fig. 75 *(below)*. Sciatic nerve, adult mouse, 12 h after injection. Myelin breakdown varies from lamellar splitting to total vesicular dissolution. *a,* Axon; *s,* Schwann's cell. TEM, × 8400

cells and oligodendrocytes is established during the 1st month of repair in the spinal cord of the cat, rat, and rabbit.

Ultrastructure

Peripheral Nervous System. Myelinolysis often begins in peri-incisural and paranodal myelin (Fig. 73), from where it spreads throughout the internodal sheath. Initial decompaction of the sheath, produced by splitting along intraperiod lines is rapidly followed by vesicular breakdown

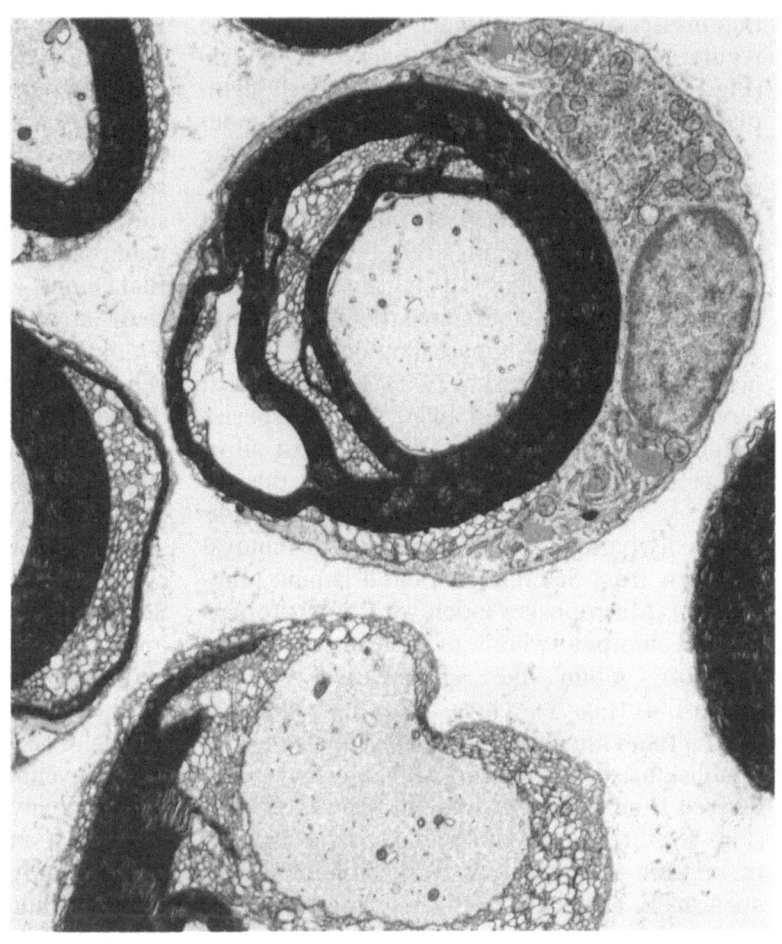

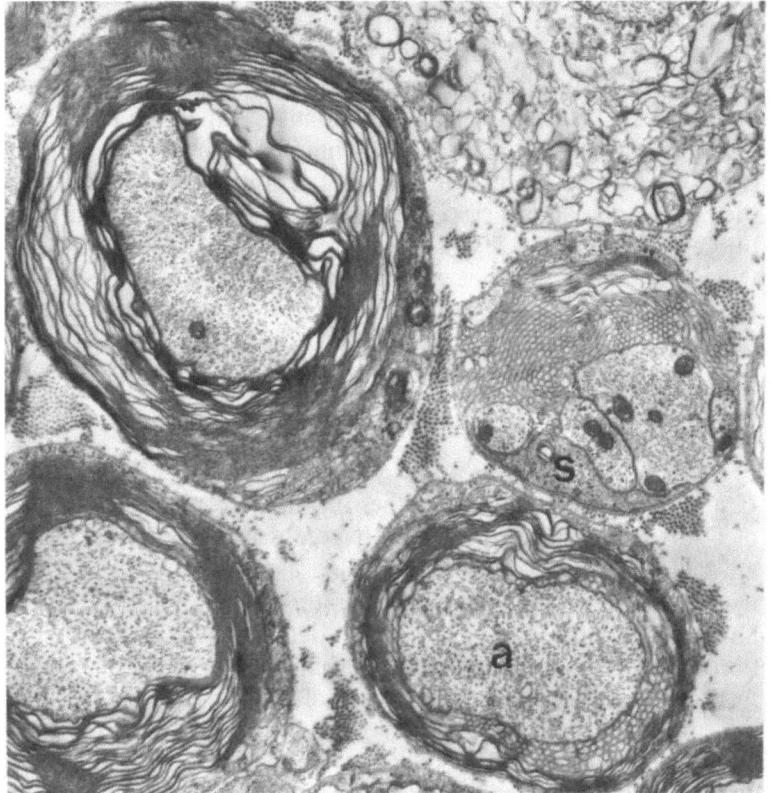

into masses of tubulo-vesicular profiles and more regular lattices of closely packed cylinders (Figs. 74, 75). Processes of Schwann-cell cytoplasm may bee seen lying between the inner aspect of the Schwann-cell basal lamina and the mass of vesicular myelin (Fig. 75). "Rarefaction" and lysis of Schwann-cell cytoplasm have been described for rat Schwann's cells (both myelinating and nonmyelinating) at the site of injection after 24 h (Mitchell and Caren 1982). Schwann-cell necrosis is less apparent in mouse sciatic nerve (Hall and Gregson 1971), a finding that serves to emphasize that there may be species differences in susceptibility. While almost all of the vesicular breakdown is initiated in the absence of mononuclear cells, macrophages undoubtedly participate in the subsequent removal of debris from Schwann-cell basal lamina tubes (Fig. 76). Macrophages laden with lipid droplets and pleomorphic whorls of lamellar debris are common within the endoneurium during weeks 1-4 (Fig. 77). Once Schwann-cell basal lamina tubes are debris free, demyelinated axons establish a 1:1 relationship with Schwann's cells derived from the original parent Schwann's cells (Fig. 78): these promyelinated axons subsequently become remyelinated. Remyelinating axons are usually associated with the processes of supernumerary Schwann's cells. The latter arise during the reactive gliosis that follows demyelination; they remain associated with the remyelinating Schwann-cell/axon units and with any collateral axon sprouts which issue from the parent axons for several months following injection (Fig. 79). As with other demyelinating lesions in the peripheral nervous system, a number of morphologic features may be seen that are consistent with the hypothesis that remodeling of internodes occurs during the early stages of remyelination after induced demyelination, e.g., very short intercalated internodes, excessive myelin wrinkling, staggered nodes, and "pseudonodes" (Hall 1973; Hildebrand et al. 1986).

Central Nervous System. All studies of the effects of lysolecithin in the spinal cord have described an acute edematous lesion comprising a central necrotic portion containing degenerating axons and glia, circumscribed by an area of demyelination. The earliest response of the myelin sheaths in this outer zone is seen within 1 h after injection and consists of changes in lamellar periodicity such that in some regions the original 10-11 nm lamellar repeat collapses to 4-6 nm, while in others the intraperiod line splits, and the

intraperiod line gap widens within the range 25-55 nm. Progressive disorganization of the sheaths continues during days 1-3 (Fig. 80) until all compact myelin has been replaced by a foam-like mass of vesicular material similar to that seen in the peripheral nervous system after exposure to lysolecithin. Myelin debris is removed by macrophages in mouse, rat, and cat spinal cord: Blakemore (1978) described macrophage-deficient areas in which debris persisted up to 6 months following injection in the rabbit. Remyelination by both Schwann's cells and oligodendrocytes is seen after this induced demyelination in the spinal cord. When remyelination is effected by oligodendrocytes, myelin has central nervous system periodicity, is thin, and characteristic small inner and outer loops of oligodendrocyte cytoplasm are present.

Schwann-cell remyelination results in thicker myelin sheaths with peripheral nervous system periodicity, an abaxonal layer of Schwann-cell cytoplasm and an enveloping Schwann-cell basal lamina. Collagen fibers are usually seen near axons remyelinated by Schwann's cells. The patterns of remyelination that have been described for rat, cat, and rabbit differ in terms of the distribution of remyelinating Schwann's cells. In the rat, remyelination by Schwann's cells is limited to the center of the lesion and the pial surface, whereas in the cat it occurs in small groups or singly. In the rabbit, many axons remain demyelinated. These differences may be correlated with the degree of Schwann-cell invasion that occurs during repair and with the responsiveness of the astrocyte population. Blakemore (1978) has speculated that the failure of the astrocytic response, coupled with a diminished number of macrophages, accounts for the areas of persistent demyelination observed in rabbit spinal cord.

Fig. 76 *(above).* Sciatic nerve, adult mouse, 7 days after injection. Debris-laden macrophage lies next to promyelinated axon, within a common Schwann-cell basal lamina tube *(arrow).* TEM, ×7300

Fig. 77 *(below).* Sciatic nerve, adult mouse, 2 weeks after injection. Endoneurium contains debris-laden macrophages and promyelinated axons. TEM, ×2250

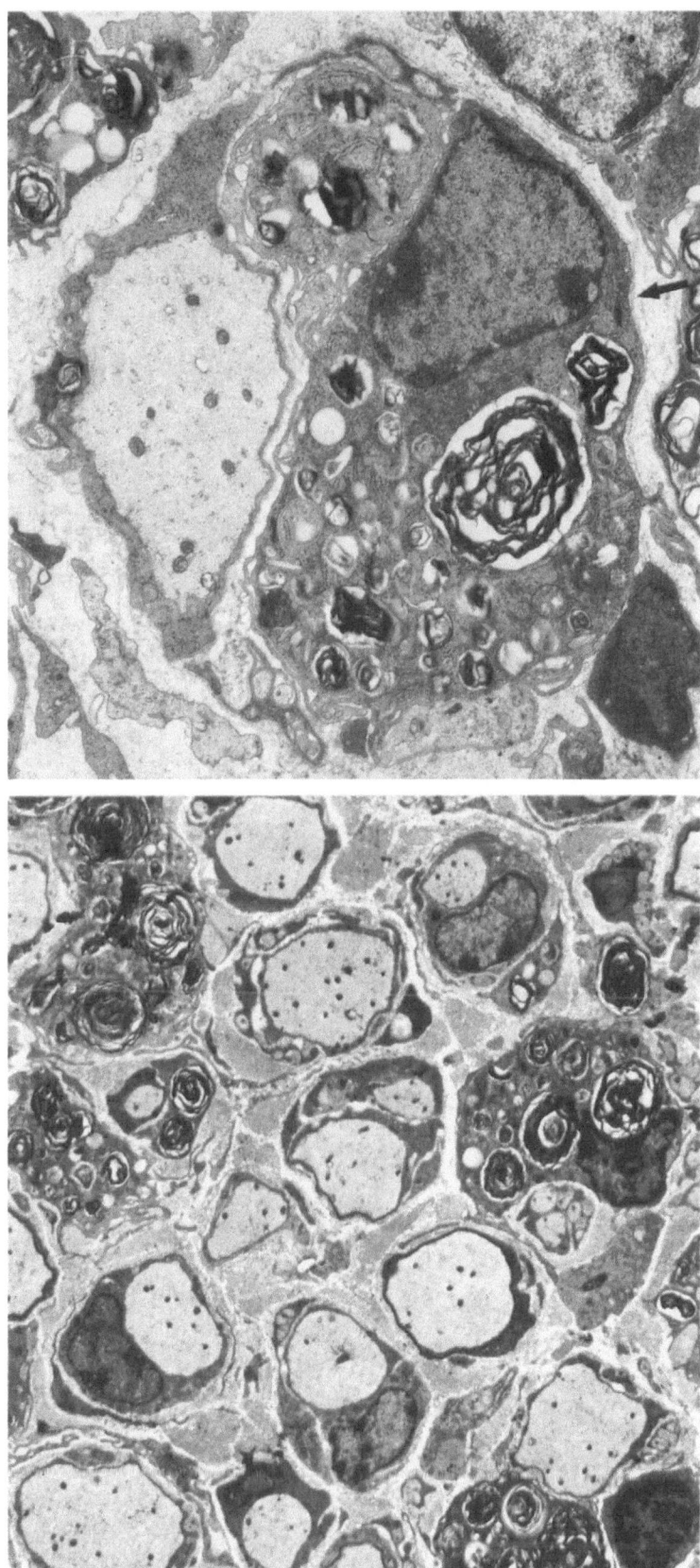

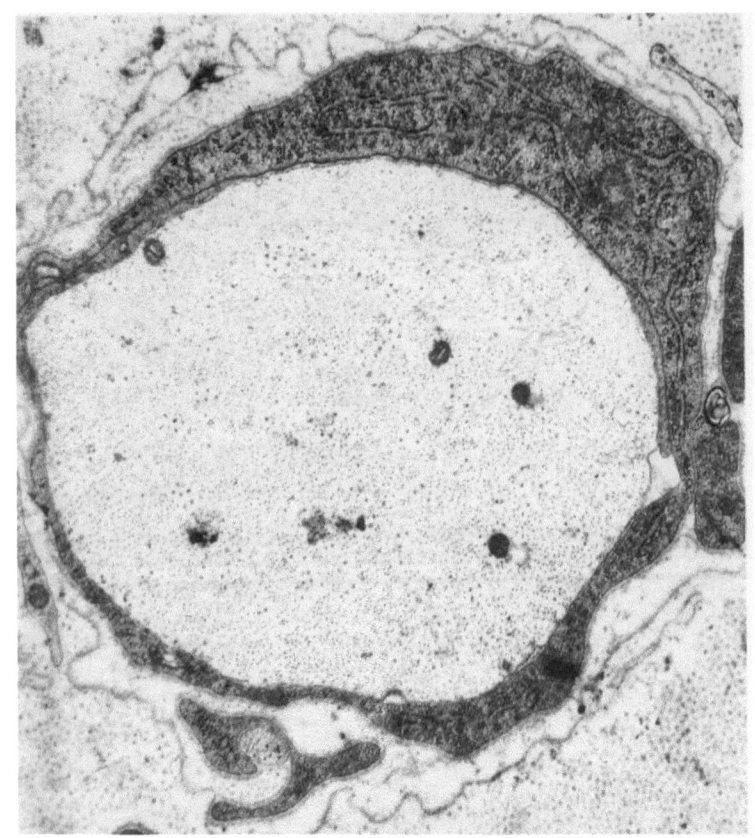

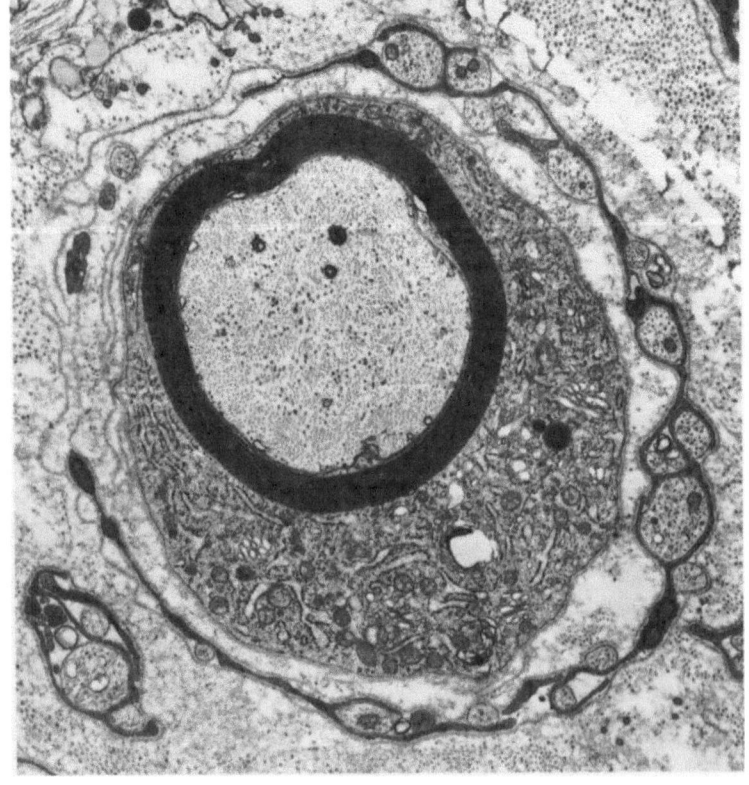

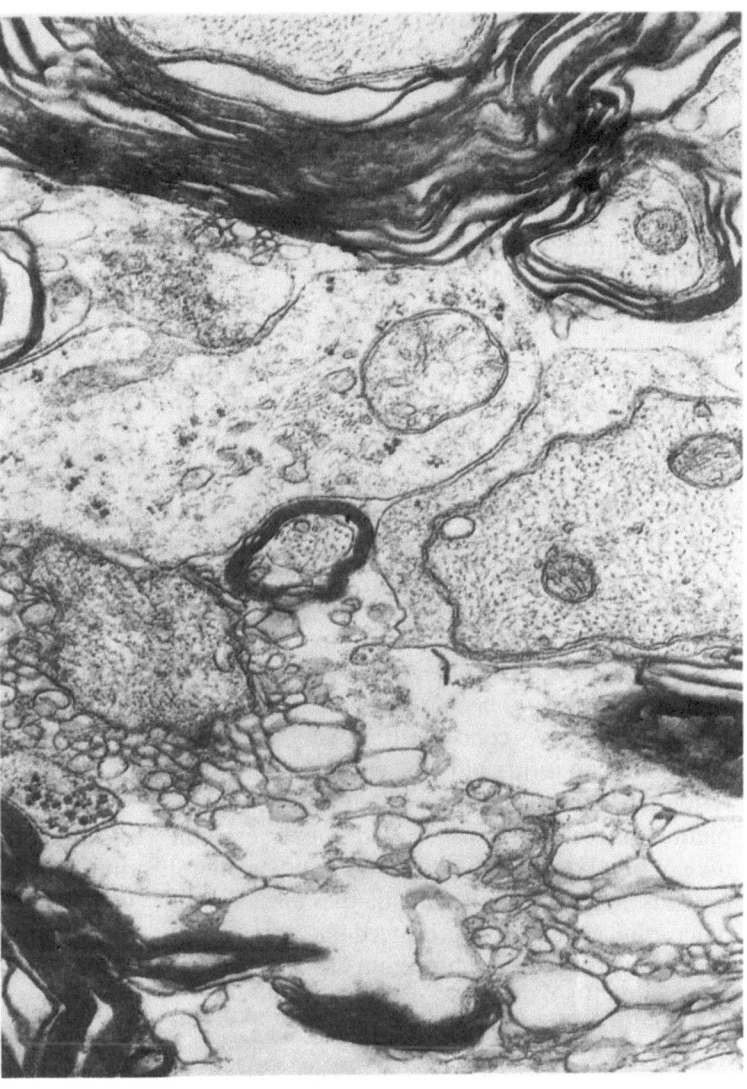

Fig. 80. Dorsal column, adult mouse, 48 h after injection. Some axons are completely demyelinated and surrounded by vesicular myelin or processes of astrocyte cytoplasm. Myelin persists around other axons, but exhibits widening of the intraperiod line gap. TEM, × 31 500

◀ **Fig. 78** *(above)*. Sciatic nerve, adult mouse, 2 weeks after injection. Promyelinated axon is surrounded by processes of Schwann-cell cytoplasm and a newly synthesized basal lamina. Notice collapsed, serpentine basal lamina that has persisted throughout the period of cellular repair: this would have been associated with the original myelinating Schwann's cell. TEM, × 14 400

Fig. 79 *(below)*. Sciatic nerve, adult mouse, 3 weeks after injection. Remyelinating axon is surrounded by processes of supernumerary Schwann cell cytoplasm and associated collateral axon sprouts. TEM, × 12 250

Differential Diagnosis

Vesiculation of the myelin sheath has been reported after intraneural injection of phospholipase A_2 (the enzyme that hydrolyzes phosphatidyl choline to lysolecithin) (Hall and Gregson 1971), in vivo or in vitro after exposure of peripheral nerve fibers to the calcium ionophores A23187 (Schlaepfer 1977; Smith et al. 1985) and ionomycin (Smith et al. 1985), during complement-mediated demyelination that follows intraneural injection of experimental allergic neuritis serum (Saida et al. 1978) or antigalactocerebroside serum (Saida et al. 1979), after intraneural injection of antimyelin serum (Hahn et al.

1980), in experimental allergic encephalomyelitis (Lampert 1965), in experimental allergic neuritis (Dal Canto et al. 1975), in Guillain-Barré syndrome (Prineas 1972), after experimental traumatic spinal cord injury (Balentine 1978; Blight 1985), in the presence of processes of macrophage cytoplasm which insinuate into the myelin sheath during cell-mediated demyelination by "stripping" in autoimmune conditions (Raine 1984).

It is interesting that in a number of these reports the spatio-temporal distribution of vesicular change correlates closely with that described after intraneural injection of lysolecithin, namely, spreading from peri-incisural and paranodal regions of the sheath. It is tempting to speculate that myelin vesiculation may be the inevitable outcome of any event capable of triggering phospholipase A_2 activation and the subsequent liberation of myelinolytic lysocompounds. In Schwann's cells an increase in endogenous phospholipase A_2 would be one consequence of a rise in cytosolic Ca^{2+} concentration, such as might result from an influx of Ca^{2+} via a plasmalemma rendered leaky by cationic ionophores or complement-mediated damage. Additional vesicular myelin breakdown in both central and peripheral nervous system that occurs in the presence of macrophages may be produced as a result of macrophage-derived phospholipase A_2 (Trotter and Smith 1986).

Biologic Features

Lysolecithin produces a demyelinating lesion when small volumes are injected into the sciatic nerve of the adult mouse (Hall and Gregson 1971); rat (Mitchell and Caren 1982); corpus callosum of the rabbit (Waxman et al. 1979); ventral roots of rat (Smith et al. 1983); spinal cord of mouse (Hall 1972), rat (Blakemore 1976), cat (Blakemore et al. 1977), and rabbit (Blakemore 1978). The local action of myelinolytic factor(s) has long been implicated in the pathogenesis of demyelination (e.g., Marburg 1906; Thompson 1961). Moreover, the effects of phospholipases and lysophosphatides on nerve lipids has attracted particular attention since the 1950s (Morrison and Zamecnik 1950; Birkmayer and Neumayer 1957; Webster 1957; Smith and Benjamins 1977). The ability of lysolecithin to solubilize membranes is dependent upon the chemical composition and source of the membranes: there is evidence that it binds to membrane components

principally via the alkyl residues. The binding of lysolecithin to central myelin has been shown to be a two-stage process. Isopyknic centrifugation of solubilized myelin of the central nervous system reveals that discrete lipoprotein complexes are released at each stage and include a high-density group containing basic protein and a low-density component containing predominantly proteolipid (Gregson 1976). Since lysolecithin has a general detergent action on membranes, it is perhaps surprising that the characteristic pattern of damage produced on exposure to lysolecithin is demyelination. Gregson and Hall (1973) proposed that nonmyelin membranes in the peripheral nervous system were apparently "spared" because, unlike myelin, they were able to reacylate lysolecithin: when reacylation was blocked, all membranes were progressively solubilized on exposure to lysolecithin. Its lytic effect on structures other than myelin within the nervous system has been reported. Mitchell and Caren (1982) have described a complete loss of nonmyelinated axons and their Schwann's cells and lysis of many myelin-associated Schwann's cells at the site of injection into the sciatic nerve of adult rats. Others have reported a lytic effect on oligodendrocytes in lesions in the central nervous system: it seems likely that demyelination is achieved not only by a direct lytic attack on the sheath but is also secondary to oligodendrocyte pathology.

In the central nervous system, where myelin sheaths are generally thinner than their peripheral counterparts, or in fascicles of the peripheral nervous system where there are many subperineurial nonmyelinated bundles, the probability that nonmyelin membranes will be exposed to excess (i.e., nonmyelin-bound) lysolecithin after injection is high. In these situations it is reasonable to assume that reacylating mechanisms would soon become saturated and therefore unable to protect cells against membranolysis.

The extent to which the morphology of a lesion induced by lysolecithin may reflect either the source of the compound, the injection technique, or species differences between experimental animals has not been examined systematically. However, work in our laboratory over 20 years has shown that differences do exist between commercially available samples of lysolecithin in terms of (a) the amount of demyelination produced with a standard intraneural injection; (b) the amount of wallerian degeneration; (c) the amount of degeneration among nonmyelinated axons. It is possible that some of the differences between samples reflect variations in fatty acid composition of lysolecithin prepared from phosphatidyl choline isolated from different sources. Injection with a glass needle held in a micromanipulator minimizes wallerian degeneration attributable to mechanical damage in the peripheral nervous system. In the central nervous system, where degeneration along the needle track and at the site of injection is inevitable, Waxman et al. (1979) have described a method to reduce degeneration, using slow injection via a needle placed stereotaxically at several levels above and below the tract under study.

References

Balentine JD (1978) Pathology of experimental spinal cord trauma. II. Ultrastructure of axons and myelin. Lab Invest 39: 254-266

Blakemore WF (1976) Invasion of Schwann cells into the spinal cord of the rat following local injection of lysolecithin. Neuropathol Appl Neurobiol 2: 21-39

Blakemore WF (1978) Observations on remyelination in the rabbit spinal cord following demyelination induced by lysolecithin. Neuropathol Appl Neurobiol 4: 47-59

Blakemore WF, Eames RA, Smith KJ, McDonald WI (1977) Remyelination in the spinal cord of the cat following intraspinal injections of lysolecithin. J Neurol Sci 33: 31-43

Blight AR (1985) Delayed demyelination and macrophage invasion: a candidate for secondary cell damage in spinal cord injury. Cent Nerv Syst Trauma 2: 299-315

Birkmayer W, Neumayer E (1957) Experimentelle Untersuchungen zur Frage der formalen Pathogenese der Multiple Sclerosia. Dtsch Z Nervenheilkd 177: 117-125

Dal Canto M, Wisniewski HM, Johnson AB, Brostoff SW, Raine CS (1975) Vesicular disruption of myelin in autoimmune demyelination. J Neurol Sci 24: 313-319

Gregson NA (1976) The chemistry and structure of myelin. In: Landon DN (ed) The peripheral nerve. Chapman and Hall, London, pp 512-604

Gregson NA, Hall SM (1973) A quantitative analysis of the effects of the intraneural injection of lysophosphatidyl choline. J Cell Sci 13: 257-277

Hahn AF, Gilbert JJ, Feasby TE (1980) Passive transfer of demyelination by experimental allergic neuritis serum. Acta Neuropathol (Berl) 49: 169-176

Hall SM (1972) The effect of injections of lysophosphatidyl choline into white matter of the adult mouse spinal cord. J Cell Sci 10: 535-546

Hall SM (1973) Some aspects of remyelination after demyelination produced by the intraneural injection of lysophosphatidyl choline. J Cell Sci 13: 461-477

Hall SM, Gregson NA (1971) The in vivo and ultrastructural effects of injection of lysophosphatidyl choline into myelinated peripheral nerve fibres of the adult mouse. J Cell Sci 9: 769-789

Hildebrand C, Mustafa GY, Waxman SG (1986) Remodelling of internodes in regenerated rat sciatic nerve: electron microscopic observations. J Neurocytol 15: 681-692

Lampert PW (1965) Demyelination and remyelination in experimental allergic encephalitis. Further electronmicroscopic observations. J Neuropathol Exp Neurol 24: 371-385

Marburg O (1906) Syringomyelie und Halsnippe. Wien Klin Wochenschr 20: 241-244

Mitchell J, Caren CA (1982) Degeneration of non-myelinated axons in the rat sciatic nerve following lysolecithin injection. Acta Neuropathol (Berl) 56: 187-193

Morrison LR, Zamecnik PC (1950) Experimental demyelination by means of enzymes, especially the alpha toxin of *Clostridium welchii*. Arch Neurol Psychiatry 63: 367-381

Prineas JW (1972) Acute idiopathic polyneuritis: an electron microscope study. Lab Invest 26: 133-147

Raine CS (1984) Analysis of autoimmune demyelination: its impact upon multiple sclerosis. Lab Invest 50: 608-635

Saida K, Saida T, Brown MJ, Silberberg DH, Asbury AK (1978) Antiserum-mediated demyelination in vivo. A sequential study using intraneural injection of experimental allergic neuritis serum. Lab Invest 39: 449-462

Saida K, Saida T, Brown MJ, Silberberg DH (1979) In vivo demyelination induced by intraneural injection of antigalactocerebroside serum. A morphologic study. Am J Pathol 95: 99-116

Schlaepfer WW (1977) Vesicular disruption of myelin simulated by exposure of nerve to calcium ionophore. Nature 26: 734-736

Smith KJ, Hall SM, Schauf CL (1983) Vesicular demyelination induced by raised intracellular calcium. J Neurol Sci 71: 19-37

Smith ME, Benjamins JA (1977) Model systems for study of perturbations of myelin metabolism. In: Morell P (ed) Myelin. Plenum, New York, pp 447-488

Thompson RHS (1961) Myelinolytic mechanisms. Symposium on disseminated sclerosis. Proc R Soc Med 54: 30-33

Trotter J, Smith ME (1986) The role of phospholipases from inflammatory macrophages in demyelination. Neurochem Res 11: 349-361

Waxman SG, Kocsis JD, Nitta KC (1979) Lysophosphatidyl choline-induced focal demyelination in the rabbit corpus callosum. Light microscopic observations. J Neurol Sci 44: 45-53

Webster GR (1957) Clearing action of lysolecithin on brain homogenates. Nature 180: 660-661

Neurotoxicity of Perhexiline Maleate in Rats

Yuzo Hyashi, Akihiko Maekawa, and Shinsuki Yoshimura

Synonyms. Drug-induced lipidosis; thesaurismosis.

Gross Appearance

No remarkable feature is seen by gross examination in the brain, spinal cord, or peripheral ganglia.

Microscopic Features

Numerous, various-sized, cytoplasmic vacuoles occur in the nerve cells of the peripheral ganglia such as the dorsal spinal ganglia, trigeminal ganglia, coeliac ganglion, and Auerbach's plexus (Fig. 81). Similar cytoplasmic vacuolation is also seen in the Purkinje's cells of the cerebellum (Fig. 82). The nerve cells with severe vacuolar changes are slightly swollen but necrotic changes occur very rarely.

Ultrastructure

Various-sized membrane-bound inclusions with concentric lamellar structures, tiny tubular structures or electron-dense amorphous materials are discernible in the cytoplasm of the nerve cells of

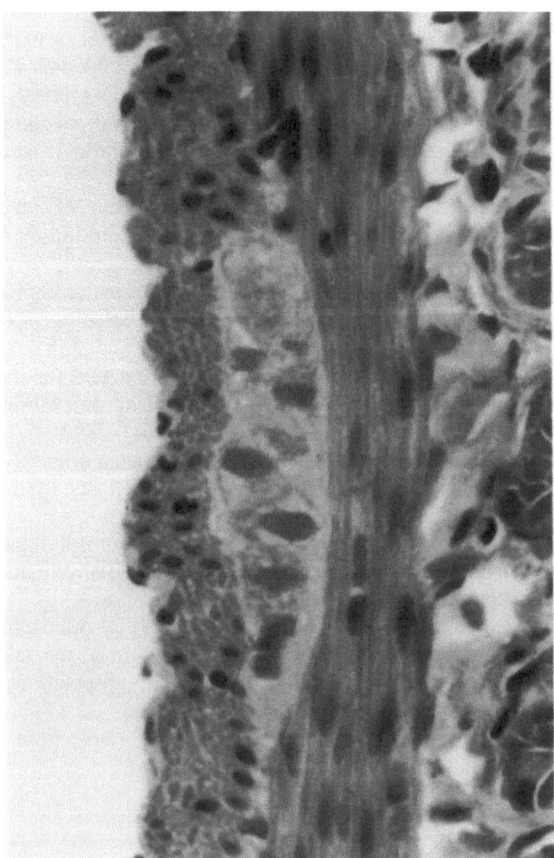

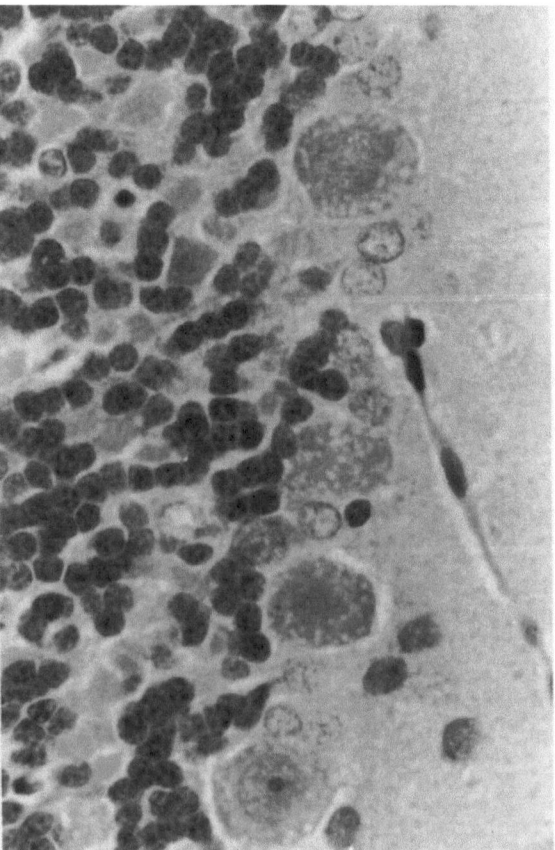

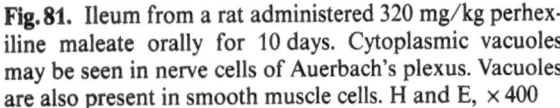

Fig. 81. Ileum from a rat administered 320 mg/kg perhexiline maleate orally for 10 days. Cytoplasmic vacuoles may be seen in nerve cells of Auerbach's plexus. Vacuoles are also present in smooth muscle cells. H and E, × 400

Fig. 82. Cerebellum from a rat administered 320 mg/kg perhexiline maleate orally for 10 days. Numerous vacuoles are present in the cytoplasm of Purkinje's cells. H and E, × 480

the peripheral ganglia (Figs. 83–85) as well as the cerebellar Purkinje's cells. Similar inclusions are also seen, though less numerous, in the cytoplasm of the Schwann's cells or satellite cells of both myelinated and nonmyelinated fibers. In addition to the occurrence of cytoplasmic inclusions, the number of lysosomes appear to be increased, but there are no remarkable alterations in other organelles (Jung and Suzuki 1978).

Biologic Features

Signs. In the case of perhexiline maleate, the main toxic signs in rats are dyspnea, neurologic disturbances, hypomotility of the intestine, and hepatic dysfunction (Hayashi et al. 1981a, b). Animals treated with perhexiline maleate exhibit an ataxic gait characterized by elevation of the forelimbs and swinging hindquarters (Hayashi et

al. 1981a, b). Peculiar movement of the head and neck, such as shaking or turning, is also frequently noticed (Hayashi et al. 1981a, b). These signs subside gradually when administration of the drug is discontinued. Toxicology studies (Hayashi et al. 1981a, b) indicate that the neurotoxicity of perhexiline maleate is dose dependent; for occurrence of typical neurologic signs, a single oral administration of 600 mg/kg for 5 days or daily oral administration of 300 mg/kg for 10 days is required. No neurologic signs appear at the dose level of 160 mg/kg for 30 days or 100 mg/kg for 6 months.

Pathogenesis. Generalized lipidosis, mostly phospholipidosis, can be induced in animals by a variety of drugs such as chloroquine, quinacrine, triparanol, and chlorphentermine (Lüllmann et al. 1975). These drugs are known to have an amphophilic chemical structure and to accumulate

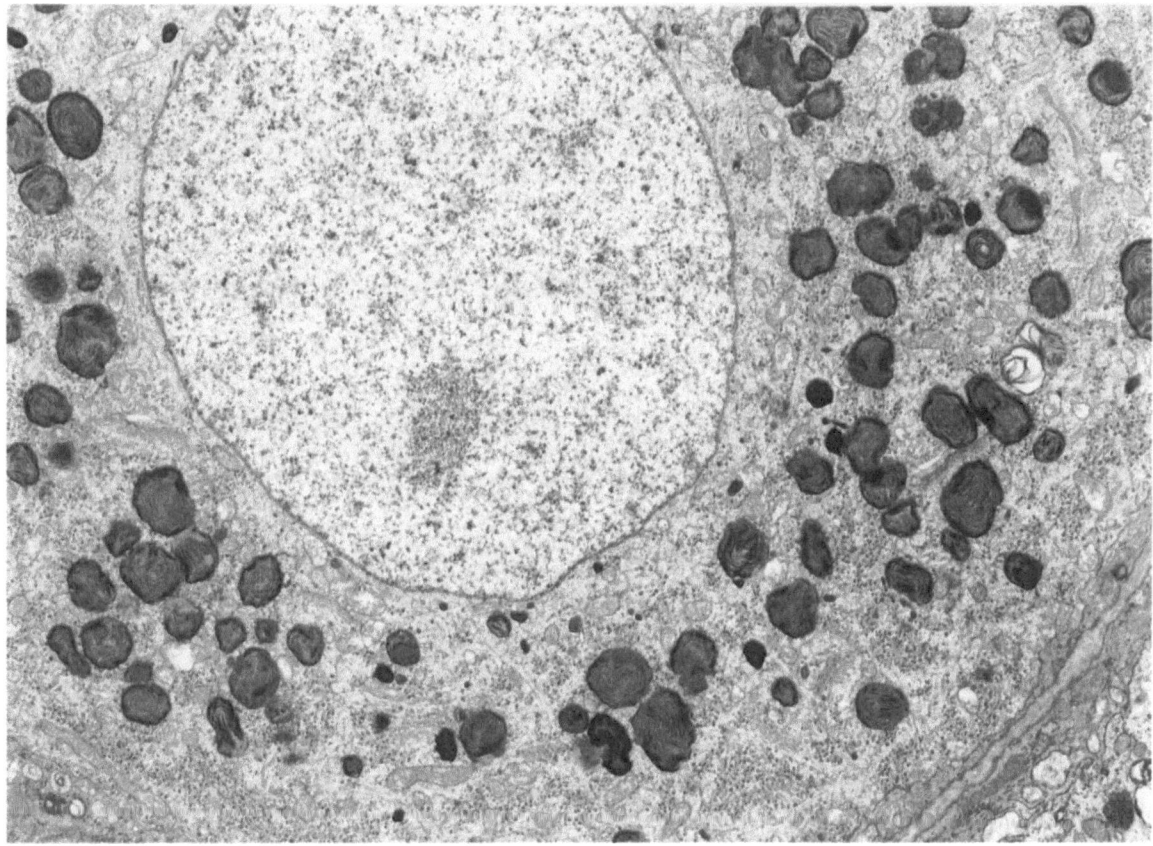

Fig. 83. A nerve cell of a dorsal spinal ganglion (L₆) from a rat administered 320 mg/kg perhexiline maleate orally for 15 days. Inclusion bodies with concentric lamellar structures are seen in the cytoplasms. TEM, × 6000

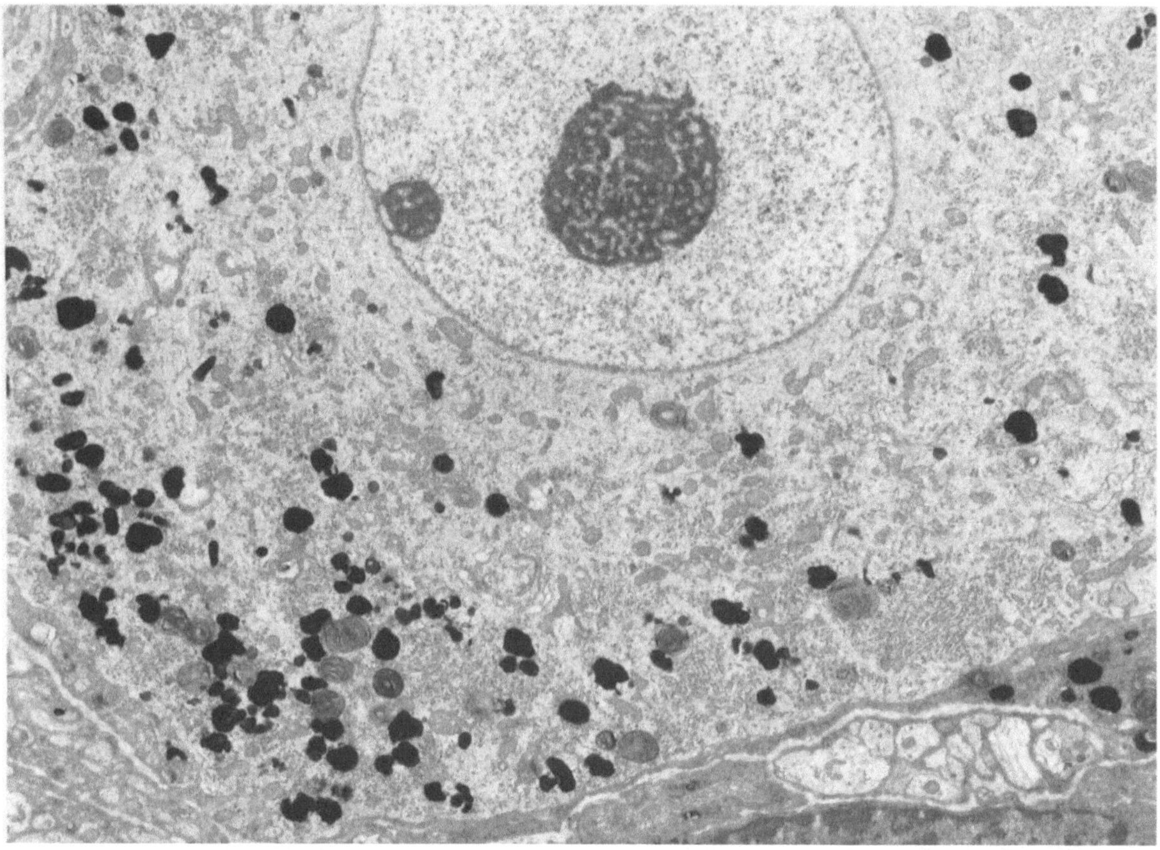

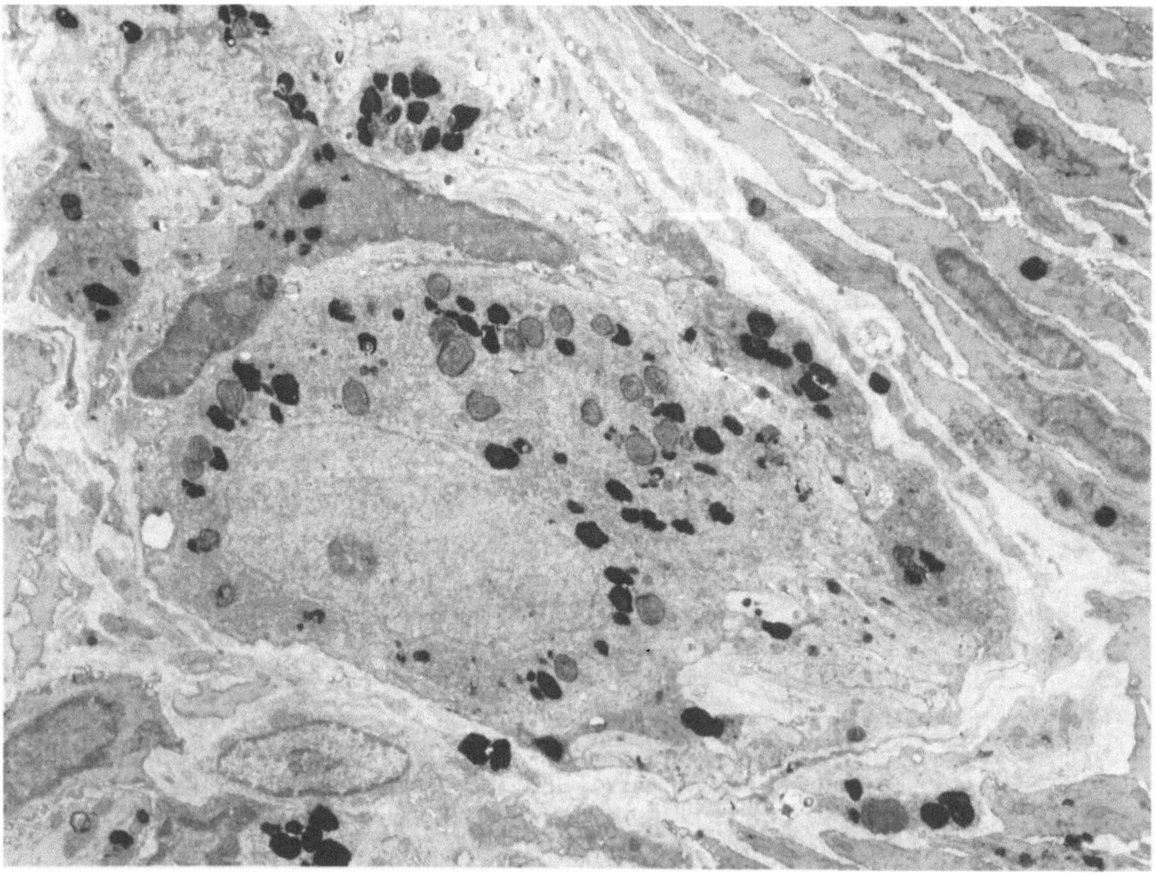

◄ **Fig. 84** *(above).* A nerve cell of the coeliac ganglion from a rat given 320 mg/kg perhexiline maleate orally for 15 days. Inclusion bodies with lamellar structure or electron-dense amorphous material are seen in the cytoplasm. Similar inclusions also appear in the cytoplasmic process of a Schwann's cell *(bottom right).* TEM, × 6000

Fig. 85 *(below).* Nerve cell of an Auerbach's plexus from a rat administered 320 mg/kg perhexiline maleate orally for 15 days. Two kinds of inclusion bodies containing concentric lamellar structures or electron-dense material are present in the cytoplasm. Electron-dense inclusion bodies are also seen in smooth muscle cells. TEM, × 6000

in various tissues. As a mechanism of the tissue accumulation, it is postulated that the amphophilic drugs enter into physiochemical interaction with the lipid moieties of the cytoplasmic membranes, thus protecting the membrane lipid from degradation enzymes present in the lysosomes. As a consequence of this impaired metabolism and for as long as the drug is present, lipids gradually accumulate within lysosomes, thus causing the transformation of lysosomes into residual bodies with lamellar internal structure (Lüllmann et al. 1975). Perhexiline maleate has a similar amphophilic structure and is thought to undergo similar tissue accumulation, eventually resulting in lipidosis with cytoplasmic inclusions (Lüllmann and Lüllmann-Rauch 1978). It must be emphasized that these amphophilic agents affect most of the organs and tissues in the body, but the toxic manifestations differ for each agent.

Comparison of Lesions in Other Species

Perhexiline maleate has been used clinically as a drug for angina pectoris. Hepatic damages and

neurologic disorders are reported to occur as side effects (Robinson 1977). Corresponding to the findings in animals, the neurologic signs in humans are ataxia, loss of tendon reflex, and paresthesia in the hands or feet. Extrapyramidal symptoms such as akinesia or tremor are also reported to occur. Peripheral neuropathy has been reported in nine patients who had taken perhexiline in doses of 200–400 mg/day for between 4 months and 2 years. Biopsy of the superficial peroneal nerve in one patient revealed the presence of inclusion bodies in the cytoplasm of the Schwann's cells (Lhermitte et al. 1976).

References

Hayashi Y, Otsuka H, Yoshimura S, Seki T, Ono H, Hashimoto K (1981a) Acute toxicity of perhexiline in rats and mice. Pharmacometrics Oyo Yakuri 21: 83–94
Hayashi Y, Yoshimura S, Yamaguchi K, Imai K, Abe F, Ono H, Hashimoto K (1981b) Subacute toxicity of perhexiline in rats. Pharmacometrics Oyo Yakuri 21: 95–122
Jung HJ, Suzuki K (1978) Morphological changes in CNS of rats treated with perhexiline maleate (Pexid). Acta Neuropathol (Berl) 42: 159–164
Lhermitte F, Fardeau M, Chedru F, Mallecourt J (1976) Polyneuropathy after perhexiline maleate therapy. Br Med J 1: 1256
Lüllmann H, Lüllmann-Rauch R, Wassermann O (1975) Drug-induced phospholipidosis. II. Tissue distribution of the amphiphilic drug chlorphentermine. CRC Crit Rev Toxicol 4: 185–218
Lüllmann H, Lüllmann-Rauch R (1978) Perhexiline induced generalized lipidosis in rats. Klin Wochenschr 56: 309–310
Robinson BF (1977) Drugs acting on the cardiovascular system. In: Dukes MNG (ed) Side effects of drugs annual, vol I. Elsevier North Holland, pp 151–163

Cycloleucine Encephalopathy, Rats and Mice

Henry C. Powell

Synonyms. Spongiform leukoencephalopathy; spongiform encephalomyelopathy, central myelinopathy.

Gross Appearance

At postmortem examination decreased muscle mass and body fat and an empty gastrointestinal tract are evident. Trypan blue dye, injected intraperitoneally 24 h prior to sacrifice does not

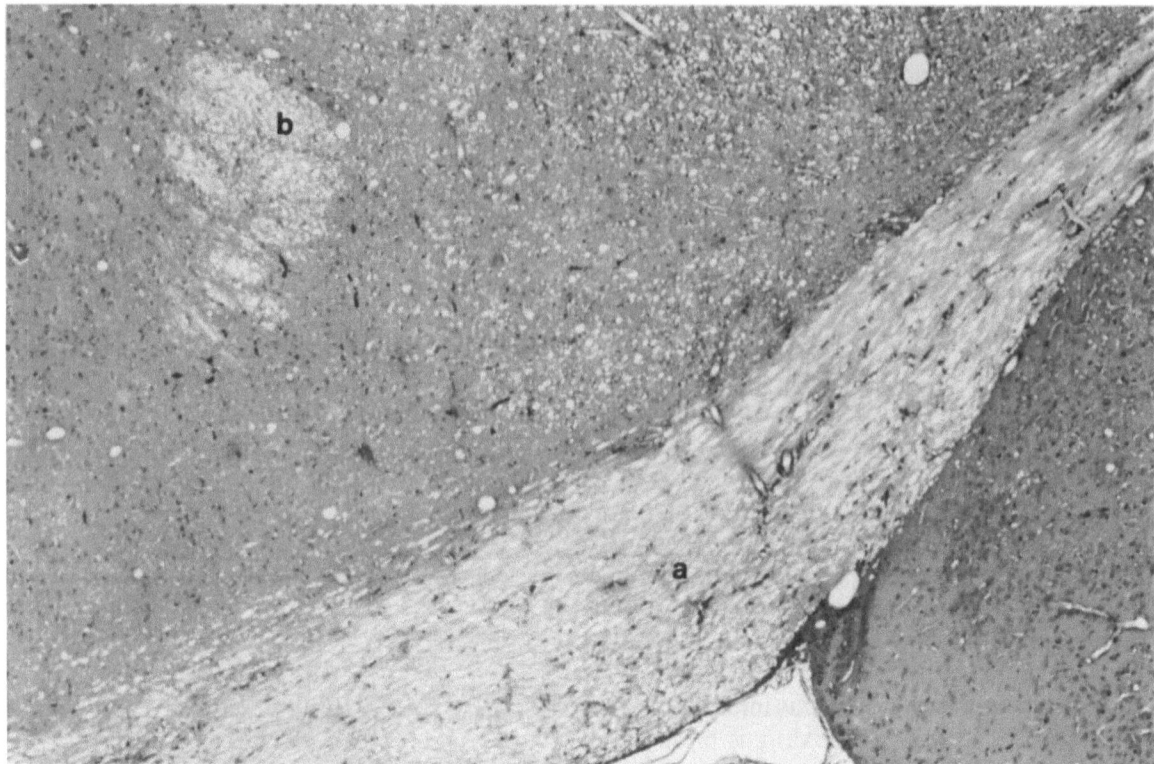

Fig. 86. Cycloleucine encephalopathy in a mouse. Status spongiosus of the white matter. Note the spongiform changes in the corpus callosum (**a**) and an adjacent myelinated tract (**b**). H and E, ×175

stain the brain, confirming the integrity of the blood-nerve barrier. Brains of mice treated with cycloleucine appear normal grossly.

Microscopic Features

Light-microscopic examination of paraffin-embedded sections reveal status spongiosus of cerebral, cerebellar, and brain stem white matter, particularly prominent in the optic tracts and columnae fornicis (Fig. 86). The spinal cord and ganglia as well as the peripheral nerves appear normal. No pathologic change is seen in the heart, kidney, thymus, spleen, or the eyes. Cytoplasmic vacuolation may be seen in occasional hepatocytes. Semi-thin sections of the white matter reveal edema characterized by vacuolar degeneration of the myelin sheaths. These changes are noted in the corpus striatum, optic tracts and chiasm, optic nerves, cerebral and cerebellar white matter. No evidence of vacuolar degeneration is evident in myelin of the spinal cord or sciatic nerves.

Status spongiosus of declining severity may be seen in recovering animals. Light-microscopic

analysis suggests that the spongiform changes are dose related (Greco et al. 1980).

Nixon (1976) described primary axonal degeneration in the cerebellum, rostral spinal cord, and peripheral nerves in C57 BL/6J mice. Myelin in these animals was stated to be normal and biochemical analyses revealed decreased protein content in the regions where histologic changes were greatest. Sulfatide deficits were also noted in these same areas whereas increases in sphingomyelin were detected (Nixon 1976). However, we were not able to reproduce spongiform degeneration of the spinal cord as reported by Jacobson et al. (1973), Gandy et al. (1973), and Nixon et al. (1974), nor did we see any changes in peripheral nerves in either of the three experimental groups we examined. In our experiments, spinal cords and sciatic nerves appeared consistently normal in both acutely and chronically intoxicated mice and rats. It was in the cerebral white matter that the characteristic changes of white matter were noted, and these changes appeared in all animals. Spongiform myelinopathy, as illustrated in Figs. 87 and 88, was observed in the spinal cords of developing rats (Ramsey and Fisher 1978). They noticed that weanling rats in-

Fig. 87 *(above).* Corpus callosum in a mouse with chronic cycloleucine intoxication. Note the swollen myelin sheath, massive enlargement of the interlamellar space and the compact appearance of the adjacent neuropil. TEM, × 12 000

Fig. 88 *(below).* Rat corpus callosum after 4 weeks of cycloleucine intoxication. Development of interlamellar spaces occurred after splits of the minor dense lines. TEM, × 90 000

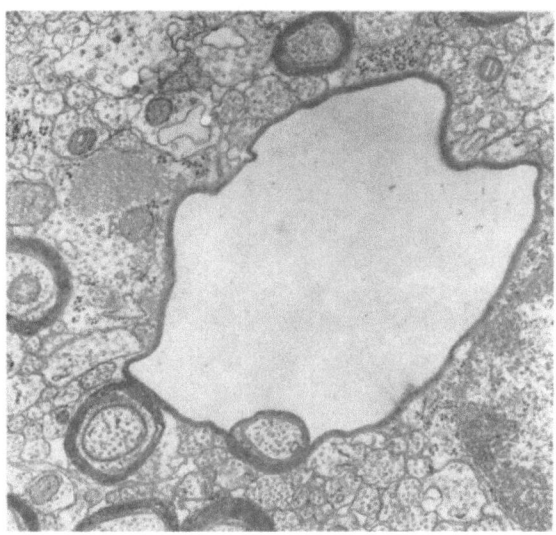

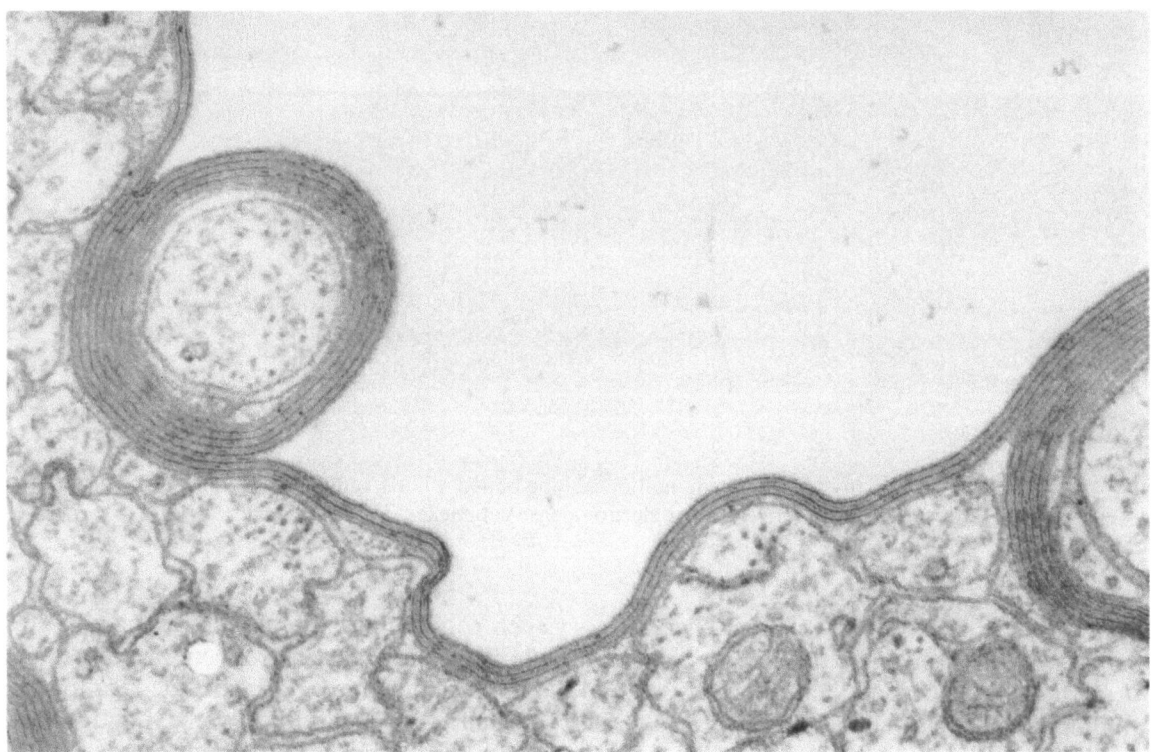

toxicated with cycloleucine at 7 days of age had the characteristic vacuolar changes of myelin. It is likely that factors such as age and species differences play an important part in the topography of the neuropathologic changes.

Ultrastructure

Intramyelinic edema with splitting of myelin lamellae along intraperiod lines may be seen with the electron microscope (Fig. 87). Extracellular edema is not observed, and the neuropil adjacent to myelin sheaths is also free of edema. Reactive changes of oligodendrocytes may be noted, including marked increase in cytoplasmic volume and prominent Golgi apparatus. The cytoplasm of astrocytes contains increased numbers of glycogen granules. No changes are seen in neurons or their processes. The vascular endothelium appears intact throughout the nervous system, and ultrastructural examination of the

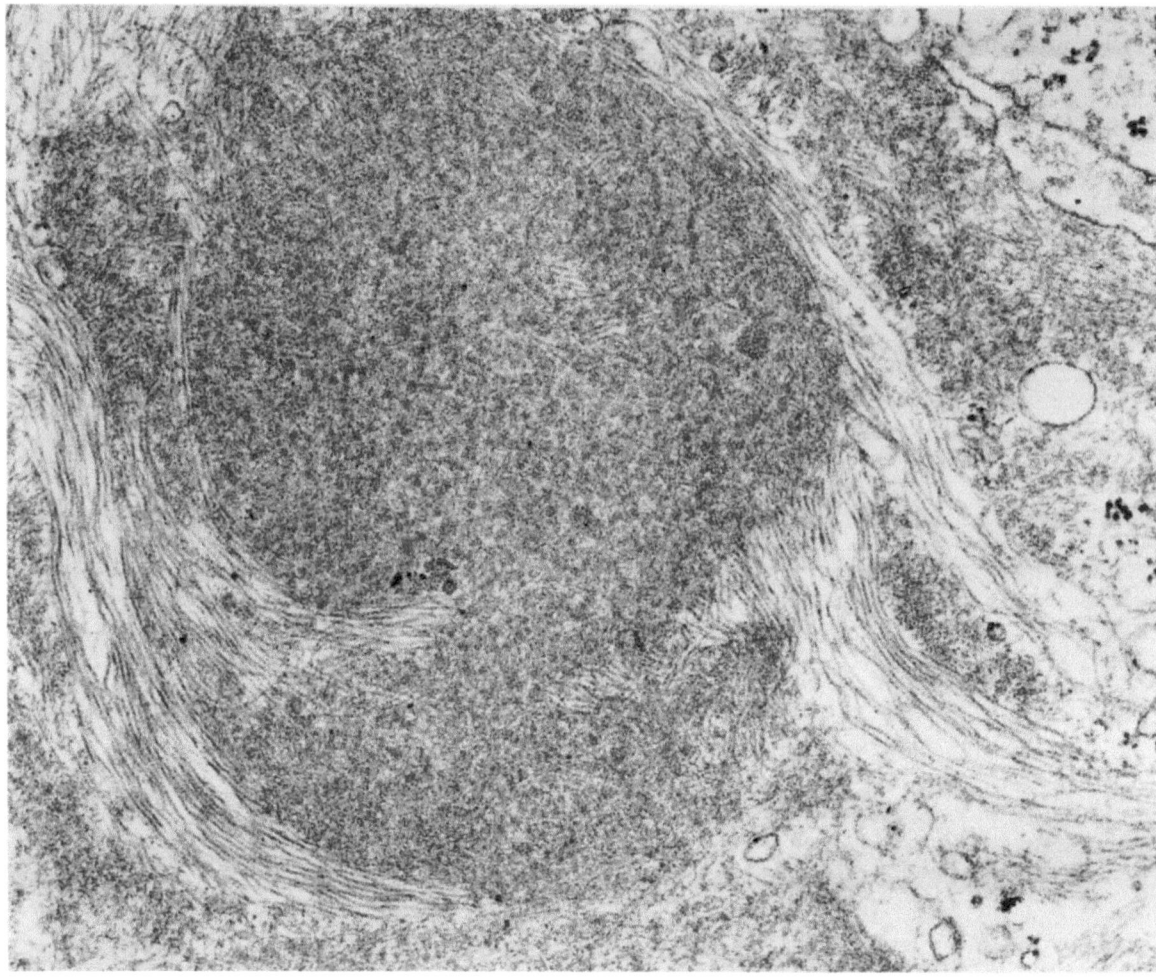

Fig. 89. Cytoplasm of an astrocyte containing non-membrane-bound whorls composed of 9-nm filaments. Note the convergence of filament whorls to form granular electron-dense complexes. TEM, ×73 600

sciatic nerves discloses no pathologic change.

The effects of chronic intoxication are similar to acute neurotoxic changes and the ultrastructural findings involving myelin are identical. However, reactive glial changes are prominent, and reactive astrocytes contain inclusions with distinctive morphologic appearance. Two types of inclusion are observed; the first consisting of non-membrane-bound whorls of filaments (Fig. 89) and the second of granular amorphous, membrane-bound inclusions. The filaments that form the non-membrane-bound inclusions measure 9 mm in diameter (Fig. 89).

Differential Diagnosis

Status spongiosus of cerebral white matter seen with cycloleucine encephalopathy resembles such conditions as triethyltin poisoning (Aleu et al. 1963) and hexachlorophene (Lampert et al. 1973), isonicotinic acid hydrazide (Lampert and Schochet 1968), cuprizone (Suzuki and Kikkawa 1969), actinomycin D (Rizzuto and Gambetti 1976), ethidium bromide (Yajima and Suzuki 1979), and acetylethyltetramethyl tetralin (AETT) (Spencer et al. 1980). The prototype of these neurotoxins is triethyltin while a clinically relevant example is hexachlorophene, an antibacterial agent with iatrogenic effects on the nervous system of low birthweight newborn infants (Powell and Lampert 1979). The basis for spongy change in each of these models of neurotoxic injury is a great affinity for the myelin sheath which becomes severely edematous. Cammer (1980) has suggested that damage to enzymes in the myelin sheath may alter myelin permeability to cations, allowing the interlamellar spaces to fill with electrolyte-rich fluid. The changes described in tri-ethyltin and hexachlorophene poisoning very closely resemble cycloleucine intoxication. However, the glial changes described in the latter have not been reported in either of the above types of neurointoxication. Other forms of status spongiosus cited above involve injury to oligodendrocytes which remain unaffected in cycloleucine encephalopathy.

Experimental studies of cycloleucine were undertaken as part of a search for an experimental model for vitamin B_{12} deficiency (Siddens et al. 1975; Gandy et al. 1973). However, the experimental model appears to resemble homocystinuria more closely, a condition in which status spongiosus of the cerebral white matter was observed (Chou and Waisman 1965), and gliosis was also noted. Homocystinuria is a rare inherited disorder of metabolism for which no animal model had previously existed.

Biologic Features

Signs

Acute Toxicity. Adult rats and mice receiving a single dose of 1–3 g/kg cycloleucine by intraperitoneal injection develop anorexia, weakness, and weight loss and die 5–7 days after inoculation.

Subacute Toxicity. Adult Swiss Webster mice that receive a single intraperitoneal injection of doses ranging from 250–900 mg/kg body weight become anorexic and weak and may undergo muscle wasting, but those that survive this illness progress to complete clinical recovery.

Chronic Toxicity. Chronic intoxication may be achieved by repeated injections at weekly intervals of doses ranging from 100–500 mg/kg. In adult rats and mice, as well as in weanling mice, repeated weekly doses of 100–500 mg/kg cycloleucine result in weakness, while those receiving lesser doses experience less loss of weight and are slightly less active, but within 2 weeks resume normal appearance and activity. Animals injected with doses greater than 250 mg/kg each week eventually die.

Natural History. Cycloleucine (1-aminocyclopentane-1-carboxylic acid), an alpha-substituted nonmetabolizable amino acid, was synthesized first in the early 1960s for use as an antitumor drug (Ross et al. 1961). It seems to function as an amino acid antagonist, being itself an unnatural type of amino acid (Berlinguet et al. 1962) that can inhibit protein synthesis in vivo and in vitro (Scholefield 1961; Sterling and Henderson 1963). Although it was effective against solid tumors in mice and against leukemia and lymphoma in both rats and mice, it was far less effective in human beings with advanced solid tumors (Ross et al. 1961). However, cycloleucine was more efficacious in treating patients with multiple myeloma and leiomyosarcoma. The drug has also been used to prevent malaria (Aviado and Reuter 1969) and as an immunosuppressant (Frisch 1969; Levine and Sowinski 1977). Unfortunately, neurotoxic injury was observed both in experimental animals and in humans that received cycloleucine. Demyelination was reported in the central nervous system of tumor-bearing animals treated with the drug. Symptoms considered to be secondary to degeneration of the spinal cord and peripheral nerves were noted in patients receiving doses in excess of 220 mg/kg daily. In a group of 140 patients who where given 300 mg/kg daily for 8–10 days, 41% experienced neurologic problems (Carter 1970). Regrettably no histopathologic information is available in any of these patients.

Cycloleucine is a synthetic amino acid that competes with certain naturally occurring amino acids for transport across the blood-brain barrier (Pardridge and Oldendorf 1975). Amino acid transport across the blood-brain barrier can be inhibited and competitive inhibition of other amino acids is one of the factors implicated in reducing protein synthesis in this disorder. Nixon (1976) found that in all regions of the central nervous system protein content was reduced. These changes were pronounced in the cerebellum and spinal cord. The sulfatide content of both the spinal cord and peripheral nerves was reduced. Also cycloleucine was found to be toxic to cerebellar tissue cultures (Nixon et al. 1976), but these effects could be mitigated by supplementing the media with a variety of amino acids.

Pathogenesis and Etiology. While the mechanism of cycloleucine neurotoxicity is unknown, two of its properties may be of particular importance. First, the drug is nonmetabolizable, and its rate of excretion is slow. It has a rather long half-life, approximately 22 days in the rat (Owen et al. 1969). Secondly, it is conceivable that capacity of cycloleucine to inhibit protein synthesis may be relevant to its toxic effects on glial cells. Cycloleucine penetrates the nervous system by facilitated diffusion across the blood-brain barrier. It

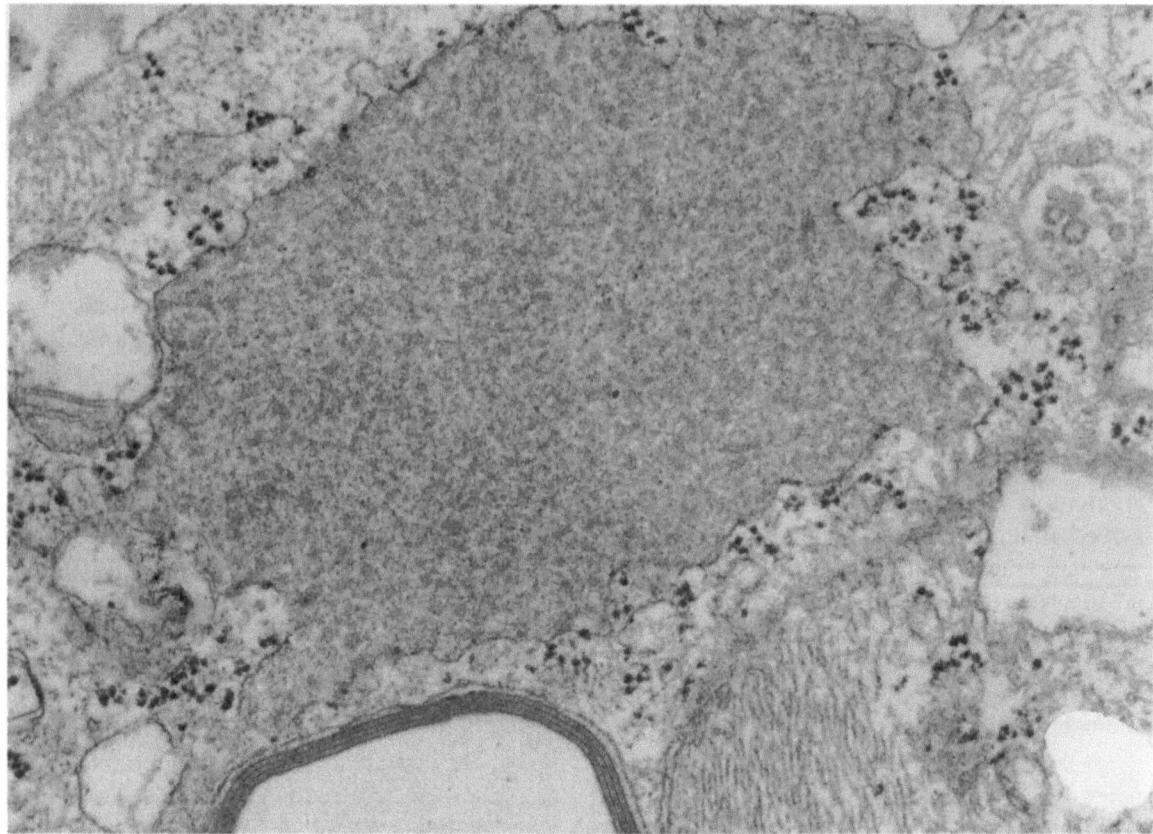

Fig. 90. Brain of a mouse with chronic cycloleucine intoxication. Membrane-enclosed intra-astrocytic inclusion. TEM, × 73 600

competes for facilitated transport with certain other amino acids, including phenylalanine and valine, and in fact cycloleucine uptake has been employed to evaluate toxic damage to the barrier system (Steinwall and Snyder 1969). In animals intoxicated with cycloleucine, Machlin et al. (1963) have shown that addition of valine to the diet alleviated the growth inhibition induced by the toxin. It seems that addition of valine in part offsets the preferential transport of this agent across the barrier. Cycloleucine has also been shown to interfere with renal transport of amino acids and has in fact been proposed as an experimental model for cystinuria (Craan and Bergeron 1978) because of its toxic effects on renal tubular epithelium, leading to efflux of dibasic amino acids and cystine. Caboche and Bachellerie (1977) and Caboche and Mulsant (1978) have noted interference by cycloleucine with the process of ribosomal RNA maturation. This process may be relevant to the glial changes reported here (Figs. 89, 90).

Acknowledgements. The work in this report was supported in part by NS 14162, NS 07078, and NS 09053 from the National Institute of Neurological and Communicative Disorders and Stroke and by a Basil O'Connor Starter Grant from the March of Dimes Birth Defects Foundation.

References

Aleu FP, Katzman R, Terry RD (1963) Fine structure and electrolyte analyses of cerebral edema induced by alkyltin intoxication. J Neuropathol Exp Neurol 22: 403–413

Aviado DM, Reutter HA (1969) Pathologic physiology and chemotherapy of plasmodium berghei. IX. Gastric secretion and the influence of 1-amino cytopentane carboxylic acid (WR 14, 997 or cycloleucine). Exp Parasitol 26: 314–322

Berlinguet L, Begin N, Sarkar NK (1962) Mechanism of antitumour action of 1-amino-cyclopentane carboxylic acid. Nature 194: 1082–1083

Caboche M, Bachellerie JP (1977) RNA methylation and control of eukaryotic RNA biosynthesis. Effects of cycloleucine, a specific inhibitor of methylation, on ribosomal RNA maturation. Eur J Biochem 74: 19–29

Caboche M, Mulsant P (1978) Selection and preliminary characterization of cycloleucine-resistant CHO cells affected in methionine metabolism. Somatic Cell Genet 4: 407–421

Cammer W (1980) Toxic demyelination: biochemical studies and hypothetical mechanisms. In: Spencer PS, Schaumburg HH (eds) Experimental and clinical neurotoxicology. Williams and Wilkins, Baltimore, pp 239–256

Carter SK (1970) 1-Aminocyclopentanecarboxylic acid (NSC-1026). A review. Chemotherapy fact sheet, July. National Cancer Institute, pp 1–9

Chou SM, Waisman HA (1965) Spongy degeneration of the central nervous system: case of homocystinuria. Arch Pathol 79: 357–363

Craan AG, Bregeron M (1978) Experimental cystinuria: the cycloleucine model. II. Amino acid efflux from intestinal and renal tissues. Metabolism 27: 1613–1625

Frish AW (1969) Inhibition of antibody synthesis by cycloleucine. Biochem Pharmacol 18: 256–260

Gandy G, Jacobson W, Sidman R (1973) Inhibition of a transmethylation reaction in the central nervous system – an experimental model for subacute combined degeneration of the cord. J Physiol (Lond) 233: 1P–3P

Greco CM, Powell HC, Garrett RS, Lampert PW (1980) Cycloleucine encephalopathy. Neuropathol Appl Neurobiol 6: 349–360

Jacobson W, Gandy G, Sidman RL (1973) Experimental subacute combined degeneration of the cord in mice (abstr). J Pathol 109: PXIII–PXIV

Lampert PW, Schochet SS (1968) Electron microscopic observations on experimental spongy degeneration of the cerebellar white matter. J Neuropathol Exp Neurol 27: 210–220

Lampert P, O'Brien J, Garrett R (1973) Hexachlorophene encephalopathy. Acta Neuropathol (Berl) 23: 326–333

Levine S, Sowinski R (1977) Effects of cycloleucine on macrophages and on experimental allergic encephalomyelitis. Exp Mol Pathol 26: 103–112

Machlin LJ, Gordon RS, Puchal F (1963) Alleviation of 1-aminocyclopentane-1-carboxylic acid toxicity by valine. Nature 198: 87–88

Nixon RA (1976) Neurotoxicity of a non-metabolizable amino acid, aminocyclopentane-1-carboxylic acid: regional protein levels and lipid composition of nervous tissue. J Neurochem 27: 237–244

Nixon RA, Jacobson W, Sidman RL (1974) Methyltransferase activity in an experimental mouse disease resembling human subacute combined degeneration (abstr). J Neuropathol Exp Neurol 33: 172

Nixon RA, Suva M, Wolf MK (1976) Neurotoxicity of a nonmetabolizable amino acid, 1-aminocyclopentane-1-carboxylic acid antagonism by amino acids in cultures of cerebellum. J Neurochem 27: 245–251

Owen G, Ruelius HW, Janssen F, Pollock JJ (1969) Species differences in the disposition of cycloleucine (abstr). Toxicol Appl Pharmacol 14: 630

Pardridge WM, Oldendorf WH (1975) Kinetic analysis of blood-brain barrier transport of amino acids. Biochim Biophys Acta 401: 128–136

Powell HC, Lampert PW (1979) Hexachlorophene toxicity. In: Vinken PJ, Bruyn GW (eds) Intoxication of the nervous system. Part II. North Holland, Amsterdam, pp 479–509 (Handbook of clinical neurology, vol 37)

Ramsey R, Fisher VW (1978) Effect of 1-aminocyclopentane-1-carboxylic acid (cycloleucine) on developing rat central nervous system phospholipids. J Neurochem 30: 447–457

Rizzuto N, Gambetti PL (1976) Status spongiosus of rat central nervous system induced by antinomycin D. Acta Neuropathol (Berl) 36: 21–30

Ross RB, Noll CI, Ross WCJ et al. (1961) Cycloaliphatic amino acids in cancer chemotherapy. J Med Pharm Chem 3: 1–23

Scholefield PG (1961) Competition between amino acids for transport into Ehrlich ascites carcinoma cells. Can J Biochem 39: 1717–1735

Siddons RC, Spence JA, Dayan AD (1975) Experimental models of vitamin B_{12} deficiency in the baboon. Adv Neurol 10: 239–252

Spencer PS, Foster GV, Sterman AB, Horoupian D (1980) Acetyl ethyl tetramethyl tetralin. In: Spencer PS, Schaumburg HH (eds) Experimental and clinical neurotoxicology. Williams and Wilkins, Baltimore, pp 296–308

Steinwall O, Snyder SH (1969) Brain uptake of C_{14} cycloleucine after damage to blood-brain barrier by mercuric ions. Acta Neurol Scand 45: 369–375

Sterling WR, Henderson JF (1963) Studies of the mechanism of action of 1-aminocyclopentane-1-carboxylic acid. Biochem Pharmacol 12: 303–316

Suzuki K, Kikkawa Y (1969) Status spongiosus of CNS and hepatic changes induced by cuprizone (biscyclohexanone oxalyldihydrazone). Am J Pathol 54: 307–325

Yajima K, Suzuki K (1979) Ultrastructural changes of oligodendroglia and myelin sheaths induced by ethidium bromide. Neuropathol Appl Neurobiol 5: 49–62

Neurotoxic Effects of Amoscanate, Rat

Georg J. Krinke

Synonyms. Periventricular necrosis; toxic ependy-mopathy.

Gross Appearance

The brains containing this lesion exhibit no re-markable macroscopic alteration.

Microscopic Features

The changes occur in the lateral wall of both lateral brain ventricles in the area facing the surface of the choroid plexus (Fig. 91).

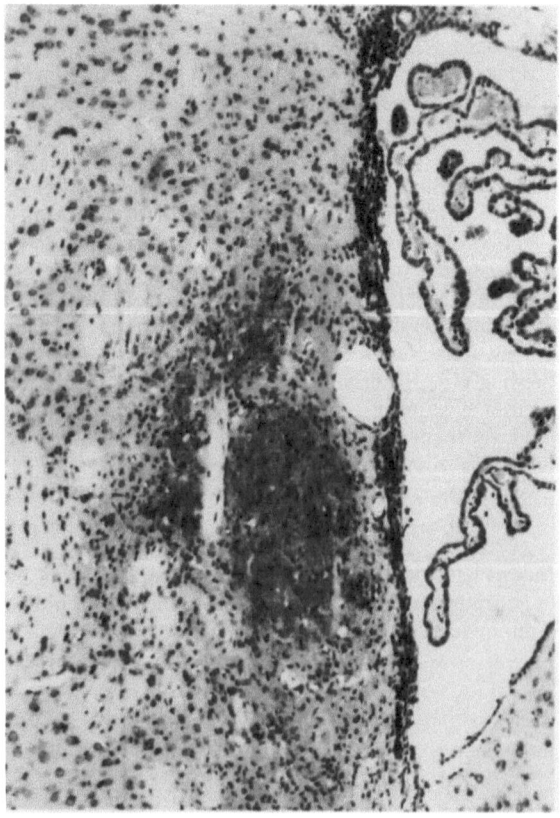

Fig. 91. Ependymal and periventricular necrosis in the wall of lateral ventricle, brain of a rat administered 125 mg/kg of absorbable amoscanate for 10 days. A well-preserved bundle of white matter forms the white streak within the darkly stained necrotic zone. Paraffin section, cresyl violet, × 100

Mild lesions are confined to the ventricular wall. The ependymal and subependymal cells reveal signs of necrosis such as shrinkage, darker stain-ing, and nuclear fragmentation. Their damage re-sults in focal erosion showing occasional poly-morphs, monocyte-derived "Kolmer cells," and lymphocytes together with sloughed ependymal cells.

Damage to the nerve tissue beneath the ependy-mal lining occurs in the more severe lesions. The affected zone, generally the caudatoputamen, is pervaded with microgranular material which is deposited within the areas of the gray matter; the bundles of myelinated fibers in the white matter are spared (Fig. 91). The microgranules are sur-rounded by scavenger cells and reactive astro-cytes, while the neurons are destroyed and disap-pear. Striking metachromasia of the deposited material may be demonstrated with the Nissl stain (cresyl violet), as well as mineralization with the von Kossa's stain.

Other areas in the brain, especially the blood vessels, the choroid plexus, and the tissues around the third and fourth brain ventricle reveal no ab-normality.

Ultrastructure

Electron microscopy is the best method for de-monstrating the mild changes which are re-stricted to the wall of the lateral ventricles. Some ependymal cells exhibit disruption of the cell membrane with loss of microvilli and cilia, and leakage of cytoplasm; other ependymal cells and the subependymal cells appear shrunken and electron-dense (Figs. 92, 93). Occasional reactive astrocytes are formed at the border of the dam-aged area (Krinke et al. 1983).

The microgranules, in the areas of periventricular necrosis, are characterized by an amorphous, electron-dense structure occasionally showing a pattern of concentric lines; some of them may contain lamellar structures resembling mitochon-dria (Clark et al. 1982). They are situated extra-cellularly, partly engulfed by mononuclear scav-enger cells and invariably surrounded by reactive astrocytes (Fig. 94).

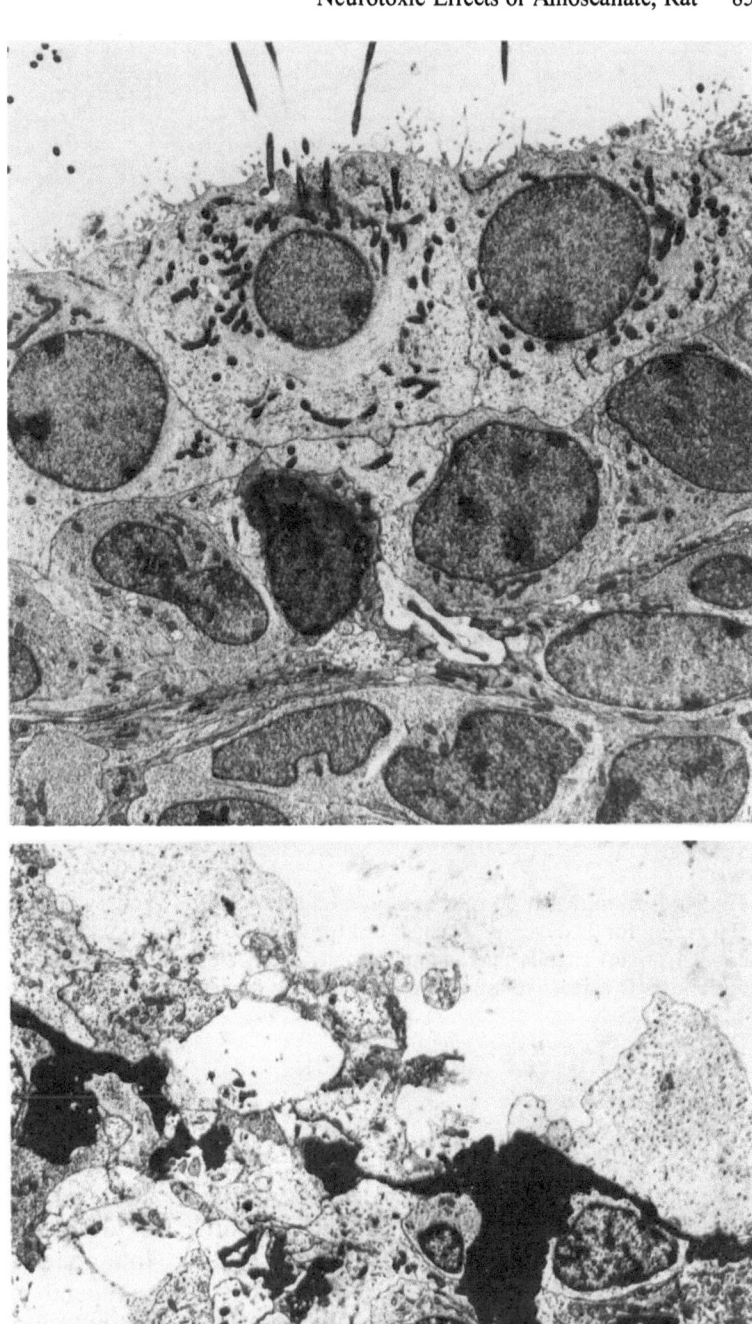

Fig. 92 *(above)*. Surface of the lateral brain ventricle of an untreated control rat. The ependymal cells at the surface, equipped with well-preserved microvilli and cilia, are attached to each other at the zonulae adherentes. TEM, uranyl acetate and lead citrate, × 4100

Fig. 93 *(below)*. Same area as in Fig. 92 from a rat which received three consecutive daily doses at 125 mg/kg. The ventricle is lined by fragments of destroyed ependymal cells, some of them shrunken and electron dense. TEM, uranyl acetate and lead citrate, × 3900

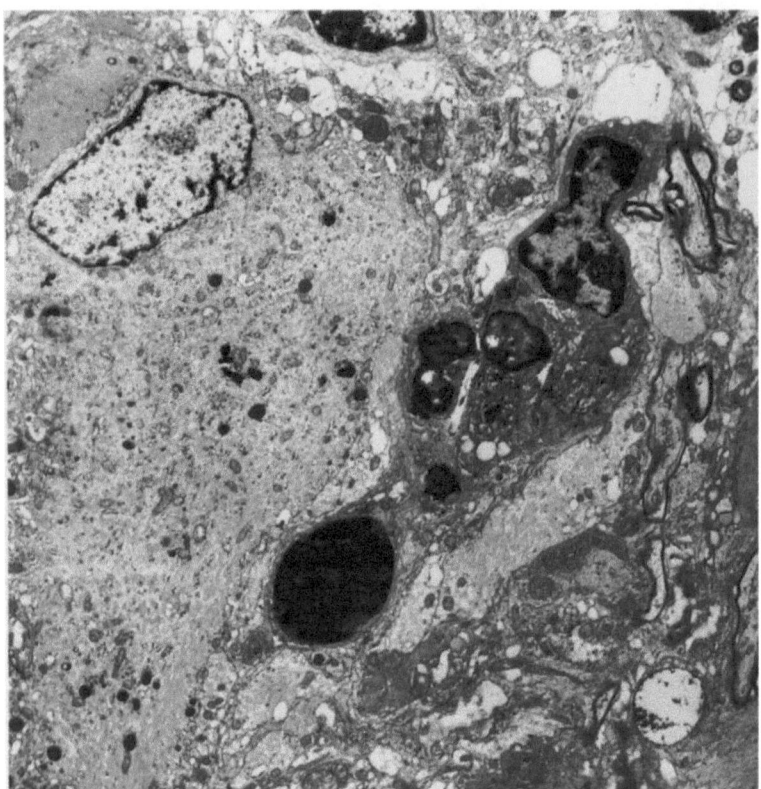

Fig. 94. Periventricular necrotic zone in a rat treated with 500 mg/kg for 28 days. A scavenger cell (possibly of microglial origin) engulfs microgranular material. In close apposition is a reactive astrocyte with eccentric nucleus and cytoplasm filled with numerous glial filaments and dense bodies. Uranyl acetate and lead citrate, TEM, × 4600

Differential Diagnosis

The topography of the amoscanate lesion in the rat brain is unique in toxicology. Local damage to the ependymal cell lining of the lateral ventricles, with subependymal edema and necrosis, has been observed in rats with congenital hydrocephalus (Kohn et al. 1981). This change, however, occurred at the parieto-occipital level above the white matter, whereas the amoscanate lesion affects the ependymal lining and gray matter at the more rostral level and does not appear to be associated with increased cerebrospinal fluid pressure.

Transplacentic exposure of embryonic mice to the cytostatic compound 5-azacytidine had induced pyknotic degeneration of the ventricular cells. This condition, in contrast to the amoscanate lesion, neither progressed to periventricular necrosis, nor was restricted to specific ventricular areas (Seifertová et al. 1972).

Bilateral deposits of mineralized material (also known as "pseudocalcification") may occur spontaneously in various regions of the rat brain, including the caudatoputamen. This age-related lesion has no connection with the brain ventricles and lacks an associated glial reaction (Burek 1978).

Inflammatory changes of the ependymal and subependymal zones, which may be encountered in the course of infectious diseases in various species, are generally associated with meningitis and diffusely affect the ventricular circumference.

Biologic Features

Etiology and Pathogenesis. The antiparasitic compound amoscanate is one of the isothiocyanates (4-isothiocyanato-4'-nitrodiphenylamine), a group of biologically highly active agents which are able to uncouple oxidative phosphorylation (Miko and Chance 1975). The occurrence of circumscribed lesions in the rat brain could possibly be attributed to an excessive, selective periventricular accumulation of amoscanate or one of its metabolites. Preservation of structures such as the choroid plexus and the white matter within the necrotic zone indicate a high susceptibility to the compound of the ependymal cells and the underlying gray matter of the caudatoputamen.

Amoscanate is available in two forms: the first, poorly absorbed from the gastrointestinal tract, is used against hookworm infection (Doshi et al. 1977); the second, which is well absorbed, is highly effective against schistosomiasis even when administered as a single oral dose (Striebel 1976). Neuropathologic lesions in the rat brain have only been observed when the absorbable form was repeatedly administered at high dosages; at least three consecutive daily (oral) doses of 125 mg/kg or 500 mg/kg were required to damage the ependymal cell lining, and periventricular necrosis occurred following a 10-day treatment (Krinke et al. 1983).

Behavioral Observations. During the first few hours following the administration of amoscanate in high doses to rats, there is a transient decrease in exploratory and locomotor activity; those individuals developing severe periventricular necrosis display a waxy rigidity such that they remain in an abnormal position (catalepsy).

Comparison with Other Species

Although signs of impaired motor activity were observed in cats and dogs exposed to high doses of absorbable amoscanate, examination of their brain showed no changes attributable to amoscanate toxicity. Monkeys tolerate exposure to between 50 mg/kg and 500 mg/kg for 28 days without developing neurotoxicity (Clark et al. 1982). There is no evidence of brain damage in man.

References

Burek JD (1978) Pathology of aging rats. CRC, West Palm Beach, p 139

Clark AW, Kiel SM, Parhad IM (1982) Neuropathology of the antischistosomal agent amoscanate administered in high oral doses to rats. Neurotoxicology 3: 1–11

Doshi JC, Vaidya AB, Sen HG, Mankodi NA, Nair CN, Grewal RS (1977) Clinical trials of a new anthelminitic, 4-isothiocyanato-4′-nitrodiphenylamine (C 9333-Go/CGP 4540), for the cure of hookworm infection. Am J Trop Med Hyg 26: 636–639

Kohn DF, Chinookoswong N, Chou SM (1981) A new model of congenital hydrocephalus in the rat. Acta Neuropathol (Berl) 54: 211–218

Krinke G, Graepel P, Krueger L, Thomann P (1983) Early effects of high-dosed absorbable amoscanate on rat brain. Toxicol Lett 19: 261–266

Miko M, Chance B (1975) Isothiocyanates. A new class of uncouplers. Biochim Biophys Acta 396: 165–174

Seifertová M, Veselý J, Čihák A, Šorm F (1972) Pyknotic degeneration of ventricular cells in embryonic brain following transplacental exposure to 5-azacytidine. Experientia 28: 841–842

Striebel HP (1976) 4-Isothiocyanato-4′-nitrodiphenylamine (C9333-Go/CGP4540), an anthelminthic with an unusual spectrum of activity against intestinal nematodes, filariae, and schistosomes. Experientia 32: 457–458

Neurotoxic Effects of 2-Chloroprocaine and Other Local Anesthetics, Rat

Robert R. Myers, Michael W. Kalichman, and Henry C. Powell

Synonyms. Chloroprocaine, Nesacaine-CE.

Gross Appearance

This report focuses on the lesions resulting from extraneural, in vivo application of clinical concentrations of pure local anesthetics. Needle trauma and injection of drug directly into nerves causes immediate nerve injury and magnifies the pathologic findings of the local anesthetics themselves which are reported below (Kalichman et al. 1986a).

Nerves bathed with 2-chloroprocaine or other local anesthetic solutions following a 1-ml injection of the solution in the soft tissue spaces adjacent to the nerves will be severely swollen, appearing slightly darker in overall color owing to substantial quantities of edema in the subperineurial space. The overall diameter of the nerve may be twice the norm, but this can be an effect localized to the injection site. Topically applied local anesthetics can damage the epineurial circulation producing gross evidence of hemorrhage and local inflammation. Long-standing lesions may also be associated with fibrosis at the injection site in response to local tissue irritation.

Microscopic Features

Edema is the most striking microscopic finding in affected nerves and is maximal 48 h after nerves have been bathed in clinical concentrations of 2-chloroprocaine or other local anesthetics (Myers et al. 1986b). The volume of edema present is directly related to the concentration of anesthetic applied (Kalichman et al. 1986b). The distribution of edema in a transverse section of nerve is not uniform, rather it follows a progression in its appearance that is related to local differences in the physical characteristics of the interstitial matrix. Edema first appears in the subperineurial region where there is a relative lack of collagen in the interstitium. Since the perineurium is elastic, edema can accumulate in large volumes in the potential space between nerve fibers and the perineurium. Low concentrations of anesthetic produce edema that is limited to this space. More serious injury seems to result in edema that appears successively in perivascular areas, along the endoneurial partitions within fascicles and between individual nerve fibers (Fig. 95). Light microscopy also reveals disruption of the perineurium consistent with its increased permeability to macromolecular tracers. Lipid droplets can be seen in the endoneurium, usually in Schwann's cells or fibroblasts. Fibroblasts are increased in numbers in the subperineurial space. If the injury is minor, these findings are transient and may be resolved within 7–14 days. Otherwise, wallerian degeneration is a characteristic secondary pathologic finding (Fig. 96).

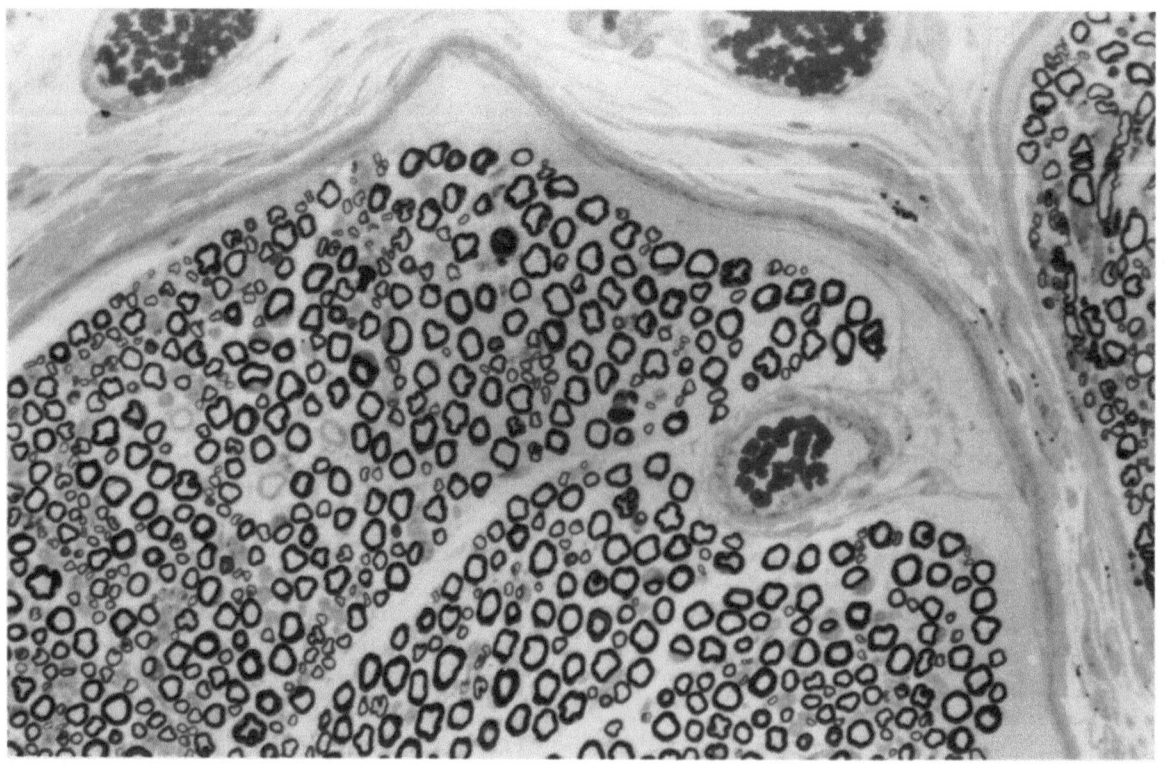

Fig. 95. Endoneurial edema in rat sciatic nerve 48 h following topical application of 5% procaine. Note substantial subperineurial accumulation of edema. Edema is also seen in perivascular space and along the endoneurial partition within the nerve. Paraphenylenediamine, × 120

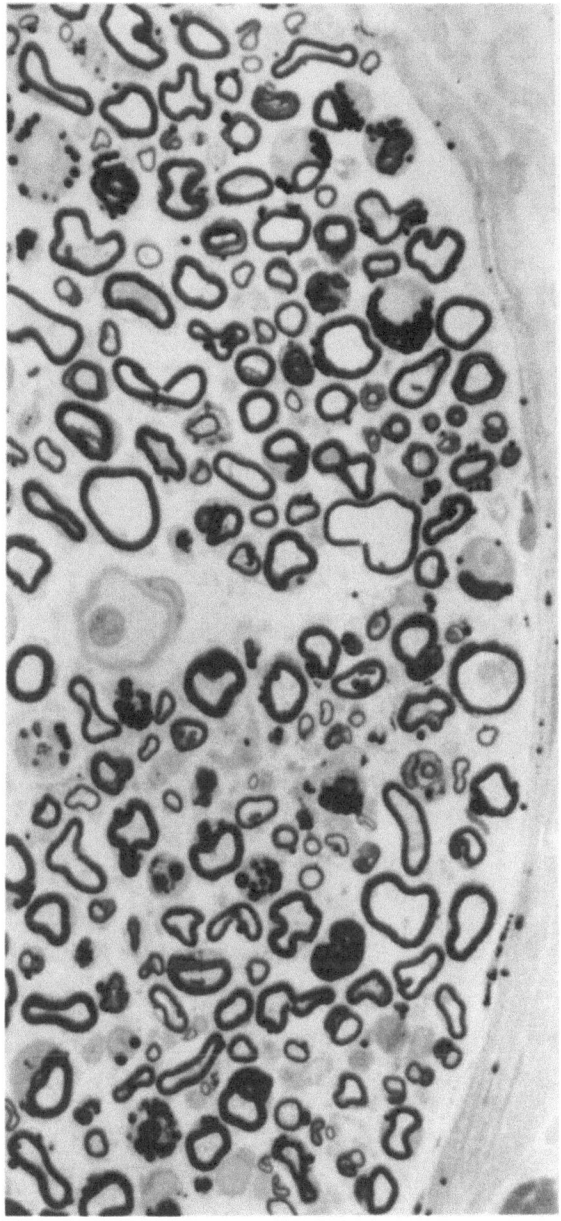

Fig. 96. Lipid accumulation is seen in the endoneurium, in Schwann's cells of myelinated fibers and in perineurial fibroblasts 48 h following topical application of 3% lidocaine to the rat sciatic nerve. Paraphenylenediamine, ×240

Ultrastructure

Electron microscopy 24–48 h after application of 2-chloroprocaine or other local anesthetics confirms the presence of edema which appears as structureless space in the endoneurial interstitium. In affected regions subjacent to the site of extraneural application, nerve injury is manifest-ed by both mast cell degranulation and reactive fibroblasts which often characteristically include arrays of thin cytoplasmic processes as well as increased endoplasmic reticulum and abnormal cellular configurations. Additionally, a peculiar abnormality noted in nerves exposed to local anesthetic is the appearance of eosinophils in the endoneurium. These cells are seen particularly in the subperineurial space and appear in areas where edema is most pronounced. Neutrophils and other inflammatory cells can also be seen.

Both dystrophic axonal changes and demyelination can be seen by electron microscopy (Fig. 97). Axonal degeneration is manifested by swelling and accumulation of masses of darkly staining organelles, vesicles, and filaments. Reactive changes consisting of increased amounts of endoplasmic reticulum can also be seen in Schwann's cells. Disintegrating cells contain swollen, degenerating organelles and membranous debris. Schwann's cells often include homogeneous, pale-staining, intracytoplasmic inclusions characteristic of Elzholz's bodies and may represent a reaction to injury rather than a primary neurotoxic effect (Jortner and Blaker 1987). The Schwann's cells of unmyelinated fibers are particularly susceptible to injury although they lack these lipid inclusions.

Lipid inclusions can be seen in both normal-appearing Schwann's cells and in disintegrating Schwann's cells. They are also observed in perineurial cells and endoneurial macrophages and fibroblasts but not in axons (Fig. 98). Lipid deposits in Schwann's cells are conspicuous and represent a distinctive morphologic finding. Schwann-cell cytoplasm that is packed with lipid droplets is often characteristic of disintegrating cells. Lipid droplets may appear in normal Schwann's cells, but they are infrequent and usually solitary. The large numbers of such deposits suggest a direct toxic effect.

In addition to the presence of lipid droplets in perineurial cells, other perineurial abnormalities can be noted, including disaggregation of perineurial cells and separation of the basement membrane. Tight junctions between perineurial cells are interrupted in affected regions. The temporal course of pathologic change is summarized in Table 5.

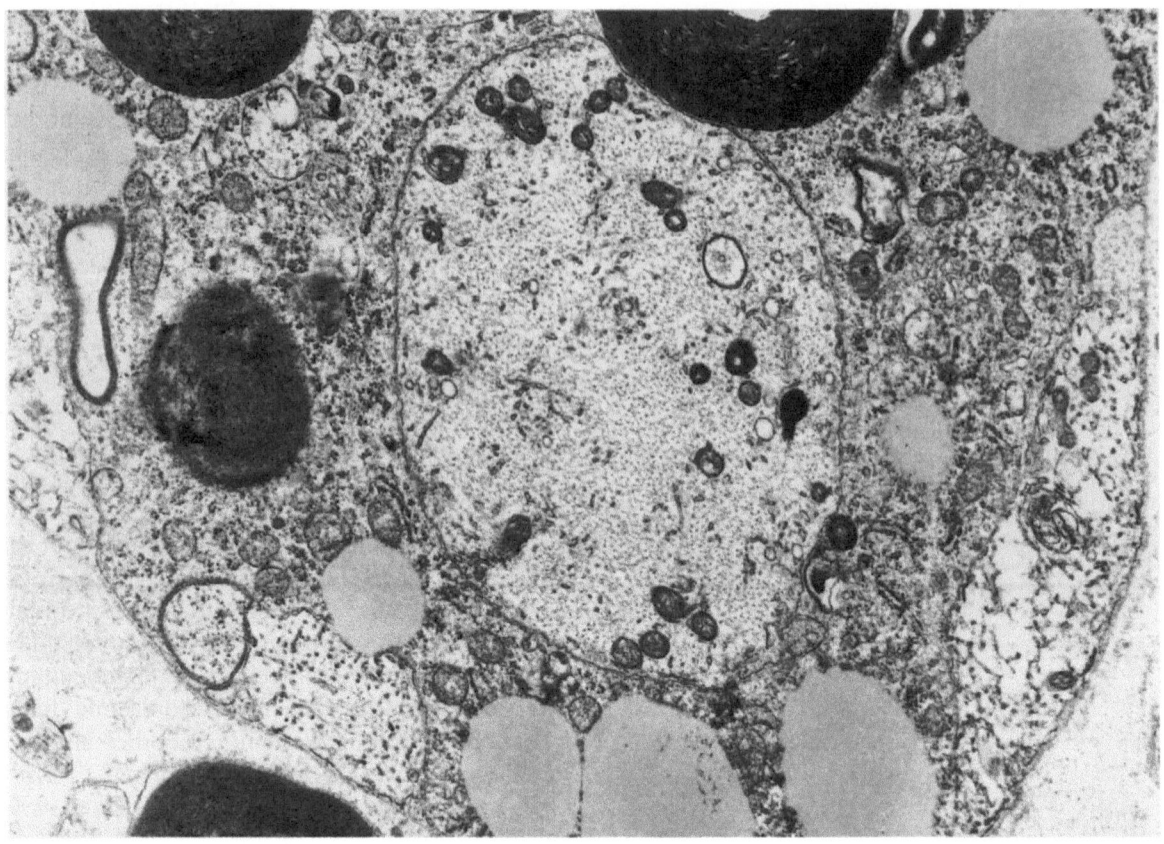

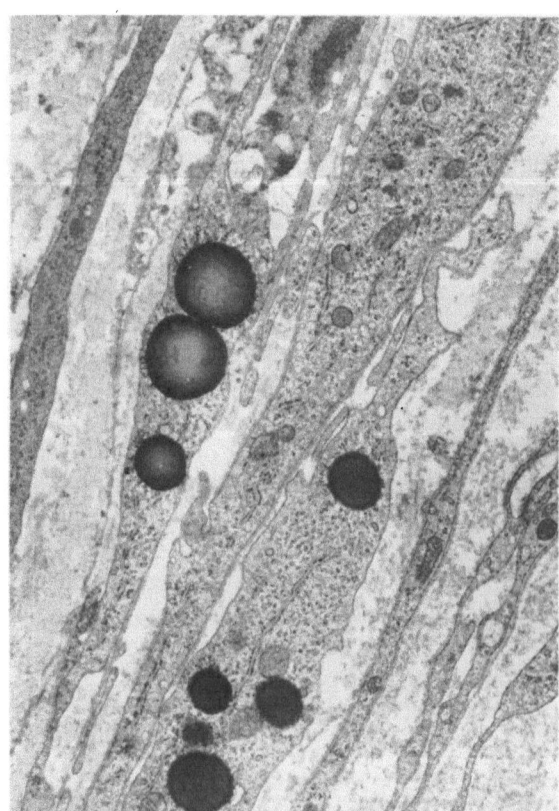

Fig. 97 *(above)*. Demyelinated axon 48 h following topical application of 2% 2-chloroprocaine. Enveloping Schwann's cell is undergoing necrosis and contains numerous lipid inclusions and myelin debris. Uranyl acetate and lead citrate, TEM, ×6000

Fig. 98 *(below)*. Separation of perineurial fibroblasts 48 h after topical application of 3% 2-chloroprocaine. Note lipid inclusions. Uranyl acetate and lead citrate, TEM, ×6000

Table 5. Temporal sequence of anesthetic-induced nerve injury following extraneural application of drug

Time	Observation
0 h	Anesthetic distribution due to lipid solubility
	Reduced nerve conduction velocity
	Increased perineurial permeability
6 h	Vascular congestion
	Endoneurial edema
1 day	Increased threshold for compound action potential
	Axonal swelling
	Schwann-cell swelling
	Lipid droplet accumulation
	Reactive fibroblasts
2 days	Increased threshold for compound action potential
	Maximal edema
	Axonal degeneration
	Demyelination
	Mast cell degranulation
	Reactive fibroblasts
	Perineurial cell disaggregation
	Separation of perineurial cell basement membrane
	Eosinophils in endoneurium
	Increased endoneurial fluid pressure
	Perineurial vessel compression
	Reduced nerve blood flow in subperineurial space
7 days	Wallerian degeneration
14 days	Remyelination
	Fibrosis
90 days	Fibrosis
	Perineurial thickening

Differential Diagnosis

The prominent pathologic feature of neurotoxic injury with local anesthetics is edema associated with disruption of the perineurial barrier and subsequent wallerian degeneration in severely injured nerves. However, the presence of edema by itself is of little value in differential diagnosis since it is frequently seen in many other toxic and traumatic injuries to nerves. Ultrastructural examinations of the perineurium may be useful since local anesthetics are the only documented agent to alter perineurial permeability as a primary mechanism of edema formation. The distribution of injured cells in local anesthetic injuries is sometimes limited to the subperineurial space, presumably reflecting perineurial damage and a relatively higher subperineurial concentration of the agent. Focal pathology may also be distributed in a crescent or pie-slice shape in transverse sections of tissue. The inclusion of lipid droplets in the endoneurium is seen with other neurotoxic injuries and is therefore not useful in the differential diagnosis of neurotoxic injuries due to local anesthetics although their incidence can be very high in anesthetic injuries.

Biologic Features

Endoneurial edema is a common, acute result of local anesthetic application which we interpret as an important pathologic finding since it is directly associated with increased endoneurial fluid pressure and reduced nerve blood flow. Increased endoneurial fluid pressure is a consequence of edema and the semi-elastic characteristics of the perineurium. The normal endoneurial fluid pressure of 2.0 ± 1.0 cm water can quadruple following topical application of local anesthetics. This, in turn, can be associated with reduced nerve blood flow to nerve fibers. The reduction is thought to be effected through a "pathological valve mechanism" that occludes anastomotic vessels traversing the perineurium which has been stretched to accommodate the edema (Myers et al. 1986a).

Etiology and Frequency. Modern usage of local anesthetic solutions is quite safe, although historically that has not always been the case (Thorsen 1947). Refinements in the solutions themselves and in the techniques of administration have been responsible for a reduced frequency of complications (Swerdlow 1980). The incidence of major complications ranges from none in 78000 cases (Scarborough 1958) to 0.16% in 65677 cases (Sadove et al. 1961). No permanent neurologic sequela was reported in a series of over 500000 spinal anesthetics reviewed by Lund and Cwik (1968). 2-Chloroprocaine for spinal anesthesia seemed to be an exception to these statistics after a rash of clinical reports were published in the early 1980s (Moore et al. 1982; Ravindran et al. 1980; Reisner et al. 1980). While definitive proof is lacking, it is thought that the complications were due to inadvertent injection of epidural volumes into subdural spaces. Laboratory studies in a peripheral nerve model have not implicated 2-chloroprocaine as more neurotoxic than other local anesthetics of the same comparable clinical concentrations.

Comparison with Other Species

These lesions should be manifested similarly in other mammalian species.

References

Jortner BS, Blaker WD (1987) Reversal of riboflavin-deficiency induced neuropathy. A model of peripheral nerve remyelination. J Neuropathol Exp Neurol 46: 353

Kalichman MW, Powell HC, Reisner LS, Myers RR (1986a) The role of 2-chloroprocaine and sodium bisulfite in rat sciatic nerve edema. J Neuropathol Exp Neurol 45: 566-575

Kalichman MW, Powell HC, Myers RR (1986b) Local anesthetic-induced nerve edema is dose-dependent (abstr). J Neuropathol Exp Neurol 45: 367

Lund PC, Cwik JC (1968) Modern trends in spinal anaesthesia. Can Anaesth Soc J 15: 118-134

Moore DC, Spierdijk J, van Kleef JK, Coleman RL, Love GF (1982) Chloroprocaine neurotoxicity: four additional cases. Anesth Analg 61: 155-159

Myers RR, Murakami H, Powell HC (1986a) Reduced nerve blood flow in edematous neuropathies. A biomechanical mechanism. Microvasc Res 32: 145-151

Myers RR, Kalichman MW, Reisner LS, Powell HC (1986b) Neurotoxicity of local anesthetics: altered perineurial permeability, edema, and nerve fiber injury. Anesthesiology 64: 29-35

Ravindran RS, Bond VK, Tasch MD, Gupta CD, Luerssen TG (1980) Prolonged neural blockade following regional analgesia with 2-chloroprocaine. Anesth Analg 59: 447-451

Reisner LS, Hochman BN, Plumer MH (1980) Persistent neurologic deficit and adhesive arachnoiditis following intrathecal 2-chloroprocaine injection. Anesth Analg 59: 452-454

Sadove MS, Levin MJ, Rant-Sejdinaj I (1961) Neurological complications of spinal anesthesia. Can Anaesth Soc J 8: 405-416

Scarborough RA (1958) Spinal anesthesia from the surgeon's standpoint. JAMA 168: 1324-1326

Swerdlow M (1980) Complications of local anesthetic neural blockade. In: Cousins MJ, Bridenbaugh PO (eds) Neural blockade in clinical anesthesia and management of pain. Lippincott, Philadelphia, pp 526-542

Thorsen G (1947) Neurological complications after spinal anaesthesia (and results from 2493 follow-up cases). Acta Chir Scand [Suppl] 95: 21

Systemic Degenerative Disorders of Primary Sensory Neurons in Rats Induced by 4-Hydroxyaminoquinoline 1-Oxide

Yuzo Hayashi, Michihito Takahashi, and Toshiaki Hasegawa

Gross Appearance

No remarkable features are seen in the brain, spinal cord, or peripheral ganglia by gross examination.

Microscopic Features

Nerve Fibers. Axonal degeneration, as demonstrated by precipitation of blackish grains or spherules in the Nauta or Fink-Heimer silver impregnation occurs in the brain and spinal cord of the rats given eight weekly injections of 4-hydroxyaminoquinoline 1-oxide (HAQO) (Hayashi and Toyoshima 1975). The lesions appear preferentially to affect the primary afferent fibers, especially the posterior funiculus (Figs. 99, 100) and the trigeminal nerve, and the grades as expressed by density and extent of precipitation are consistent with the severity of the neurologic signs.

In the rats examined 1 week after the last injection, staining with blackish silver grains or spherules is observed in Goll's nuclei and Goll's tract at the upper cervical cord. At the 3rd week, precipitates appear in the Burdach's tract at the upper cervical cord and the Goll's tract of the thoracic cord. At the 6th week, the posterior funiculus of the lumbodorsal cord is found to be involved. These findings indicate that the degeneration occurs first at the axonal tip and proceeds retrogressively toward the perikarya. This type of axonal degeneration, termed "dying-back process," is known to occur in man as well as in animals under certain conditions, such as triorthocresyl phosphate poisoning, long-term exposure to isoniazide or chronic thiamine deficiency (Cavanagh 1964a, b).

In examinations at the 14th and 34th week, alterations are found in the various primary sensory pathways in the spinal cord, medulla, and pons including Lissauer's tracts, substantia gelatinosa,

Fig. 99 *(above).* Cross section of upper cervical cord from ▶ a rat 4 weeks after eight weekly injections of HAQO. Axonal degeneration, expressed by precipitation of silver grains, is seen in Goll's tract *(G)* and less extensively in Burdach's tract *(B).* Fink-Heimer silver impregnation, × 130

Fig. 100 *(below).* Longitudinal section of Goll's tract of the cervical cord from a rat 4 weeks after eight weekly injections of HAQO. Some axons appear swollen *(arrow)* with precipitation of blackish-silver grains. Fink-Heimer silver impregnation, × 400

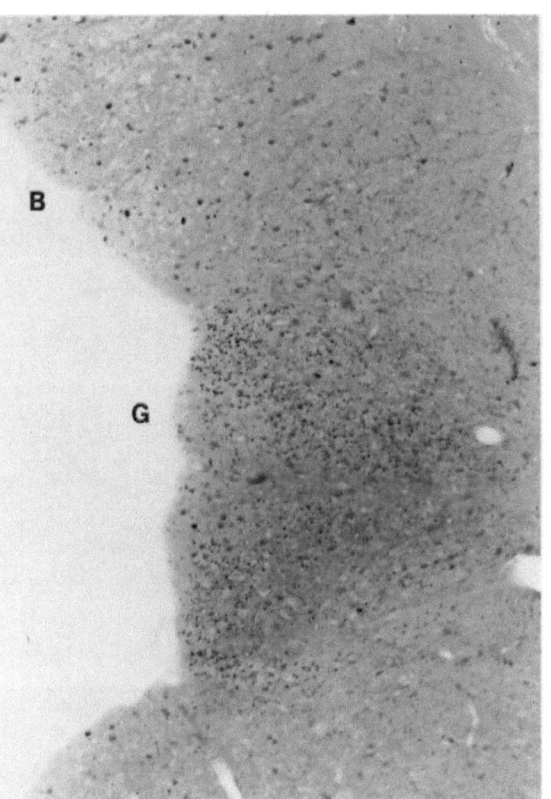

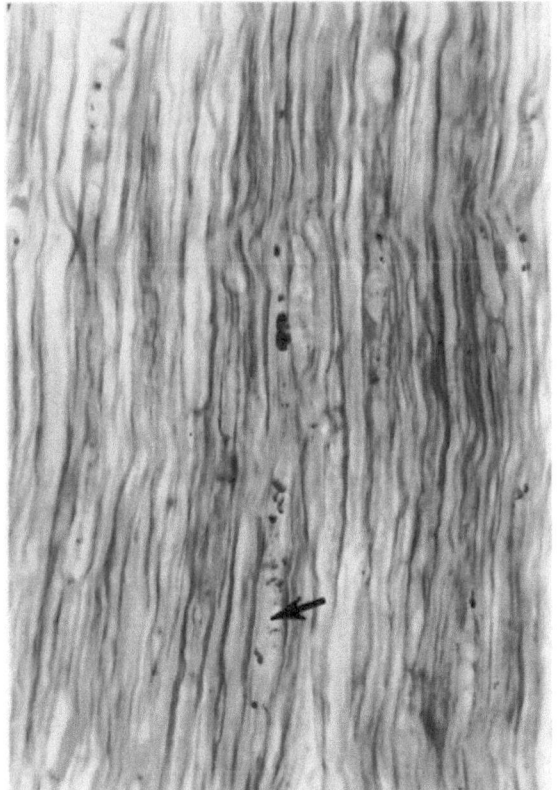

and funicular grays (Fig. 101). In contrast, no axonal degeneration occurs in the secondary sensory neurons or motor neurons. Therefore, the ataxia as noted clinically is thought to be a sign secondary to disturbance of the proprioceptive sensation.

Swelling or slight disintegration of the myelin sheaths is occasionally noted in the areas in which the axonal degeneration is severe. However, conspicuous demyelination or isolated internodal breakdown of myelin sheaths is not seen, and neither glial reaction nor inflammatory cell infiltration is found associated with the axonal degeneration.

Perikarya. Degenerative changes occur in the nerve cell bodies of the dorsal spinal ganglia and trigeminal ganglia (Hayashi and Toyoshima 1975). After 1–3 weeks following the last injection, central chromatolysis appears in some of the large-sized nerve cells (Fig. 102). At the 6th week, most of the nerve cells are reduced in size and exhibit various grades of chromatolysis with frequent occurrence of small vacuoles and periodic acid Schiff-positive granules in the cytoplasm (Fig. 103). These alterations become more conspicuous with time, and at a later stage the nerve cells show necrosis with karyolysis and marked cytoplasmic vacuolation. The satellite cells appear to be thickened though inflammatory cell infiltration is not seen.

Differential Diagnosis

Pathologic alterations of nerve fibers by HAQO are hardly distinguishable from those caused by certain other chemicals such as clioquinol or tri-orthocresyl phosphate in terms of either microscopic features or localization of the lesions, but degenerative changes of perikarya occur more prominently in HAQO-induced diseases than in

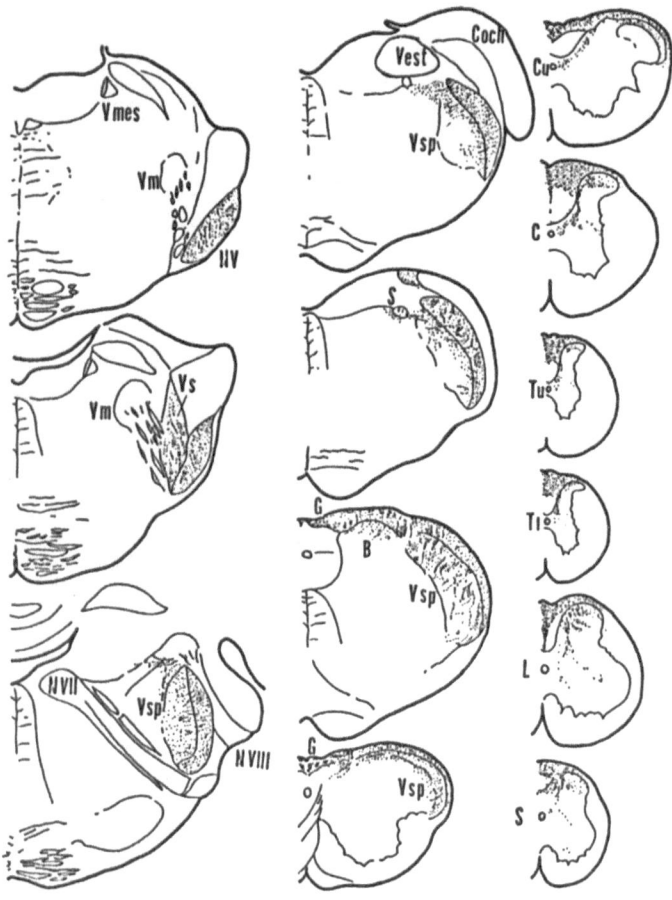

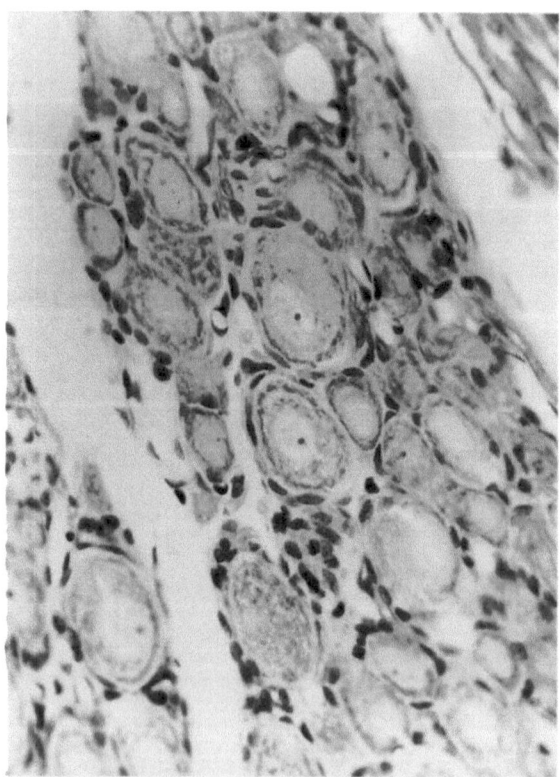

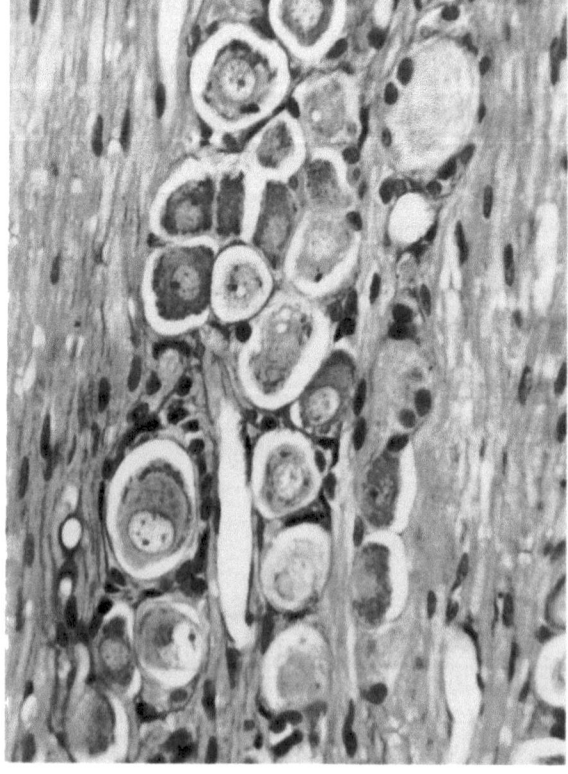

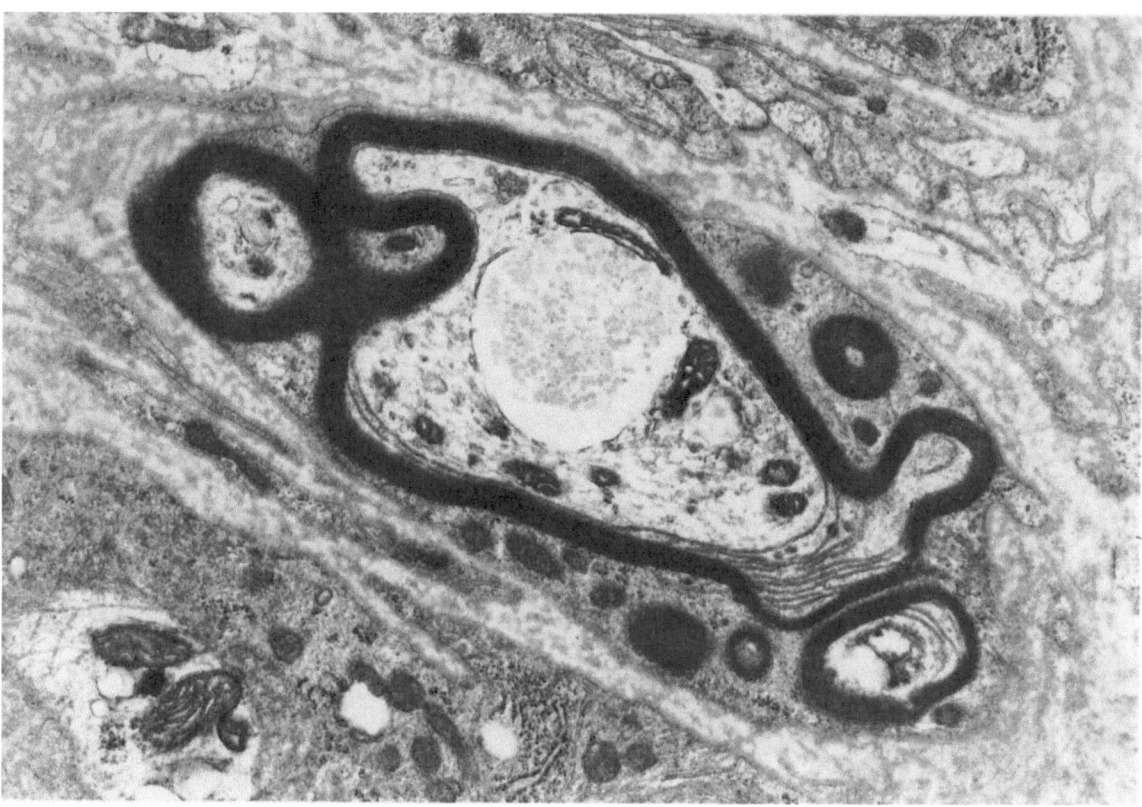

Fig. 104. A nerve fiber in the trigeminal ganglion from a rat 19 weeks after eight weekly injection of HAQO. A membrane-bound, large vacuole containing granules is seen in the axon. Myelin sheaths are well preserved. Uranyl acetate and lead citrate, TEM, × 28 000

◄ **Fig. 101** *(above).* Distribution of axonal degeneration in the pons, medulla oblongata, and spinal cord in a rat 14 weeks after eight weekly injection of HAQO. Axonal degeneration *(black dots)* occur preferentially in the primary sensory pathways. *NV,* sensory root of the trigeminal root; *Vmes,* mesencephalic tract and nucleus of trigeminal nerve; *Vm,* motor nucleus of trigeminal nerve; *Vs,* chief sensory nucleus of trigeminal nerve; *Vsp,* spinal tract of trigeminal nerve; *NVII,* root of facial nerve; *NVIII,* root of statoacoustic nerve; *Vest,* vestibular nuclei; *Coch,* cochlear nucleus; *So,* solitary tract and nucleus; *G,* Goll's tract; *B,* Burdach's tract; *Cu,* upper cervical cord; *C,* cervical enlargement; *Tu,* upper thoracic cord; *Ti,* middle thoracic cord; *L,* lumbar cord; *S,* sacral cord

Fig. 102 *(lower left).* An area of the dorsal spinal ganglion (L₆) from a rat 1 week after eight injections of HAQO. Central chromatolysis appears in large-sized nerve cells. Kluver-Barrera staining, × 520

Fig. 103 *(lower right).* Part of the dorsal spinal ganglion (L₆) from a rat 19 weeks after eight weekly injections of HAQO. Nerve cells are shrunken with central chromatolysis, vacuoles, and PAS-positive granules in the cytoplasm. Satellite cells are increased in number. PAS stain, × 520

the other conditions. In contrast to methylmercury poisoning, there is no alteration of motor neurons in HAQO-induced neurologic disorders.

Ultrastructure

Ultrastructurally, nerve fibers are seen to contain various-sized, membrane-bound vacuoles and electron-dense granules and amorphous materials in the axoplasm (Figs. 104, 105). Lipofuscin granules are also frequently found, and the number of neurofilaments appears to be decreased. The myelin sheaths are usually well preserved. Numerous membrane-bound aggregates of lipid droplets, vacuoles, and dense granules (lipofuscin granules) are seen ultrastructurally in the perinuclear area of the cytoplasm where the population of ribosomal granules are diffuse or focally decreased, and neurofilament bundles appear to be disarranged (Fig. 106). Nuclear envelopes have unusually shaped contours with frequent deep indentations. These findings resemble age-related morphologic alterations of nerve cells.

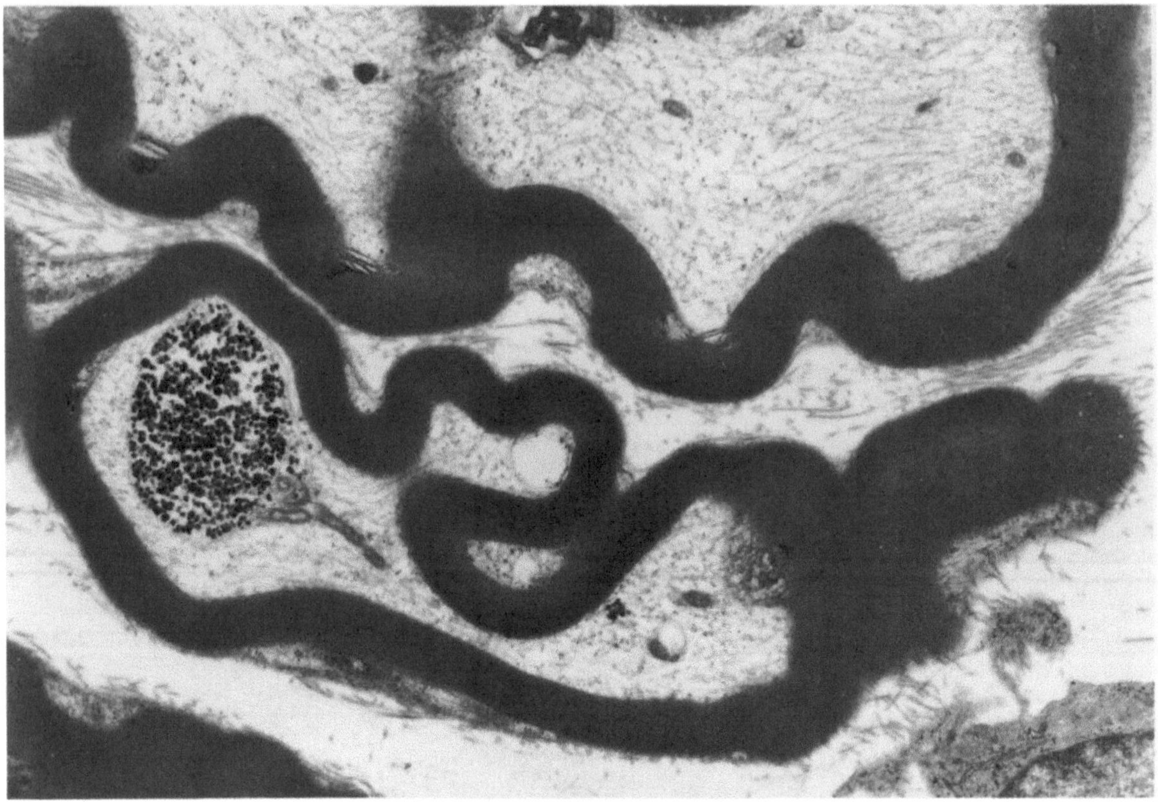

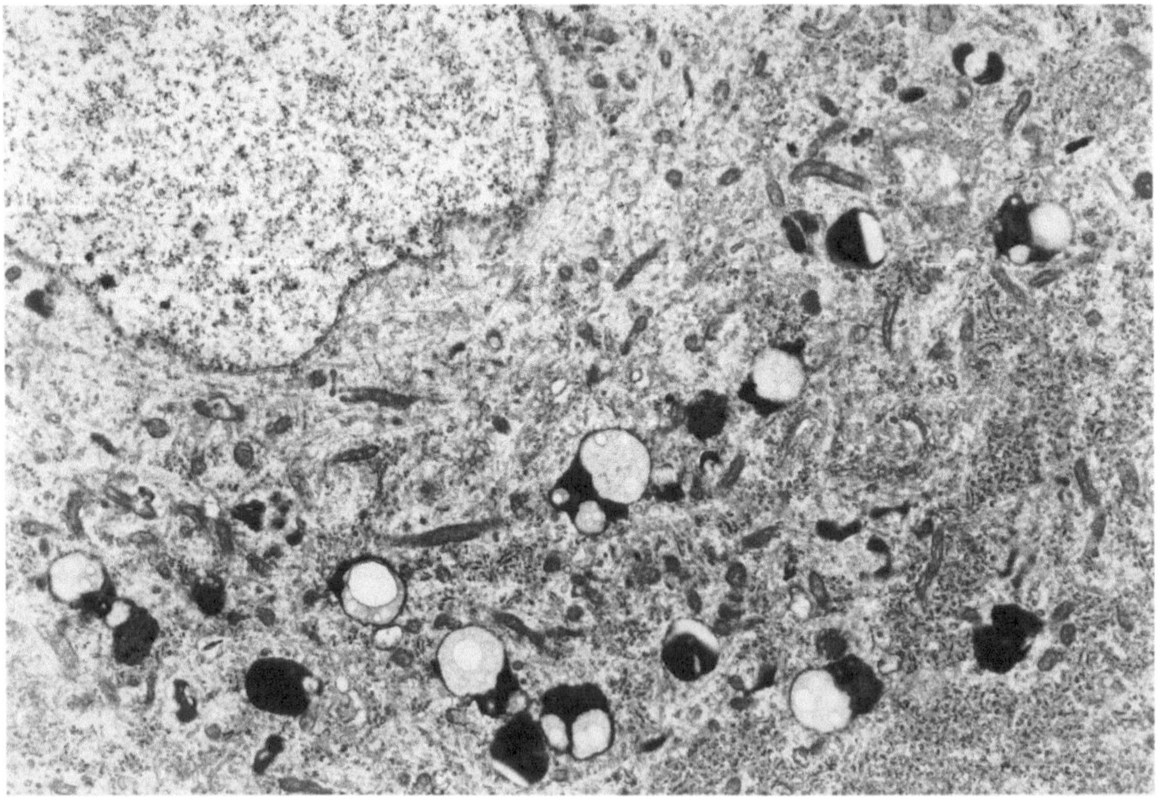

◄ **Fig. 105** *(above).* Nerve fibers in the dorsal spinal ganglion (L_6) from a rat 16 weeks after eight weekly injection of HAQO. A membrane-bound vacuole containing electron-dense granules is seen in the axon. Neurofilaments appear to be disrupted while myelin sheaths are well preserved. Uranyl acetate and lead citrate stain, TEM, ×28000

Fig. 106 *(below).* A nerve cell of the trigeminal ganglion from a rat 14 weeks after eight weekly injections of HAQO. Membrane-bound granules and vacuoles containing osmiophilic materials (lipofuscin granules) appear in the cytoplasm. Number of ribosomes and neurofilaments appears to be decreased around the nucleus. Uranyl acetate and lead citrate, TEM, ×16000

Biologic Features

Experimental Protocol. Male Sprague-Dawley rats, approximately 5–6 weeks of age, are used in studies on the neurotoxicity of HAQO. Aqueous solutions of HAQO for intravenous injections are prepared by dissolving 40 mg HAQO hydrochloride (available from Tokyo Kogyo Co. Ltd., Tokyo) in 1 ml 0.1 N HCl and diluting with physiologic saline to a volume of 10 ml (Hayashi et al. 1971). This solution is injected into a tail vein of rats once a week for 8 weeks at a dose of 5 mg HAQO HCl/kg body weight (about 2/5 of LD_{50}). During the period of administration, nearly 30% of the rats die with hemorrhage of the intestine and disruption of the lymphatic tissues; the survivors develop neurologic disorders.

Clinical Signs. The rats which tolerate eight weekly injections of HAQO exhibit ataxia and sensory disturbances of the hindlimbs 2–3 weeks after the last injection (Hayashi and Toyoshima 1975). The neurologic disorders become more severe with time. The first sign is a slow gait, excessive swaying of the hindquarters and uncoordinated toe movement. They also show an increased reactivity to touch or pain sensation. Six weeks following the last injection, they develop a "goose-stepping" gait characterized by exaggerated lifting of the hind feet and falling sideways when trotting. At this stage, hypalgesia (determined by pricking of the hindlimbs and tails with a needle) occurs in some rats.

Within 14 weeks from the onset of the neurologic signs, most of the animals are dragging their paralyzed hindlimbs, and analgesia of the hindlimbs and tails is also demonstrable. The forelimbs are less severely affected and, even at the 20th week, there is only slight hypalgesia and uncoordinated toe movement.

Mode of Action. HAQO was first synthesized in 1957 by Ochiai et al. and 6 years later was shown to be a potent carcinogen by Endo and Kume (1963) who demonstrated that subcutaneous injections of this compound induced fibrosarcomas at the injection site in mice. Subsequently, oral or intravenous injections of HAQO were found to produce tumors of the glandular stomach, lung, intestine, and pancreas in rats (Hayashi et al. 1971) or mice (Mori and Ohta 1967). A series of short-term tests indicated that HAQO possessed mutagenic potential in microorganisms (Okabayashi et al. 1964). The interaction of HAQO with DNA in vivo has been shown by means of fluorescence spectroscopy (Matsushima et al. 1967) or incorporation of ^{14}C-labeled HAQO (Ikegami et al. 1970). At present, HAQO is used solely as a laboratory chemical for experimental studies of carcinogenesis or mutagenesis.

By analyzing the reaction products of polyadenylic acid with HAQO, Kawazoe et al. (1975) have indicated that the chemical structure of the quinoline-adenine adduct is either 3-(N^6-adenyl)-4-aminoquinoline 1-oxide or 3-(N^1-adenyl)-4-aminoquinoline 1-oxide. An acute ultrastructural effect on cells induced by HAQO both in vivo and in vitro is known to be a peculiar type of nucleolar alteration characterized by disintegration of nucleolonemal structures and segregation of the granular, fibrillar, and amorphous components into separate zones. Reynolds et al. (1964) have mentioned that such nucleolar alterations, called "nucleolar segregation," can be used as a morphologic marker for a special type of cell injury involving DNA.

Pathogenesis. Some experimental evidence has been reported regarding the mechanism of HAQO neurotoxicity. First, Hayashi et al. (1971) demonstrated that a single intravenous injection of HAQO in rats could induce nucleolar segregation in nerve cells of the spinal and trigeminal ganglia. This finding indicates that HAQO can interact with DNA of the nerve cells. Secondly, a study on the chemical structure-activity relationship showed that no neurologic disorders occurred in rats treated with allied non-carcinogenic quinoline compounds (Table 6). Thirdly, it was found further that no neurologic disorders appeared in rats following two or four weekly injections of 5 mg/kg HAQO-HCl though these dose levels are sufficient for tumor induction (Hayashi and Hasegawa 1971). Therefore, the neurotoxicity of HAQO is definitely dose dependent with

Table 6. Structure-activity relationship of 4-hydroxyami-noquinoline 1-oxide and its related compounds

Compounds	Carcino-genicity	Induction of nucleolar segregation	Neuro-toxicity
4-Hydroxyamino-quinoline 1-oxide	+	+	+
4-Hydroxyamino-quinoline	−	−	−
Quinoline 1-oxide	−	−	−
4-Aminoquinoline 1-oxide	−	−	−
4-Hydroxyamino-pyridine 1-oxide	−	−	−

eight weekly injections of 5 mg/kg being required. On the basis of these findings, it is postulated that accumulation of DNA damage in the nerve cells underlies the pathogenesis of HAQO neurotoxicity.

References

Cavanagh JB (1964a) Peripheral nerve changes in ortho-cresyl phosphate poisoning in the cat. J Pathol Bacteriol 87: 365–383

Cavanagh JB (1964b) The significance of the "dying back process" in experimental and human neurological disease. In: Richter GW, Epstein MA (eds) International review of experimental pathology, 3rd edn. Academic, New York, pp 219–267

Endo H, Kume F (1963) Comparative studies on the biological actions of 4-nitroquinoline 1-oxide and its reduced compound, 4-hydroxyaminoquinoline 1-oxide. Jpn J Cancer Res 54: 443–453

Hyashi Y, Hasegawa T (1971) Experimental pancreatic tumor in rats after intravenous injection of 4-hydroxy-aminoquinoline 1-oxide. Jpn J Cancer Res 62: 329–330

Hayashi Y, Toyoshima K (1975) Carcinogenic activity and neurotoxicity. In: Kusama T, Nakazawa T (eds) Degeneration and regeneration in nervous system: the basic and clinical studies. Igaku-Shoin, Tokyo, pp 205–226

Hayashi Y, Hasegawa T, Toyoshima K (1971) Nucleolar alterations of peripheral nerve cells in rats following administration of 4-hydroxyminoquinoline 1-oxide. Experientia 27: 925–926

Ikegami S, Nemoto N, Sato S, Sugimura T (1970) Binding of ^{14}C-labeled 4-nitroquinoline 1-oxide to DNA in vivo. Chem Biol Interact 1: 321–330

Kawazoe Y, Araki M, Huang GF, Okamoto T, Tada M (1975) Chemical structure of QA$_{11}$, one of the covalently bound adducts of carcinogenic 4-nitroquinoline 1-oxide with nucleic acid bases of cellular nucleic acids. Chem Pharm Bull (Tokyo) 23: 3041

Matsushima T, Kobuna I, Sugimura T (1967) In vivo interaction of 4-nitroquinoline 1-oxide and its derivatives with DNS. Nature 216: 508

Mori K, Ohta A (1967) Carcinoma of the glandular stomach of mice induced by 4-hydroxyaminoquinoline 1-oxide. Jpn J Cancer Res 58: 551–554

Ochiai E, Ohta A, Nomura H (1957) Über das 4-Hydroxyaminochinolin N-oxide. Chem Pharm Bull (Tokyo) 5: 310–313

Okabayashi T, Yoshimoto A, Ide M (1964) Mutagenic activity of 4-hydroxyaminoquinoline 1-oxide. Chem Pharm Bull (Tokyo) 12: 257–261

Reynolds RC, Montgomery P O'B, Hughes B (1964) Nucleolar "caps" produced by actinomycin D. Cancer Res 24: 1269–1277

Inorganic Mercury Poisoning, Rat

Kenneth R. Reuhl

Synonyms. Mercurialism; mercurial erethism.

Gross Appearance

There is no consistent gross lesion which characterizes inorganic mercury intoxication in the rat.

Microscopic Features

The extent to which an inorganic mercurial may enter the brain and thereby damage neurons or glia depends upon the form of mercury to which the animal is exposed. Mercurous (Hg^+) and mercuric (Hg^{2+}) mercury do not readily cross the blood-brain barrier; however, high concentrations (10–20 ppm) of intravenously injected mercuric chloride will damage the blood-brain barrier, causing increased barrier permeability (Steinwell and Olsson 1969). Inhaled mercury vapor (Hg°), being lipophilic, rapidly crosses the blood-brain barrier and accumulates within the brain.

Once past the blood-brain barrier, inorganic mercury in any form may damage neurons of the cerebral and cerebellar cortices and the dorsal root ganglia (Chang 1977). In most cases, neuronal loss resulting from inorganic mercury exposure takes the form of widely scattered, single pyknotic neurons in the cerebrum and especially the cerebellar cortex. This lesion may be extremely subtle and may easily be overlooked unless thorough examination, including quantitative determinations of neuron density, is performed. Berlin and Ullberg (1963), using radio-labeled mercuric chloride (HgCl₂), demonstrated mercury in the hypothalamus and in areas poorly protected by the blood-brain barrier, such as the area postrema. However, it is not yet known whether inorganic mercury causes damage to neurons or glia in these regions.

In an attempt to bypass the protective effects of the blood-brain barrier and to examine the direct effects of inorganic mercury, several investigators (Venable and Mills 1977; Gallagher et al. 1982) injected or iontophoresed mercuric chloride directly into the cerebrum. Lesions induced by intracranial mercuric chloride were similar to those induced by methylmercury administered in the same fashion. Large numbers of swollen neurons were found along the needle path within 24 h of treatment. Neurons in the area of mercury diffusion eventually became pyknotic (Gallagher et al. 1982). Virtually nothing is known regarding the neuropathic effects of mercury vapor in rats.

Ultrastructural Features

The ultrastructural features of inorganic mercury poisoning in the central nervous system have not been well described. Despite the recognized neurologic effects (micromercurialism, mercurial tremor, and erethism), resulting from exposure to mercury vapor (Skerfving and Vostal 1972), no systematic studies have been undertaken to document the ultrastructural basis of these signs and symptoms. Similarly, the ultrastructural effects of

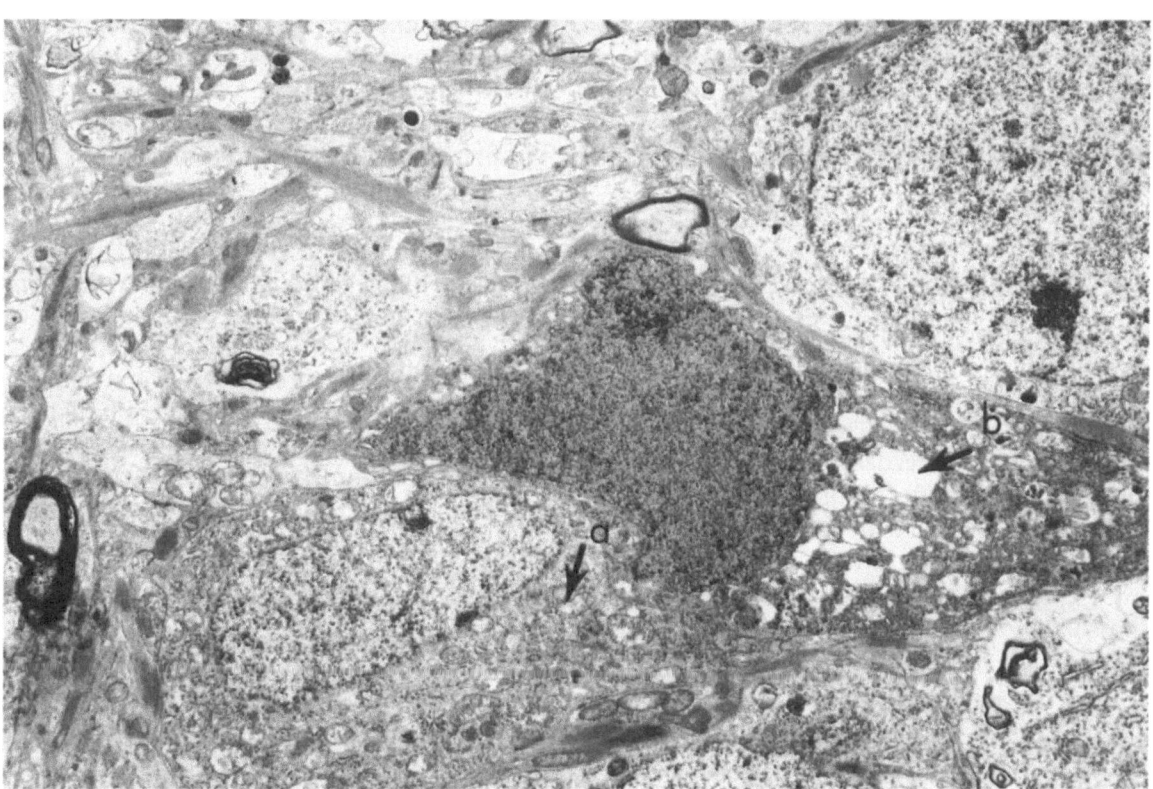

Fig. 107. Hippocampal pyramidal neuron of a rat following 40 days of exposure to mercuric chloride. Mitochondria are swollen *(a)* and cisternal organelles *(b),* such as endoplasmic reticulum and Golgi apparatus, are dilated. TEM, × 4600

mercurous or mercuric compounds on the central nervous system have received scant attention. Chang and Hartmann (1972) described neuronal damage in the cerebellum and dorsal root ganglia of the rat after injecting 1 mg $HgCl_2$/kg subcutaneously daily for 50 days. Within the dorsal root ganglia, vacuoles formed between neurons and satellite cells, eventually deforming the neurons. Changes in hippocampal neurons included detachment of ribosomes from endoplasmic reticulum and vacuolation of mitochondria (Fig. 107). In the cerebell, granule cells and Purkinje's cells underwent similar degenerative changes. Some rodent species appear resistant to chronic, low-level administration of inorganic mercury salts. For example, Ganser and Kirschner (1985) were unable to induce neurologic signs in mice despite more than 100 days of treatment with 1.2 mg $HgCl_2$/kg daily.

Gallagher et al. (1982) compared the ultrastructural effects of mercuric chloride and methylmercury upon intracerebral injection of the toxicant. Progressive swelling of mitochondria, dilatation of the cisternal organelles such as smooth and rough endoplasmic reticulum, and edema of the cell matrix resulted in a marked increase in neuronal volume. Edema increased progressively and eventually led to neuronal degeneration and death. There do not appear to be any pathognomonic ultrastructural features of mercury-induced neuropathy. The changes described above are relatively nonspecific responses to toxic cell injury.

Differential Diagnosis

Inorganic mercury poisoning is uncommon and is unlikely to be encountered outside experimental or occupational settings in which exposure is known to occur. The ill-defined histopathologic lesions make definitive diagnosis in the absence of exposure history very difficult. The presence of scattered neuronal changes in the cerebellum and perineuronal edema in the dorsal root ganglia should alert the pathologist to the possibility of mercury poisoning.

Biologic Features

Mercury vapor and mercury salts have distinctly different bioavailabilities and consequently represent distinctly different health risks. Mercury vapor, nonpolar due to its neutral valence state, may be rapidly absorbed in the lung and circulat-

ed to the brain, where it readily crosses the blood-brain barrier. Ample clinical evidence has confirmed the toxicity of mercury vapor. While it is unlikely that mercury vapor poisoning was the basis of Lewis Carroll's Mad Hatter, as has often been suggested, the clinical and behavioral changes accompanying chronic mercury vapor exposure in the felt hat, mercury mining, and other nineteenth century industries were widely recognized. As early as 1861, Kussmaul described the asthenic-vegetative and erethistic syndromes in human inorganic mercury (largely mercury vapor) toxicity (Kussmaul 1861). These syndromes are composed largely of behavioral changes such as irritability, memory loss, depression, and, occasionally, psychosis (Skerfving and Vostal 1972). Tremors also appear in humans poisoned with mercury vapor. Despite recognition of the hazards associated with mercury vapor, there are few studies of its neuropathologic effects in rats. The distribution of damage within the rat brain has been poorly documented, and ultrastructural changes underlying mercury-induced behavioral deficits in the rat have not been determined.

Inorganic mercury salts have long been regarded as relatively nonneurotoxic. This opinion is based not upon lack of neural susceptibility to inorganic mercury, but rather upon low absorption of ingested inorganic mercury by the gastrointestinal tract and the limited movement of the polar inorganic mercury compounds across the blood-brain barrier, which is relatively effective in excluding the small amounts of inorganic mercury encountered in daily life. However, at sufficiently high concentrations inorganic mercury salts may directly damage the blood-brain barrier, presumably by inhibiting endothelial enzyme systems or by direct effects upon endothelial membranes, thereby increasing vascular permeability. Once the barrier is altered, inorganic mercury and normally excluded macromolecules may enter the brain and damage neurons and glial cells (Chang 1980).

Within the neuron or glial cell, mercury disrupts a variety of biochemical processes. Inhibition of protein synthesis appears to be a consistent feature of mercury intoxication, both by inorganic and organic mercurials (Cavanagh and Chen 1971). Inorganic mercury binds avidly to sulfhydryl groups of proteins (Clarkson 1972), and inactivation of sulfhydryl-containing enzymes such as ATPase has been reported in neural tissues following inorganic mercury treatment (Chang et al. 1973).

Comparison with Other Species

Interspecies comparisons are difficult because neuropathologic lesions resulting from exposure to mercury vapor or to inorganic mercury salts have been sparsely documented. On the basis of behavioral and morphologic effects of directly injected mercuric salts, it is apparent that the rat brain responds at the cellular level to inorganic mercurials in a manner similar to that of other rodents and higher species, including man.

References

Berlin M, Ullberg S (1963) Accumulation and retention of mercury in the mouse. I. An autoradiographic study after a single intravenous injection of mercuric chloride. Arch Environ Health 6: 589–601

Cavanagh JB, Chen FC (1971) Amino acid incorporation in protein during the "silent phase" before organo-mercury and p-bromophenylacetylurea neuropathy in the rat. Acta Neuropathol (Berl) 19: 216–224

Chang LW (1977) Neurotoxic effects of mercury – a review. Environ Res 14: 329–373

Chang LW (1980) Mercury. In: Spencer PS, Schaumberg HH (eds) Experimental and clinical neurotoxicology. Williams and Wilkins, Baltimore, pp 508–526

Chang LW, Hartmann HA (1972) Ultrastructural studies of the nervous system after mercury intoxication. I. Pathological changes in the nerve cell bodies. Acta Neuropathol (Berl) 20: 122–138

Chang LW, Ware RA, Desnoyers PA (1973) A histochemical study on some enzyme changes in the kidney, liver and brain after chronic mercury intoxication of the rat. Food Cosmet Toxicol 11: 283–286

Clarkson TW (1972) The pharmacology of mercury compounds. Annu Rev Pharmacol 12: 375–406

Gallagher PJ, Mitchell J, Wheal HV (1982) Identity of ultrastructural effects of mercuric chloride and methyl mercury after intracerebral injection. Toxicology 23: 261–266

Ganser AL, Kirschner DA (1985) The interaction of mercurials with myelin: comparison of in vitro and in vivo effects. Neurotoxicology 6: 63–77

Kussmaul A (1861) Untersuchungen über den konstitutionellen Mercurialismus und sein Verhältnis zur konstitutionellen Syphilis. Stahel, Würzburg

Skerfving S, Vostal J (1972) Symptoms and signs of intoxication: an epidemiological and toxicological appraisal. In: Friberg L, Vostal D (eds) Mercury in the environment. CRC, Cleveland, pp 93–107

Steinwall O, Olsson Y (1969) Impairment of the blood-brain barrier in mercury poisoning. Acta Neurol Scand 45: 351–361

Venable HL, Mills SH (1977) Neurological and behavioral effects of intracranial administration of mercuric chloride on rats. J Toxicol Environ Health 3: 871–876

Tellurium Poisoning, Rat

Kenneth R. Reuhl

Synonym Tellurism.

Gross Appearance

In the congenital form of tellurium poisoning, the principal effects visible to the naked eye are paralysis and hydrocephalus. In the adult, acute toxicity due to tellurium does not result in any gross lesions. Chronic toxicity results in diffuse, dark gray discoloration of the cerebral cortex.

Microscopic Features

Congenital. Pregnant rats fed high dietary concentrations of elemental tellurium (Te) give birth to pups with hydrocephalus (Garro and Pentshew 1964; Duckett 1971). At birth the pups have enlarged ventricles, but significant microscopic findings are confined to flattening of the ependyma and edema of the subependymal white matter. Until day 5, intraventricularly injected dye circulates freely in the cerebrospinal fluid indicating that the hydrocephalus is initially of the communicating type. By day 5, the cerebral aqueduct has become stenotic, and there is microscopic evidence of cortical compression by the cerebrospinal fluid (Duckett 1971). Cortical thinning is pronounced, particularly in the occipital region. Neuronal degeneration and subependymal phagocytosis is observed beneath areas of cortical edema. Hemorrhage is a contributing cause of death in animals throughout the 1st week of life and is presumably the result of elevated intracranial pressure (Garro and Pentschew 1964) although direct injury to the blood vessels by tellurium may also contribute. By day 7, a ventriculostomy forms by the rupture of the occipital cortex, permitting the flow of CSF between the ventricular system and the subarachnoid space. This communication permits extended survival of the hydrocephalic animal. Nevertheless, brains of surviving animals display extensive cortical necrosis. In adult animals which survive the congenital hydrocephalus, the cortical mantle is thin, the cerebral aqueduct is stenotic, and the ventriculostomies patent.

Adult. Tellurium poisoning in the adult is microscopically characterized by lipofuscinosis of cortical neurons, particularly pyramidal cells, cerebellar Purkinje's cells, neurons of brain stem nuclei, and motor neurons of the spinal cord (Miyoshi and Takauchi 1977). The lipofuscin is apparently due to accumulation of tellurium within organelles, leading to accelerated organelle degeneration and digestion by lysosomes. Proliferation of lysosomes can be demonstrated by electron microscopy or by enzyme histochemistry. Despite the intraneuronal accumulation of substantial amounts of tellurium, little central nervous system damage has been reported in rats exposed as adults.

Tellurium administered in the diet during the 1st month of life causes an unusual transient peripheral neuropathy. The neuropathy is characterized by a segmental demyelination appearing 1–3 weeks after the initiation of dietary exposure and lasting 1–2 weeks. Remyelination occurs despite the continued administration of tellurium and is generally complete at 3–6 months of age (Miyoshi and Takauchi 1977).

Ultrastructure

Congenital. Most of the ultrastructural changes present in congenitally exposed pups examined postnatally appear attributable to edema. When examined on postnatal day 1, extracellular edema and swelling of cell bodies and processes are pronounced. By 3 days of age, when hydrocephalus is recognizable grossly, the cortical mantle is thin, the ependymal layer flattened, and ependymal cells vacuolated. On day 5 compression of the cortex by the expanding cerebrospinal fluid results in severe damage to the ependyma and underlying cortical neurons and processes. These changes are more advanced in day-7 animals. The ependyma consists of overlapping layers of undifferentiated-appearing flat cells containing lipofuscin and bundles of fibrils (Duckett 1971).

Adult. The gray-black discoloration of the brain following tellurium poisoning results from the accumulation of the element within neuronal organelles. Needle-shaped crystals measuring 100–200 nm in length were reported by Duckett and White (1974) in neuronal mitochondria, residual bodies, membrane-delineated vacuoles, and lipofuscin; analysis by energy-dispersive X-ray spectrometry confirmed the presence of tellurium in these organelles. These results were confirmed to some extent by Miyoshi and Takauchi (1977), who found tellurium in lysosomes, but not in mitochondria.

The tellurium granules are highly persistent in the neuron. Isotopic ^{127m}tellurium has been identified in rat brain more than 200 days after injection. Hollins (1969) and Yeun et al. (1975) identified abundant tellurium-induced discoloration in brains of rats more than 1 year after tellurium exposure ceased. It has been shown by Duckett and White (1974) and others (Miyoshi and Takauchi 1977) that the tellurium-containing lysosomes are eventually processed to form the abundant lipofuscin noted in the perikarya of tellurium-treated animals.

Tellurium-induced peripheral neuropathy is first manifested by changes in Schwann's cells of the sciatic nerves and spinal roots. Dilation of endoplasmic reticulum and sequestration of cytoplasm by membranous whorls appear within the 1st week of tellurium consumption. The Schwann's cells degenerate, and myelin splits along the interperiod line, resulting in intramyelinic vacuoles (Lampert et al. 1970; Lampert and Garrett 1971). Eventually the myelin fragments and is removed by macrophages. At this time, the animal characteristically displays transient hindlimb weakness or even paralysis. Remyelination begins rapidly, and by 6 months after the paralytic episode, myelination of the peripheral nerves appears normal.

Differential Diagnosis

Tellurism is not a naturally occurring disease in animals and is unlikely to be a diagnostic alternative in most circumstances. Interest in the toxic effects is therefore confined to its use in the laboratory as a cause of hydrocephalus or intracellular absorption of the chemical.

It must be differentiated from the effects of other agents capable of discoloring the brain, such as acetyltetramethyl tetralin (AETT) (Spencer et al. 1979).

Biologic Features

Tellurium, like many other metals, may affect a variety of biochemical processes. Consequently, the neuropathy associated with tellurium exposure depends, in part, upon the age of the animal at the time of exposure. Tellurium administered to the pregnant rat rapidly passes into the fetus and may result in hydrocephalic offspring. The time period of gestation during which the exposure occurs is important. Tellurium given prior to gestational day 10 or after day 16 results in a low number of hydrocephalic pups, but exposure on gestational days 10–15 causes a high incidence of the malformation. Despite the relative ease with which hydrocephalus can be induced with tellurium, the mechanisms underlying the development of tellurium-induced hydrocephalus are not known. Tellurium accumulates in the choroid plexus and may interfere with the production and/or resorption of cerebrospinal fluid (Braheny and Lampert 1980). The subsequent steps leading to aqueductal stenosis and ventricular rupture have not been characterized.

Tellurium-associated peripheral neuropathy is most easily induced in weanling animals. The period of vulnerability corresponds to the period of active myelination, indicating the vulnerability of the Schwann's cell. The biochemical target of tellurium in the Schwann's cell has yet to be identified.

The adult animal appears comparatively refractory to major neural damage induced by tellurium. There is no evidence that the lipofuscinosis has major functional effects in the chronically exposed animal.

Comparison with Other Species

There are few examples of tellurium exposure in humans; consequently, it is not possible to compare the toxic effects of the metal in rats and in man. Tellurium is toxic to rats, mice, rabbits, and ducklings, but systematic comparisons of the associated neuropathology between these species have not been performed.

References

Braheny SL, Lampert PW (1980) Tellurium. In: Spencer PS, Schaumburg HH (eds) Experimental and clinical neurotoxicology. Williams and Wilkins, Baltimore, pp 558–569

Duckett S (1971) The morphology of tellurium-induced hydrocephalus. Exp Neurol 31: 1–16

Duckett S, White R (1974) Cerebral lipofuscinosis induced with tellurium. Electron dispersive X-ray spectrophotometry analysis. Brain Res 73: 205–214

Garro F, Pentschew A (1964) Neonatal hydrocephalus in the offspring of rats fed during pregnancy non-toxic amounts of tellurium. Arch Psychiatr Nervenkr 206: 272–280

Hollins JG (1969) The metabolism of tellurium in rats. Health Phys 17: 497–505

Lampert PW, Garrett MS (1971) Mechanism of demyelination in tellurium neuropathy. Electron microscopic observations. Lab Invest 25: 380–388

Lampert P, Garro F, Pentschew A (1970) Tellurium neuropathy. Acta Neuropathol (Berl) 15: 308–317

Miyoshi K, Takauchi S (1977) Chronic tellurium intoxication in rats. Folia Psychiatr Neurol Jpn 31: 111–118

Spencer PS, Foster GF, Sterman AB, Horoupian D (1979) Acetyl ethyl tetramethyl tetralin. In: Spencer PS, Schaumberg HH (eds) Experimental and clinical neurotoxicology. Williams and Wilkins, Baltimore, pp 296–308

Yeun TG, Agnew WF, Carregal EJ (1975) Lysosomal handling of tellurium by the choroid plexus following chronic administration: an ultrastructural study. Exp Neurol 47: 213–228

Cadmium Poisoning, Rat

Kenneth R. Reuhl

Synonyms. Cadmiosis.

Gross Appearance

Congenital. When exposure occurs in utero, hydrocephalus and cortical hemorrhage are the significant gross findings.

Neonatal. Diffuse hemorrhage of cerebrum and cerebellum, affecting both cortex and white matter, appears during the neonatal period. Hemorrhage in the brain is most severe if exposure to cadmium occurs during first 10 days of life and is rarely encountered if exposure occurs after 30 days of age.

Adult. Adults exposed to cadmium manifest hemorrhagic necrosis of trigeminal and spinal sensory ganglia.

Microscopic Features

Congenital. Administration of cadmium during gestation may result in fetal hydrocephalus, involving the lateral and third ventricles. The overlying cerebral cortex is often compressed, and neuronal necrosis is common.

Neonatal. Treatment of rat pups with cadmium before 20 days postpartum may cause extensive hemorrhage in both the cerebrum and cerebellum. The hemorrhages appear primarily as petechiae in both the cerebral cortex (particularly on the surface) and in cerebral white matter. In the most severe manifestation, the hemorrhages are confluent. The hemorrhagic diathesis may be associated with extensive neuronal and glial necrosis and disruption of neural fiber pathways. The cerebellum and caudatoputamen are particularly vulnerable when cadmium treatment occurs during the first days of postnatal life (Gabbiani et al. 1967a; Wong and Klaassen 1982). Damage to the caudatoputamen and corpus callosum, induced by treatment on day 4, may result in bilateral cystic cavities lined with glial cells. These cavities may extend from the anterior to the posterior commissure and appear to be the residue of infarcts resulting from cadmium-induced vas-

cular injury. Hydrocephalus may result from cadmium exposure during the 1st week of life (Fig. 108). Exposure to cadmium at this time also causes extensive loss of cerebellar neurons in the internal granule cell layer and among Purkinje's cells (Webster and Valois 1981). The developing neurons of the cerebellar external granule cell layer are less extensively involved although they, too, may show variable degrees of damage (Arvidson 1983).

The severity of brain hemorrhage and encephalomalacia are decreased substantially in more mature animals. Gabbiani et al. (1967a) found that rat pups treated with 10 mg cadmium per kilogram between the ages of 1 and 20 days had a 60%-100% incidence of cerebral hemorrhage and a 100% incidence of cerebellar hemorrhage. This incidence decreased to 0% in both regions of the brain when treatment occurred on day 30 postpartum. The incidence of damage to sensory spinal ganglia, however, increased from 0% following treatment on day 10 to 100% following treatment on day 30. Dose dependence and thresholds for cadmium-induced hemorrhage and encephalomalacia have not been precisely determined in the rat.

Adult. In contrast to the broad distribution of brain hemorrhage characteristic of neonatal cadmium neurotoxicity, cadmium-induced lesions in adult rats tend to be highly localized to the trigeminal ganglion and spinal sensory ganglia of the peripheral nervous system (Gabbiani 1966; Gabbiani et al. 1967a, b). Extensive hemorrhage in these structures results from injury to the endothelia of small vessels, including arterioles (Gabbiani et al. 1967b), capillaries and venules (Schlaepfer 1971). Secondary neuronal loss may accompany the hemorrhage.

The effects of subchronic or chronic cadmium administration to rodents have been poorly documented. Behavioral (Nation et al. 1983) and biochemical (Hrdina et al. 1976) changes have been reported following such exposures, but associated lesions in the central nervous system have not been identified. A neuropathy involving demyelination of spinal nerve roots and sciatic nerves and loss of spinal ganglion cells occurs following exposure of rats to 10–40 ppm cadmium in drinking water for 18–31 months. These changes are not associated with hemorrhage or histologically evident endothelial damage (Sato et al. 1978), suggesting direct toxicity to neurons and Schwann's cells. Cadmium has been identified by electron probe microanalysis in the perikarya of neurons in dorsal root ganglion cultures exposed to the metal (Tischner 1980), and it would seem probable that some cadmium accumulation would occur in both central and peripheral nervous systems after long-term exposure.

Arvidson (1986) has described the distribution of $^{109}CdCl_2$ within the brains of adult rats. The metal accumulated in those areas not protected by the blood-brain barrier, such as the choroid plexus, pineal gland, and area postrema. Cadmium was also localized in the olfactory bulbs, and the author postulated that the anosmia reported in cadmium-exposed humans may be the result of retrograde axonal transport of cadmium taken up by olfactory receptor cells after being trapped in the nasal mucosa. Retrograde movement of cadmium has been documented in the rat hypoglossal nerve (Arvidson 1985).

Ultrastructural Features

The endothelial cell of the arteriole, capillary, and venule appears to be a major target of cadmium toxicity. Indeed, virtually all of the major neural effects of cadmium exposure may be a secondary result of primary endothelial cell damage. The mechanism by which cadmium affects endothelium is not clear. Studies have shown that cadmium administration to neonatal rats results in disjuncture of endothelial cells by the broadening of interendothelial clefts. Eventually, the tight junctions rupture causing extravasation of plasma proteins and red blood cells into the brain parenchyma (Gabbiani et al. 1974). Many of the resulting neuronal and glial changes are likely secondary to hemodynamic events, such as

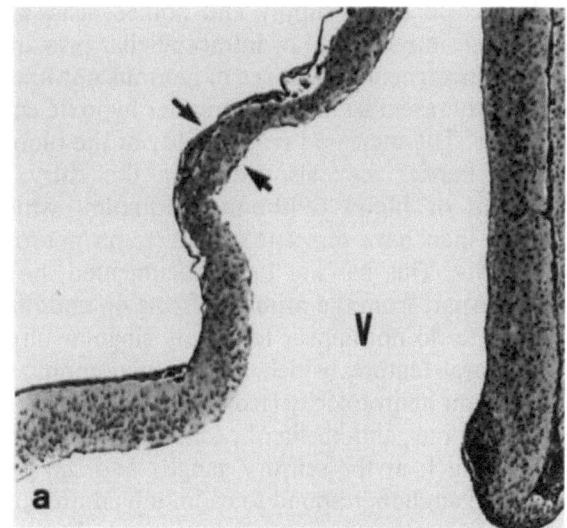

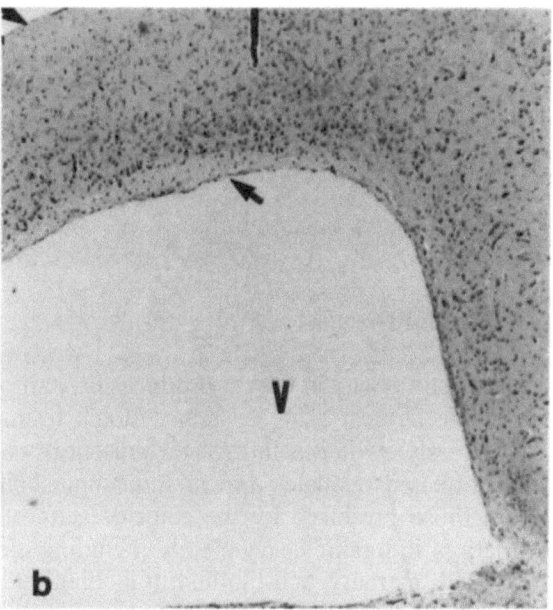

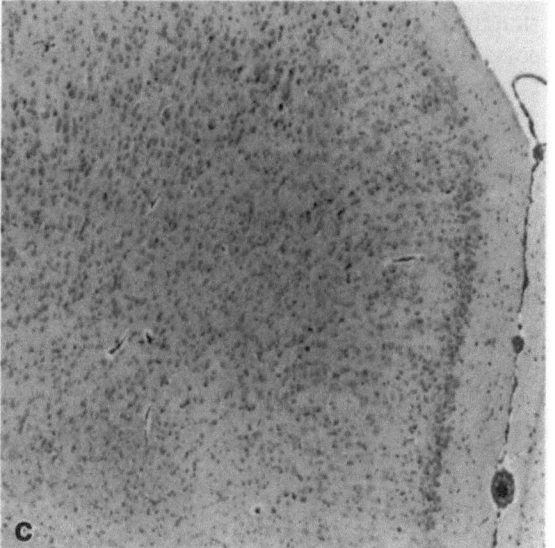

Fig. 108a–c. Neurotic effects of cadmium. Exposure to ▶ cadmium during the 1st week of life may result in variable degrees of hydrocephalus in the rat. In its most severe form (**a** 21-day-old rat), the cortex is a thin band of tissue surrounding a dilated lateral ventricle (V). Such lesions are grossly apparent. Mild hydrocephalus (**b** adult rat) has no readily apparent deleterious effects and may be found unexpectedly at autopsy. The normal cortical thickness is represented by the control section (**c** adult rat). Transverse sections at the level of the optic chiasma. (From Newland et al. 1986.) H and E, ×40

changes in blood supply and homeostasis, and elevated intracerebral or intracerebellar pressure. The ultrastructural changes of neurons not unexpectedly resemble those seen under hypoxic conditions. The increased permeability of the blood-brain barrier may also result in the entry of plasma or blood cell-bound cadmium, which could then have direct toxic effects on neurons and glia. This has not been documented, however. Apart from the primary effects on endothelia there do not appear to be any singular ultrastructural features which are pathognomonic of cadmium neurotoxicity (Rohrer et al. 1978).

In adult rats, endothelia of cadmium-sensitive regions, such as the sensory ganglia and the gassarian ganglion, respond to cadmium administration in a less pronounced manner than do endothelia in the brains of neonatal rats. In cadmium-treated adult rats, vacuoles form between endothelial cells of small vessels (Gabbiani et al. 1974), but the fate of these vacuoles is unknown. For obscure reasons, endothelium of vessels in the adult rat central nervous system appears relatively insensitive to cadmium.

Differential Diagnosis

Cadmium toxicity in the rat produces no pathognomonic clinical signs or morphologic lesions. The grossly evident hemorrhages present in cadmium-treated neonates appear indistinguishable from those produced by the chloride salts of a variety of inorganic heavy metals, including indium, lead, mercury, and thallium (Gabbiani et al. 1967a). In the adult, cadmium-induced hemorrhagic suffusion of the trigeminal and spinal sensory ganglia is distinct in appearance from trigeminal ganglion damage by other metals, such as trimethyltin, which is directly neurotoxic but which does not usually cause hemorrhage. If cadmium toxicity is suspected, careful examination of the kidney for cadmium-related tubular damage may provide supporting evidence for this diagnosis.

Biologic Features

Ample experimental evidence suggests that the primary site of the toxic activity of cadmium is the endothelial cell and, particularly, the endothelial tight junction. The degree of brain injury following cadmium exposure is inversely related to the maturity and integrity of the blood-brain barrier at the time of exposure. The barrier is not fully developed in neonatal rats, and cadmium treatment during this period of life results in extensive hemorrhage, as previously described. The immaturity of vascular endothelia in neonates not only renders the vessels particularly vulnerable to injury, but also permits greater subsequent entry of cadmium into the brain. For example, Wong and Klaassen (1980) found that the brain cadmium concentration was five times greater in 4-day-old rats than in adult rats following intravenous administration of $CdCl_2$. As the nervous system endothelium matures, it becomes more resistant to cadmium until, at 30 days of age, only the trigeminal and spinal sensory ganglia show a significant pathologic response. These latter areas appear vulnerable to other toxic metals as well, indicating that the blood-brain barrier in these areas is more permeable than in more cadmium-resistant areas (Jacobs 1980). Blood vessels of peripheral sensory and autonomic ganglia are permeable to plasma proteins due to the presence of fenestrations in the endothelial lining (Jacobs 1980). Leakage of protein-bound cadmium through these fenestrations presumably contributed to the sensitivity of these areas to cadmium. However, the exact biologic features of endothelia which determine susceptibility to cadmium are unknown.

It is not clear whether or not cadmium has significant toxicity to neurons once it has traversed the blood-brain barrier. Cadmium is toxic to organs which are not protected by an excluding barrier system, such as the kidney, and the documented antagonistic action of cadmium and other divalent cations, such as cadmium and zinc, suggests that the metal should be directly neurotoxic if sufficient quantities accumulate within neurons and/or glia. The ubiquity of cadmium in the environment and in foodstuffs ensures the potential for chronic exposure. However, renal damage or bone disease associated with cadmium-induced renal injury are more likely than neurologic injury to result from environmentally relevant levels of the metal.

Comparison with Other Species

Detailed interspecies comparisons of cadmium neurotoxicity are not available. Neonatal rabbits treated with cadmium have hemorrhagic changes in the nervous system resembling those in neonatal rats but with a slightly different distribution of injury (Gabbiani et al. 1967a). The cerebellum is more severely involved in the rabbit than in the rat; damage to the trigeminal ganglion (a hallmark of the adult neurotoxic response in the rat) is involved as early as postnatal day 5 in the rabbit. The mouse closely resembles the rat in its response to cadmium. Insufficient data are available to compare these findings to those with other species (Nomiyama 1976).

References

Arvidson B (1983) Cadmium toxicity and neural cell damage. In: Dreosti IE, Smith RM (eds) Neurobiology of the trace elements. Humana, Clifton, NJ, pp 51–78

Arvidson B (1985) Retrograde axonal transport of cadmium in the rat hypoglossal nerve. Neurosci Lett 62: 45–49

Arvidson B (1986) Autoradiographic localization of cadmium in the rat brain. Neurotoxicology 7: 89–96

Gabbiani G (1966) Action of cadmium chloride on sensory ganglia. Experientia 22: 261–262

Gabbiani G, Baic D, Deziel C (1967a) Toxicity of cadmium for the central nervous system. Exp Neurol 18: 154–160

Gabbiani G, Gregory A, Baic D (1967b) Cadmium-induced selective lesions of sensory ganglia. J Neuropathol Exp Neurol 26: 498–506

Gabbiani G, Badonnell MC, Mathewson S, Ryan GB (1974) Acute cadmium intoxication: early selective lesions of endothelial clefts. Lab Invest 30: 686–695

Hrdina PD, Peters DAV, Singhal RL (1976) Effects of chronic exposure to cadmium, lead, and mercury on brain biogenic amines in the rat. Res Commun Chem Pathol Pharmacol 15: 483–493

Jacobs J (1980) Vascular permeability and neural injury. In: Spencer PS, Schaumberg HH (eds) Experimental and clinical neurotoxicology. Williams and Wilkins, Baltimore, pp 102–117

Nation JR, Clark DE, Bourgeois AE, Baker DM (1983) The effects of chronic cadmium exposure on schedule controlled responding and conditioned suppression in the adult rat. Neurobehav Toxicol Teratol 5: 275–282

Newland MC, Ng WW, Baggs RB, Gentry GD, Weiss B, Miller RK (1986) Operant behavior in transition reflects neonatal exposure to cadmium. Teratology 34: 231–241

Nomiyama K (1976) Effects of cadmium on human health: a review of studies mainly performed in Japan. Japan Public Health Association, Tokyo

Rohrer SR, Shaw SM, Lamar CH (1978) Cadmium induced endothelial cell alterations in the fetal brain from prenatal exposure. Acta Neuropathol (Berl) 44: 147–149

Sato K, Iwamasa T, Tsuru T, Takeuchi T (1978) An ultrastructural study of chronic cadmium chloride-induced neuropathy. Acta Neuropathol (Berl) 41: 185–190

Schlaepfer WW (1971) Sequential study of endothelial changes in acute cadmium intoxication. Lab Invest 25: 556–564

Tischner K (1980) Cadmium. In: Spencer PS, Schaumberg HH (eds) Experimental and clinical neurotoxicology. Williams and Wilkins, Baltimore, pp 348–355

Webster WS, Valois AA (1981) The toxic effects of cadmium on the neonatal mouse CNS. J Neuropathol Exp Neurol 40: 247–257

Wong KL, Klaassen CD (1980) Tissue distribution and retention of cadmium in rats during postnatal development: minimal role of hepatic metallothionein. Toxicol Appl Pharmacol 53: 343–353

Wong KL, Klaassen CD (1982) Neurotoxic effects of cadmium in young rats. Toxicol Appl Pharmacol 63: 330–337

Benign and Malignant Neoplasms, Meninges, Rat

Kunitoshi Mitsumori, Steven A. Stefanski, and Robert R. Maronpot

Synonyms. Meningioma; fibroblastic meningioma; syncytial meningioma; meningothelial meningioma; psammomatous meningioma; granular cell meningioma; granular cell tumor; malignant meningioma; meningeal sarcoma.

Gross Appearance

Benign meningeal neoplasms such as meningiomas and granular cell tumors are characteristically well circumscribed, spherical, gray-white discolored masses or thickenings, intimately connected with the meninges. The meninges over the frontal, parietal, and temporal portion of the cerebrum and the dorsal and lateral portions of the cerebellum are the most frequent anatomic locations for these neoplasms. Averaging less than 3 mm in diameter, benign meningeal neoplasms range from 1 mm to 10 mm. Larger tumors grow by expansion causing compression of the adjacent brain tissue, with sharp demarcation from surrounding tissue and no invasion into the brain parenchyma.

Malignant meningeal neoplasms are generally in contact with the meninges and form spherical masses that are frequently accompanied by invasive growth into adjacent tissues. Because of adhesions between these tumors and dura mater or cranial bone, it may be difficult to remove the neoplasm and brain intact from the cranial cavity. Although meningeal sarcomas are rare, these malignant neoplasms have been observed in all sites of the brain except the temporal, occipital, and basilar portions of the cerebrum (Fitzgerald et al. 1974; Jones et al. 1973; Mitsumori et al. 1987a). In one report, it was noted that 42% of meningeal sarcomas were in the lateral portion of the cerebellum (Mitsumori et al. 1987a). The majority of malignant meningeal neoplasms discovered at necropsy are 6–10 mm in diameter.

Microscopic Features

Benign meningiomas in rats are subclassified as fibroblastic, meningothelial (syncytial), granular cell, and psammomatous. In addition, there is a mixed form of the meningothelial meningioma that contains granular cells.

Fibroblastic meningiomas are comprised of small elongated cells with pale, eosinophilic fibrillar cytoplasm, elongated nuclei, and reticulated nuclear chromatin resembling that of fibroblasts (Newman and Mawdesley-Thomas 1974; Mitsumori et al. 1987a). The neoplastic cells form irregular patterns or closely interwoven bundles with varying amounts of collagen separating individual cells and may be arranged in concentric whorls around blood vessels (Fig. 109).

Meningothelial meningiomas grow in lobulated solid masses separated by fibrous stroma and contain two types of cells (Newman and Mawdesley-Thomas 1974; Mitsumori et al. 1987a). The predominant cells are usually epithelial, but may be elongated, have abundant homogeneous, eosinophilic cytoplasm, and contain a large round to oval vesicular nucleus with one or two prominent nucleoli (Figs. 110 and 111). These cells usually have distinct cell borders and are arranged in rows. The second cell type is elongated with sparce cytoplasm, indistinct cell borders, and a small oval or elongated nucleus with dense chromatin.

Granular cell meningiomas (Krinke et al. 1985) are identical to the neoplasms that have previously been diagnosed as granular cell tumors of the brain in rats (Burek 1978; Chen and Stula 1979; Hollander et al. 1976). The typical granular cell meningioma is composed of sheets or nests of closely packed, granular cells and contains a small amount of collagen (Fig. 112). As in the meningothelial meningiomas, two cell types occur in these tumors. The predominant cells are polygonal with large round to oval vesicular nuclei. These tumor cells have pink, fine to coarse

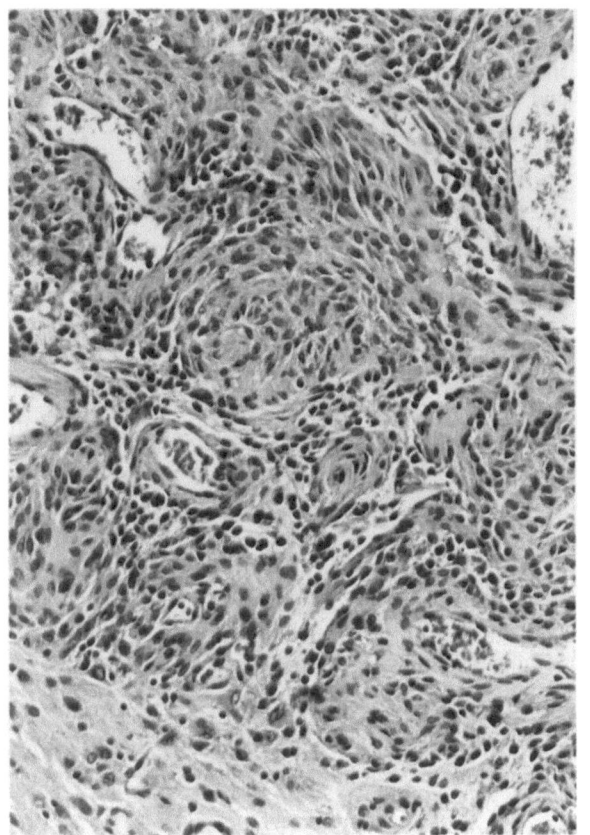

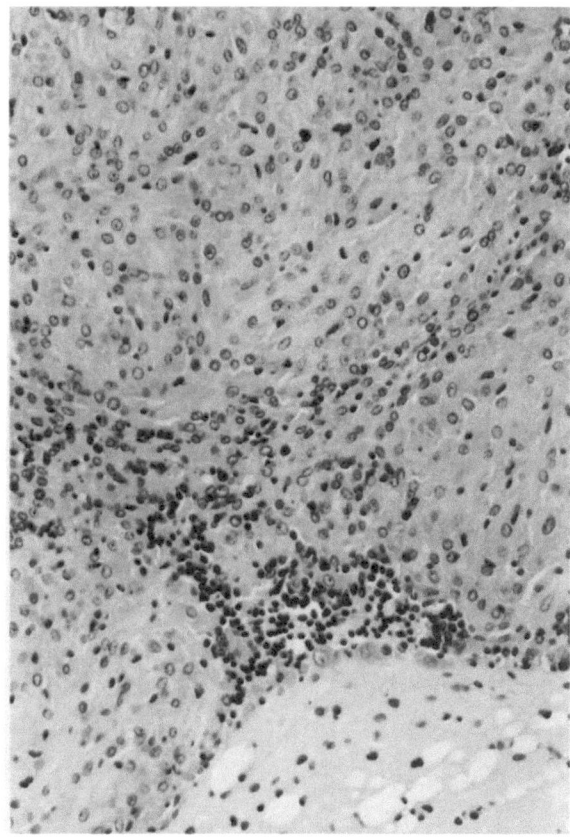

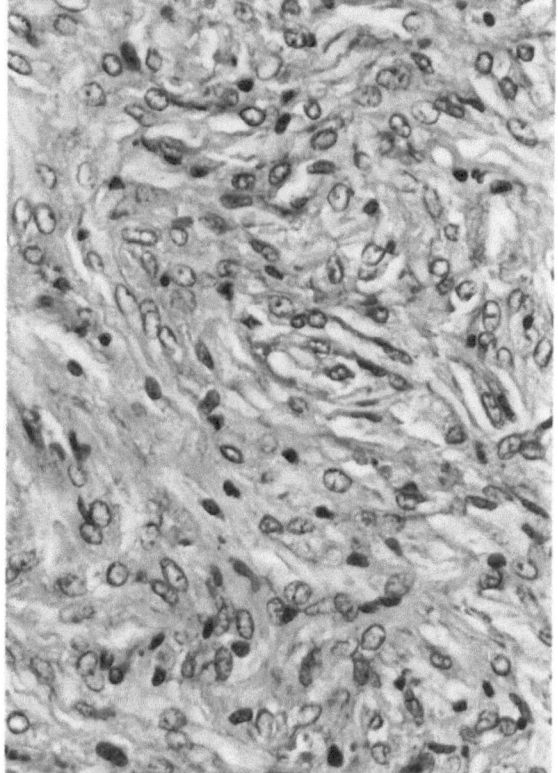

Fig. 109 *(upper left).* Fibroblastic meningioma, meninges, rat. Note fibroblastic cells and varying amounts of collagen separating individual cells. Occasional concentric whorl formation of fibroblastic cells around blood vessels. H and E, × 175

Fig. 110 *(upper right).* Meningothelial meningioma, meninges, rat. Note lobulated arrangement of tumor cells. H and E, × 175

Fig. 111 *(lower right).* Meningothelial meningioma, meninges, rat. Note two cell types: epithelial cells (meningothelial cells) with abundant cytoplasm and large vesicular nuclei, and small cells with sparce cytoplasm and small dense nuclei. H and E, × 350

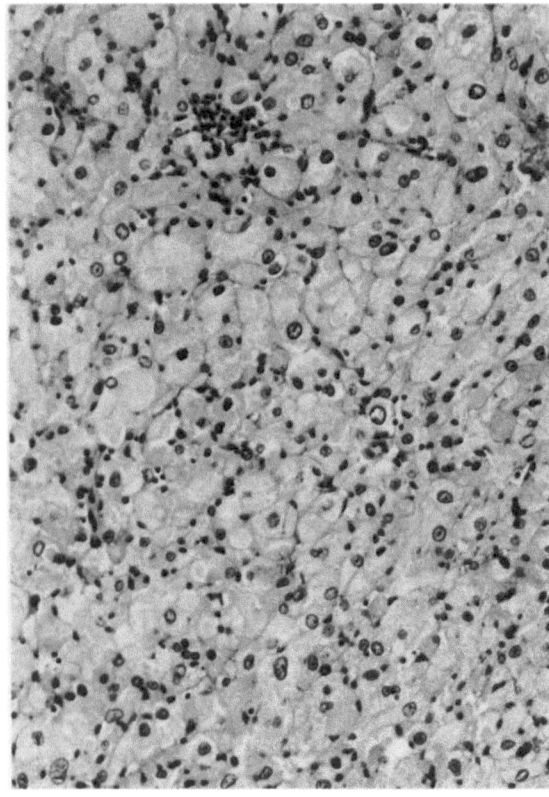

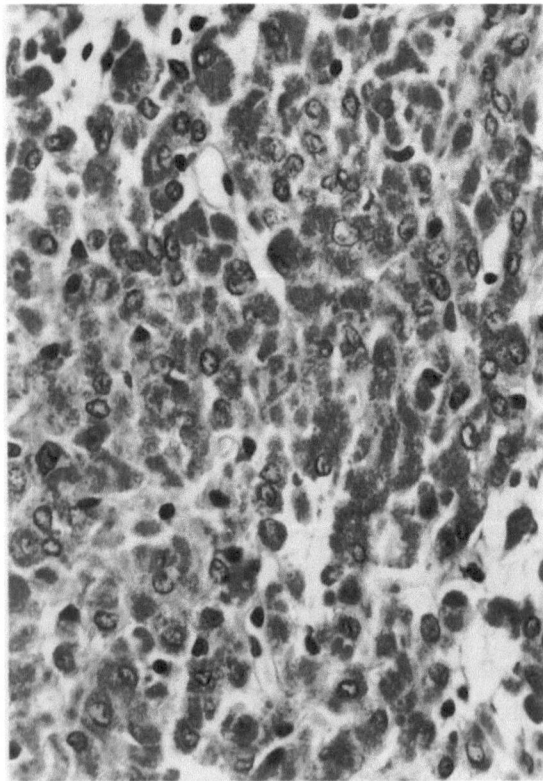

Fig. 112 *(above).* Granular cell meningioma, meninges, rat. Tumor is composed of large polygonal cells with eosinophilic granular cytoplasm and large vesicular nuclei, and small cells with scanty cytoplasm and small dense nuclei. H and E, ×175

Fig. 113 *(below).* Granular cell meningioma, meninges, rat. Cytoplasmic granules of tumor cells with PAS-positive staining. PAS, ×350

Fig. 114 *(upper left).* Meningothelial meningioma with ▶ granular cells, meninges rat. A variant of granular cell meningioma. Eosinophilic granular cells seen in the peripheral portion of the lobule *(upper left).* H and E, ×175

Fig. 115 *(lower left).* Meningothelial meningioma with granular cells, meninges, rat. PAS-positive cytoplasmic granules in tumor cells in the peripheral portion of the lobule *(upper right).* PAS, ×350

Fig. 116 *(upper right).* Granular cell meningioma, meninges, rat. Only tumor cells without cytoplasmic granules have strongly positive staining for vimentin. Immunostaining (avidin-biotin-peroxidase) of vimentin, ×350

Fig. 117 *(lower right).* Meningothelial meningioma with granular cells, meninges rat. Meningothelial cells strongly positive for vimentin in the central portion of the lobule. Immunostaining (avidin-biotin-peroxidase) of vimentin, ×350

granular cytoplasm and usually have distinct cytoplasmic boundaries. The cytoplasmic granules are strongly PAS positive (Fig. 113). The number of PAS-positive granules is variable in each polygonal cell. An occasional PAS-negative granular cell can be found. In the second, less common cell type, the tumor cells have a small, oval, hyperchromatic nucleus and scant cytoplasm often containing PAS-positive granules.

A "mixed" form of tumor, meningothelial meningiomas with varying numbers of eosinophilic granular cells identical to those in granular cell tumors (sometimes called "meningothelial meningioma with granular cells") also occurs spontaneously in rats (Mitsumori et al. 1987a). In these mixed tumors, small, discrete, eosinophilic cytoplasmic granules are seen in large epithelial cells (meningothelial cells), especially in the peripheral portions of the tumor lobules (Fig. 114). These eosinophilic cytoplasmic granules are PAS positive (Fig. 115). The majority of meningothelial cells in the central portions of the lobules do not contain these cytoplasmic granules. Neoplastic cells that are intermediate between agranular meningothelial cells and large granular cells may be seen in these neoplasms.

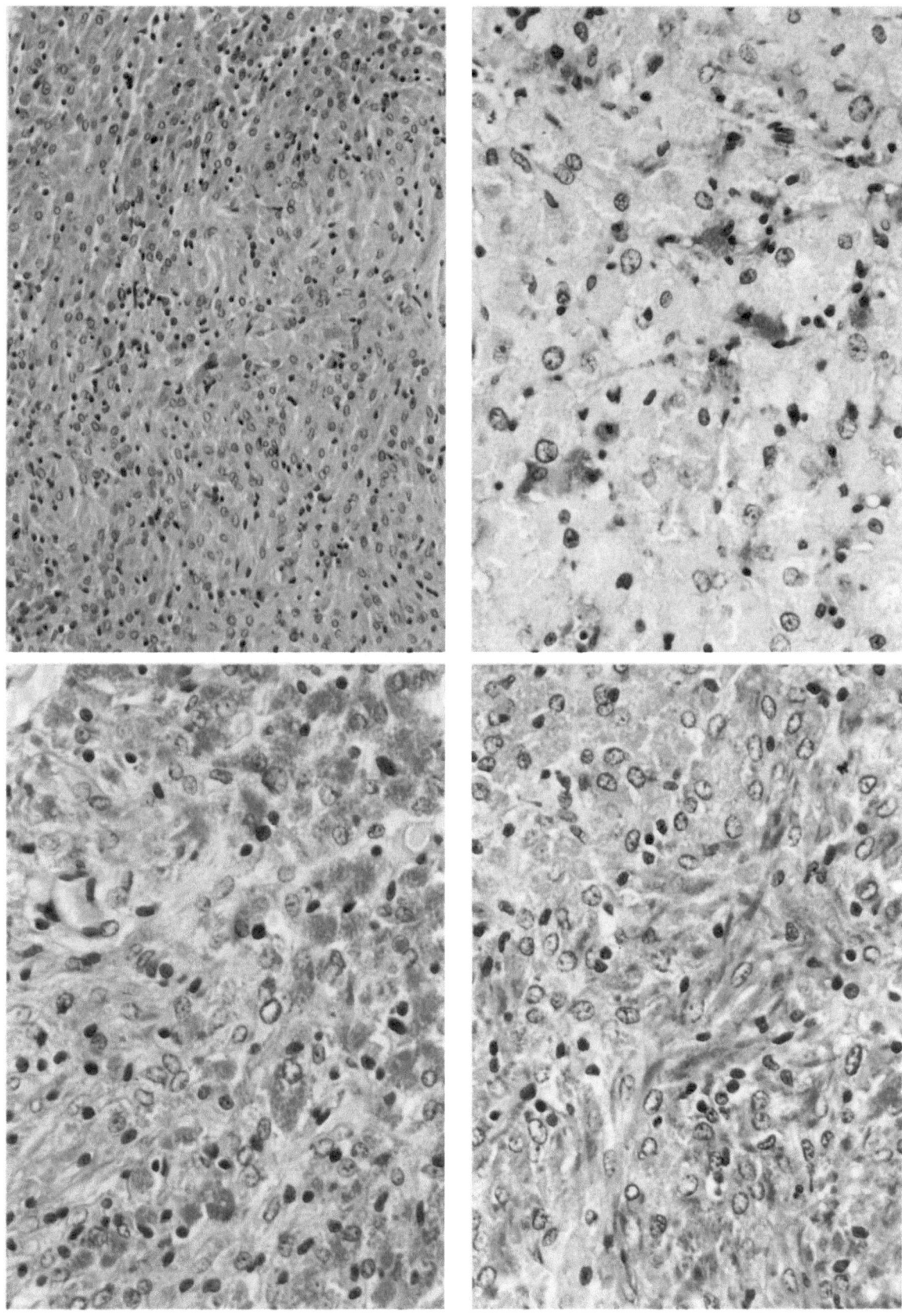

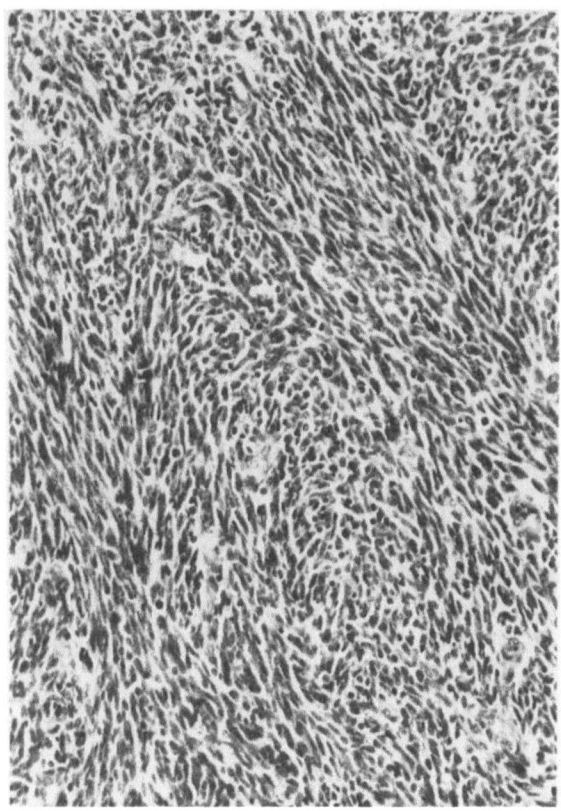

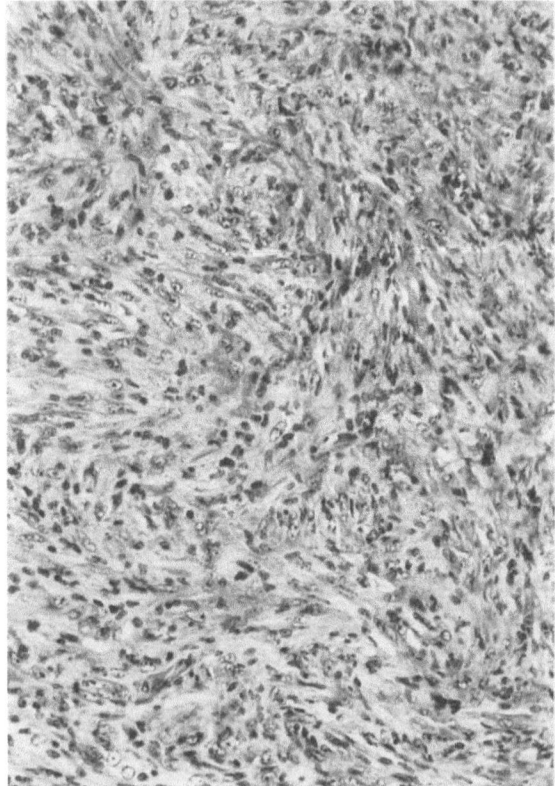

◀ **Fig. 118** *(above)*. Meningeal sarcoma (spindle cell sarcoma), meninges, rat. The tumor is composed of spindle cells with scant basophilic cytoplasm and elongated hyperchromatic nuclei. H and E, × 175

Fig. 119 *(below)*. Meningeal sarcoma (fibrosarcoma), meninges, rat. Tumor consists of elongated cells with eosinophilic fibrillar cytoplasm and large nuclei with reticulated chromatin, and abundant collagen. H and E, × 175

Immunohistochemical staining of rat granular cell meningiomas using antibodies for keratin, glial fibrillary acid protein, vimentin, and S-100 protein revealed that these tumor cells were positive only for vimentin (Mitsumori et al. 1987b). The large polygonal cells filled with granules in the granular cell tumors were weakly positive for vimentin (marker of mesenchymal cells), but the large cells without granules and the small cells with scanty cytoplasm and dense nuclei were strongly positive (Fig. 116). In the meningothelial meningiomas with granular cells, meningothelial cells in the central portion of the lobules and the small cells with dense nuclei were also strongly positive for vimentin (Fig. 117), but cells filled with granules in the peripheral portion of the lobules were weakly stained for vimentin.

One *psammomatous meningioma* has been reported in a 24-month-old male WAG/Rij rat (Burek 1978). This neoplasm consisted of cells arranged in lobulated masses and contained numerous psammoma bodies. The tumor cells were polyhedral with indistinct cell boundaries, pale pink cytoplasm, and round to oval nuclei.

Meningeal sarcomas in rats are subclassified into fibrosarcomas and spindle cell sarcomas (Mitsumori et al. 1987b). The primary distinction between the two types of meningeal sarcomas is based on the degree of cellular differentiation of the component cells. *Spindle cell sarcomas* are comprised of relatively undifferentiated spindle-shaped cells with scant, basophilic cytoplasm and elongated nuclei with coarse nuclear chromatin. Mature collagen is not observed in these sarcomas (Fig. 118).

Fibrosarcomas, on the other hand, are composed of elongated cells with eosinophilic, fibrillary cytoplasm and large elongated nuclei with reticulated chromatin and prominent nucleoli and they have a definite component of intercellular collagen (Fig. 119). The neoplastic cells in both types of meningeal sarcomas are arranged in bundles with irregular or interlacing patterns. Mitotic figures are frequent in both of these sarcomas.

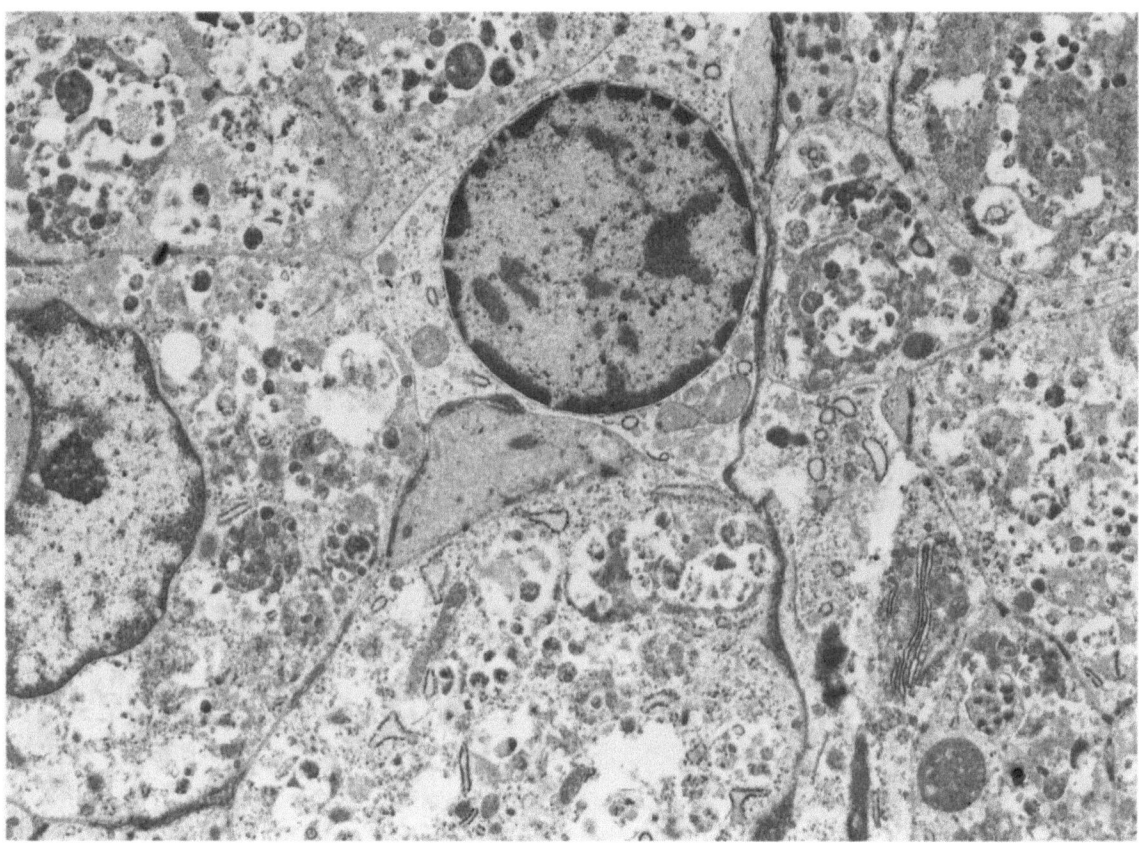

Fig. 120. Granular cell meningioma, meninges, rat. Granular cells are filled with membrane-bound dense bodies and vacuoles. Note frequent desmosomes between the membranes of adjacent cells. TEM, × 8100

Some meningeal sarcomas contain pleomorphic cells with bizarre nuclei and occasional multinucleated cells. These neoplasms frequently invade the surrounding brain parenchyma and/or cranial bone, but distant metastases are rare.

Ultrastructure

Electron-microscopic features of granular cell meningiomas in rats have been characterized (Mitsumori et al. 1987b). Ultrastructurally these neoplasms contain two cell types, viz., granular cells and filamentous cells. Although granular cells are the most frequent cell type, the ratio of filamentous cells to granular cells varies with each tumor. Granular cells are filled with variably sized heterogeneous, membrane-bound dense bodies that originate from lysosomes (Fig. 120). Other cytoplasmic components include multivesicular bodies, empty vacuoles, mitochondria, inconspicuous rough endoplasmic reticulum, and a small number of fine intermediate filaments. These granular cells have large oval to slightly irregular nuclei with a relatively narrow rim of heterochromatin and prominent nucleoli. Filamentous cells contain abundant fine intermediate cytoplasmic filaments, short cisternae of rough endoplasmic reticulum, mitochondria, and indistinct Golgi complex (Fig. 121). Small numbers of dense multivesicular bodies, identical to those in granular cells, are sometimes noted in these filamentous cells. Nuclei are similar to those in the granular cells or are small with dense chromatin.

Granular cells and filamentous cells are closely apposed to each other. Desmosomes (maculae adherentes) are frequently observed between the cell membranes of these adjacent cells (Figs. 120 and 121). The presence of desmosomes is also a salient feature of *granular cell meningiomas* in addition to the extensive accumulation of intracytoplasmic granules. No structure similar to basement membrane is seen around the tumor cells.

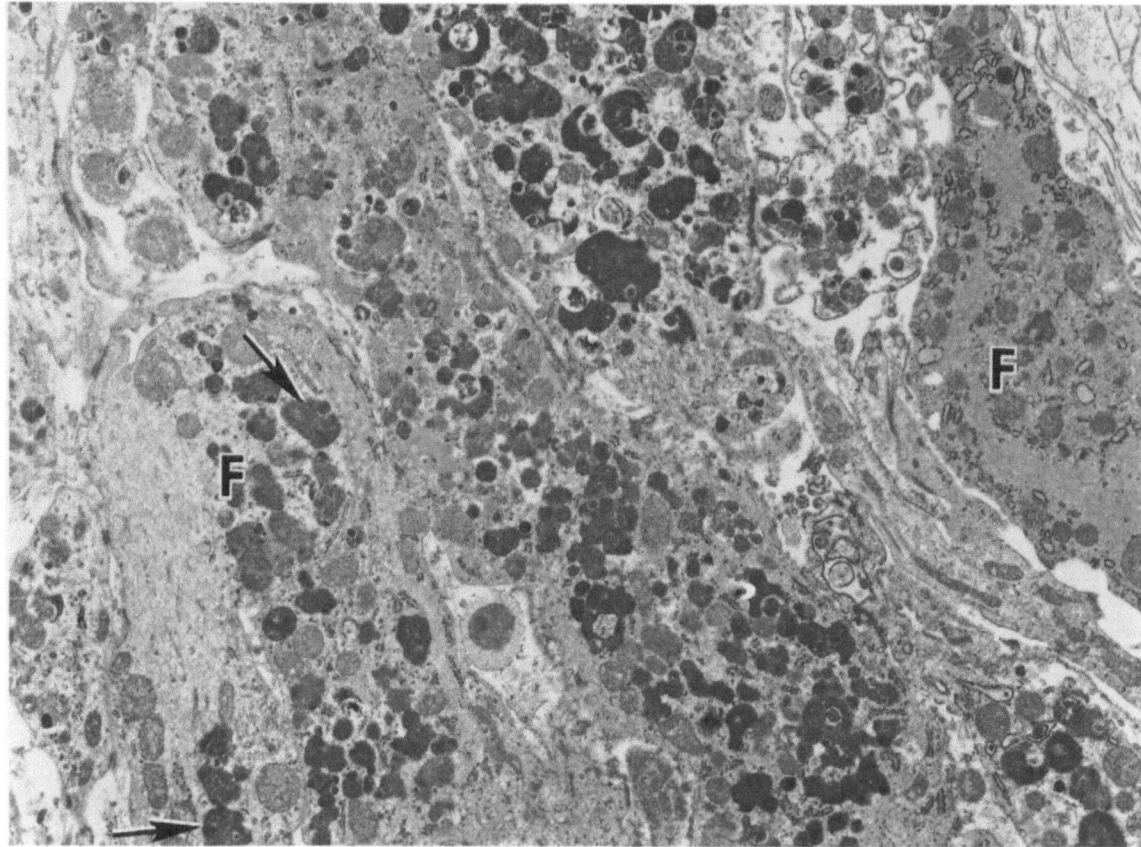

Fig. 121. Granular cell meningioma, meninges, rat. Note granular cells and filamentous cells *(F)* containing abundant intermediate filaments. Dense bodies *(arrows)* are also present in the filamentous cells. TEM, ×8100

Ultrastructural studies on other meningeal tumors such as meningothelial and fibroblastic meningiomas or meningeal sarcomas have not been reported in rats, presumably because of their rarity.

The fine structural characteristics of meningothelial meningiomas in humans (Halliday et al. 1985) and dogs (Patnaik et al. 1986) include pronounced interdigitations of the adjacent cell membranes, frequent presence of desmosomes, and presence of fine intracytoplasmic intermediate filaments identical to vimentin.

Differential Diagnosis

For benign meningeal tumors, a major diagnostic problem is the differentiation between meningiomas (fibroblastic and meningothelial) and schwannomas occurring in the cranial nerves. Schwannomas are composed of fibroblasts producing collagen and Schwann's cells and they sometimes have whorled patterns which are referred to as "Verocay bodies". These patterns are partly similar to the concentric whorl formation observed in fibroblastic meningiomas. However, the whorled pattern is always seen around blood vessels in fibroblastic meningiomas but not in schwannomas. Typical palisading arrays frequently seen in schwannomas are not observed in meningiomas.

In addition, meningothelial cells usually have a distinct cell border while neoplastic Schwann's cells do not. Since meningiomas in rats are negative for S-100 protein, demonstration of this histochemical marker of Schwann's cells is also helpful in differential diagnosis (Gough et al. 1986).

Distinguishing a granular cell meningioma from a gemistocytic astrocytoma or anaplastic astrocytoma may present a diagnostic problem. Tumor cells in some astrocytomas may have abundant, homogeneous cytoplasm that stains intensely with eosin and, thus, resembles that of the tumor cells in granular cell meningiomas (Fitzgerald et al. 1974). However, tumor cells in astrocytomas do not have the PAS-positive cytoplasmic granules that are seen in granular cell meningiomas. In addition, astrocytomas are frequently accompanied by invasive growth and are not as clearly· demarcated from the surrounding brain parenchyma as are granular cell meningiomas. Immunohistochemical demonstration of glial fibrillary acid protein (GFAP) and S-100 protein is consistent with a diagnosis of astrocytomas; granular cell meningiomas do not contain these markers.

While diagnosis of collagen-producing meningeal sarcomas is straight forward, distinguishing meningeal spindle cell sarcomas from spindle cell variants of glioblastomas may be difficult. Specific location of the neoplasm may be helpful in differentiating these neoplasms. Meningeal spindle cell sarcomas should be in anatomic proximity or in contact with the meninges while glioblastomas may be localized deep in the brain parenchyma. However, glioblastomas may also invade the leptomeninges from the brain parenchyma, making anatomic location a less reliable criterion. Although no published reports have been found, immunohistochemical staining may help with diagnosis. Theoretically, the rat glioblastoma is positive for GFAP and vimentin, while meningeal sarcomas are positive only for vimentin.

Biologic Features

Spontaneous granular cell tumors (Hollander et al. 1976; Chen and Stula 1979) and meningiomas (Fitzgerald et al. 1974; Newman and Mawdesley-Thomas 1974; Sumi et al. 1976) in the brain have been reported to occur in various strains of aged rats. Although it is widely accepted that meningiomas are derived from arachnoid cells and/or fibroblasts forming the meninges, the potential histogenesis of granular cell meningiomas in rats has only recently been proposed (Krinke et al. 1985). Based on anatomic location, ultrastructural features, and immunocytochemical characteristics, rat granular cell tumors are believed to arise from meningeal arachnoid cells (Mitsumori et al. 1987 a, b). Since granular cells with characteristic PAS-positive granules have been demonstrated in many meningothelial meningiomas (Mitsumori et al. 1987 a), it is apparent that meningothelial meningiomas and granular cell meningiomas are closely related. The available evidence suggests that tumors of the meninges containing granular cells are a variant of meningiomas and, hence, should be classified as granular cell meningiomas.

Spontaneous incidences of meningeal tumors, including granular cell varieties, vary with different rat strains (Table 7). Granular cell and other meningiomas have been described as the most common intracranial brain tumor in Sprague-Dawley (Krinke et al. 1985), Wistar (Sumi et al. 1976), and BN/Bi (Burek 1978) rats. In contrast, the incidence of granular cell meningiomas in untreated F344 rats obtained from carcinogenicity studies performed by the National Toxicology Program (NTP) and the National Cancer Institute (NCI) between 1972 and 1985 was relatively low (NTP data base as of 1985). Glial cell tumors were the most common brain tumors in F344 rats. The percentages of the pure form of benign meningioma (tumors that do not contain granular cells), granular cell meningioma (granular cell tumor and meningioma with granular cells), and meningeal sarcoma versus all menin-

Table 7. Incidence of spontaneous meningeal tumors in different strains of rats

	Sprague-Dawley (Krinke et al. 1985)		F344 (NTP data base as of 1985)		Wistar (Sumi et al. 1976)		BN/Bi (Burek 1978)	
	M	F	M	F	M	F	M	F
(a) Rats examined (–)	4480	4480	11531	11609	149	182	74	236
(b) Rats with brain tumors (–)	51	39	140	114	13	15	2	14
b/a (%)	1.1	0.9	1.2	1.0	8.7	8.2	2.7	5.9
(c) Rats with glial tumors	6	5	100	83	2	1	0	1
c/b (%)	11.8	12.8	71.4	72.8	15.4	6.7	0	7.1
(d) Rats with meningeal tumors[a]	33	22	20	15	11	14	2	11
d/b (%)	64.7	56.4	14.3	13.2	84.6	93.3	100	78.6

M, male; *F*, female; *NTP*, National Toxicology Program.
[a] Meningeal tumors, granular cell tumor including meningiomas.

Table 8. Classification of 107 granular cell and meningeal tumors in rats obtained from NTP/NCI[a] carcinogenicity studies

Tumor classification	Male	Female	Total	
			(-)	(%)
Benign meningioma				
Fibroplastic and meningothelial meningiomas	3	2	5	5
Meningothelial Meningioma with granular cells	16	5	21	20
Granular cell tumor	36	26	62	58
Meningeal sarcoma				
Spindle cell sarcoma	6	3	9	8
Fibrosarcoma	6	4	10	9
Total	67	40	107	100

[a] *NTP*, National Toxicology Program; *NCI*, National Cancer Institute.

geal tumors examined in NTP carcinogenicity studies were 5%, 78%, and 17%, respectively (Mitsumori et al. 1987a) (Table 8). Hence, granular cell meningiomas are the most common meningeal tumors in F344 rats (Solleveld et al. 1986).

Although meningeal granular cell tumors including meningiomas have been reported in aging rats as early as 15 months of age (Hollander et al. 1976) and may be as large as 10 mm in diameter (Mitsumori et al. 1987a), most benign meningeal tumors are generally observed as small nodules less than 3 mm in diameter in the rats killed at the end of 2-year toxicity and carcinogenicity studies. Meningeal sarcomas in rats are extremely rare (Fitzgerald et al. 1974; Jones et al. 1973). Because of invasive growth into brain parenchyma, they may cause death of the animal. In 2-year carcinogenicity studies conducted by the NTP and NCI, the incidence of meningeal sarcomas relative to all brain tumors was 1.5% (19/1252). We are not aware of any reports suggesting that meningeal tumors in rats are induced by chemicals.

Comparison with Other Species

Spontaneous meningeal tumors in small experimental animals other than rats are very rare. A low incidence of meningeal tumors has been reported in treated mice (Morgan et al. 1984). In man, meningiomas comprise about 15% of all primary intracranial tumors and are generally subclassified into five types: meningothelial (syncytial), transitional, fibroblastic, psammomatous, and angioblastic (Rubinstein 1972). The transitional meningioma is intermediate between the meningothelial type and the fibroblastic type, and 90%–95% of the meningiomas encountered in humans are described as meningothelial, fibroblastic or a mixture of the two (transitional). In dogs, the meningioma is the second most common brain tumor (Patnaik et al. 1986), with meningothelial and transitional types being the most frequent. Meningiomas, especially the transitional type, are the most common intracranial neoplasms observed in cats (Nafe 1979). No published description of human or animal meningiomas with eosinophilic granular cells similar to those in rat granular cell tumors was found. Predilection sites for granular cell tumors are the tongue in humans (Lack et al. 1980) and dogs (Vandergaag and Walvoort 1983) and the lung in horses (Turk and Breeze 1981). Only rare cases of meningeal granular cell tumors have been documented in humans (Markesbery et al. 1973) and dogs (Parker et al. 1978). The widely accepted theory is that granular cell tumors in humans are derived from neural crest Schwann's cells (Chimelli et al. 1984). Recently, intracerebral granular cell tumor in humans has been suggested to originate from astrocytes (Dickson et al. 1986). In either event, the available information indicates that intracerebral granular cell tumors in rats are unique.

References

Burek JD (1978) Pathology of aging rats. CRC, West Palm Beach, pp 145-148

Chen HC, Stula EF (1979) Naturally occurring granular cell tumors of the brain in rats. Toxicol Pathol 7: 15-18

Chimelli L, Symon L, Scaravilli F (1984) Granular cell tumor of the fifth cranial nerve: futher evidence for Schwann cell origin. J Exp Neurol 43: 634-642

Dickson DW, Suzuki KI, Kanner R, Weitz S, Horoupian DS (1986) Cerebral granular cell tumor: immunohistochemical and electron microscopic study. J Neuropathol Exp Neurol 45: 304-314

Fitzgerald JE, Schardein JL, Kurtz SM (1974) Spontaneous tumors of the nervous system in albino rats. JNCI 52: 265-273

Gough AW, Hanna W, Barsoum NJ, Moore J, Sturgess JM (1986) Morphologic and immunohistochemical features of two spontaneous peripheral nerve tumors in Wistar rats. Vet Pathol 23: 68-73

Halliday WC, Yeger H, Duwe GF, Phillips MJ (1985) Intermediate filaments in meningiomas. J Neuropathol Exp Neurol 44: 617-623

Hollander CF, Burek JD, Boorman GA, Snell KC, Laqueur GL (1976) Granular cell tumors of the central nervous system of rats. Arch Pathol Lab Med 100: 445-447

Jones EL, Searle CE, Smith WT (1973) Tumours of the nervous system induced in rats by the neonatal administration of N-ethyl-N-nitrosourea. J Pathol 109: 123-139

Krinke G, Naylor DC, Schmid S, Frohlich E, Schnider K (1985) The incidence of naturally-occurring primary brain tumours in the laboratory rat. J Comp Pathol 95: 175-192

Lack EE, Worsham GF, Callihan MD et al. (1980) Granular cell tumor: a clincopathologic study of 110 patients. J Surg Oncol 13: 301-316

Markesbery WR, Duffy PE, Cowen D (1973) Granular cell tumors of the central nervous system. J Neuropathol Exp Neurol 32: 92-109

Mitsumori K, Maronpot RR, Boorman GA (1987a) Spontaneous tumors of the meninges in rats. Vet Pathol 24: 50-58

Mitsumori K, Dittrich K, Stefanski S, Talley F, Maronpot RR (1987b) Immunohistochemical and electron microscopic study of meningeal granular cell tumors in rats. Vet Pathol 24: 356-359

Morgan KT, Frith CH, Swenberg JA, McGrath JT, Zulch KJ, Crowder DM (1984) A morphologic classification of brain tumors found in several strains of mice. JNCI 72: 151-160

Nafe LA (1979) Meningiomas in cats: a retrospective clinical study of 36 cases. J Am Vet Med Assoc 174: 1224-1227

Newman AJ, Mawdesley-Thomas LE (1974) Spontaneous tumours of the central nervous system of laboratory rats. J Comp Pathol 84: 39-50

Parker GA, Botha W, Van Dellen A, Casey HW (1978) Cerebral granular cell tumor (myoblastoma) in a dog: case report and literature review. Cornell Vet 68: 506-520

Patnaik AK, Kay WJ, Hurvitz AI (1986) Intracranial meningioma: a comparative pathologic study of 28 dogs. Vet Pathol 23: 369-373

Rubinstein LJ (1972) Tumors of the mesodermal tissue. Atlas of tumor pathology. Tumors of the central nervous system. Armed Forces Institute of Pathology, Washington, DC, pp 169-204

Solleveld HA, Bigner DD, Averill DR Jr, et al. (1986) Brain tumors in man and animals: report of a workshop. Environ Health Perspect 68: 155-173

Sumi N, Stavrou D, Frohberg H, Jochmann G (1976) The incidence of spontaneous tumors of the central nervous system of Wistar rats. Arch Toxicol 35: 1-13

Turk MAM, Breeze RG (1981) Histochemical and ultrastructural features of an equine pulmonary granular cell tumour (myoblastoma). J Comp Pathol 91: 471-481

Vendergaag I, Walvoort HC (1983) Granular cell myoblastoma in the tongue of a dog: a case report. Vet Q 5: 89-93

Malignant Reticulosis, Rat

Robert H. Garman

Synonyms. Neoplastic reticulosis, reticulum cell sarcoma, reticulohistiocytic sarcoma, malignant reticuloendotheliosis, primary lymphoma of the CNS, microgliomatosis, round cell sarcoma, polymorphonuclear sarcoma, sarcomatosis of the meninges (or brain), perivascular sarcoma, adventitial sarcoma, perithelial sarcoma.

Gross Appearance

Malignant reticuloses are highly infiltrative neoplasms and, in the rat, usually produce insufficient alteration in the brain's topography to allow gross detection.

Microscopic Features

Malignant reticulosis is characterized by perivascular and subarachnoid infiltrates of neoplastic cells (Figs. 122 and 123), although significant invasion of the neuropil is present as well (Figs. 124 and 125). The constituent cells may resemble lymphocytic, plasmacytic, monocytic, reticulum, or microglial cells in appearance. These cells generally have pale nuclei which tend to adopt the elongated, twisted or lobed appearance of the microglial cell when they infiltrate the neuropil (Fig. 124). The cytoplasm is often scanty, but may be moderate in amount in some cases (Fig. 126). Typically, the cells are mononuclear, but binucleate and small multinucleate giant cells are sometimes seen (Fig. 126). Varying numbers of lymphocytes may be present within the neoplastic infiltrates and are often more numerous in the perivascular infiltrates distant to the main por-

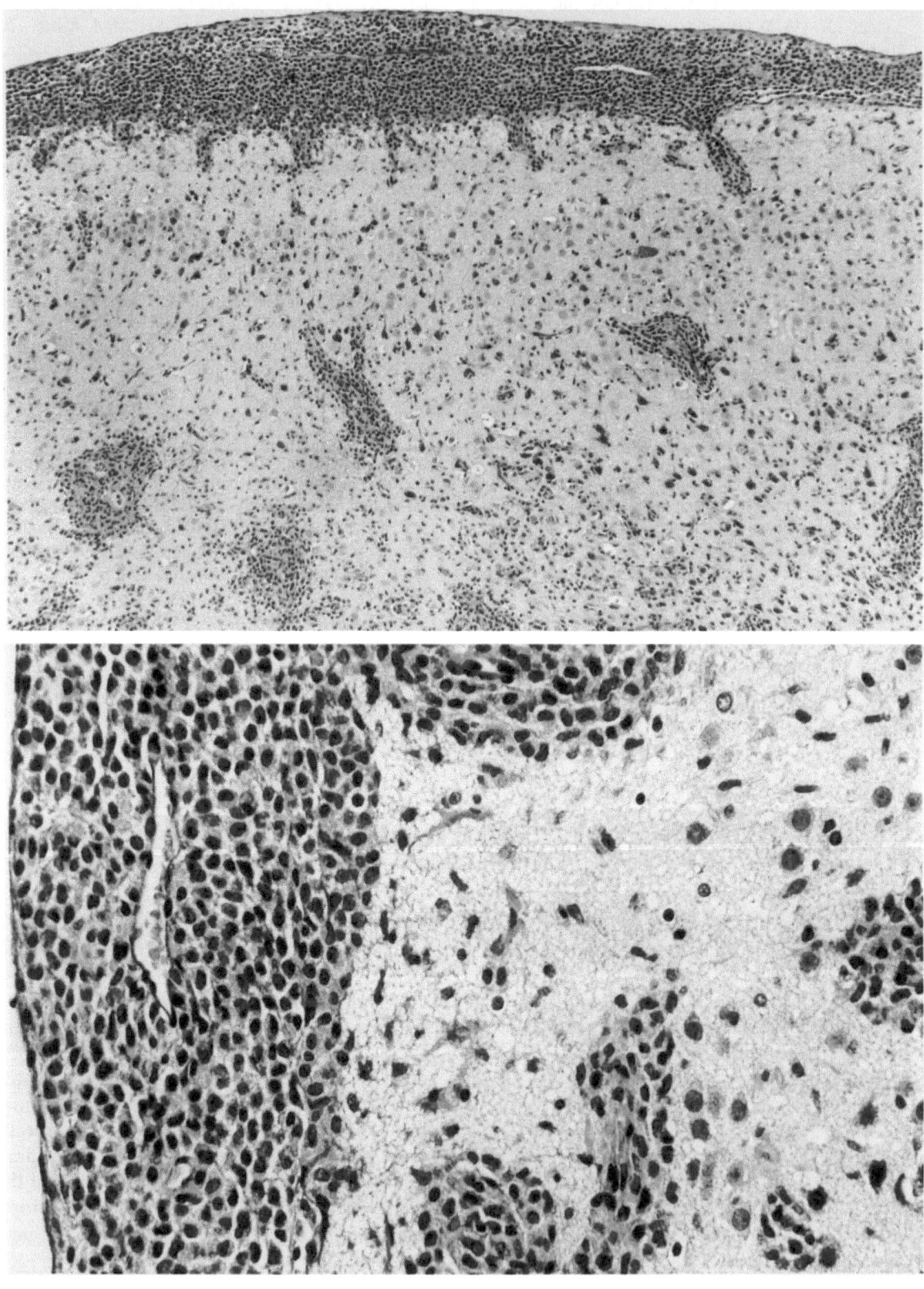

Fig. 122 *(above).* Malignant reticulosis, cerebral cortex, rat. A prominent neoplastic cell infiltrate is present within meninges *(top)* as well as within dilated Virchow-Robin spaces around the cerebral vessels. Case 1, H and E, ×80

Fig. 123 *(below).* Same neoplasm as in Fig. 122 (in this orientation, the meninges are to the left). Note that the tumor cell nuclei are round to elongated in configuration. Case 1, H and E, ×320

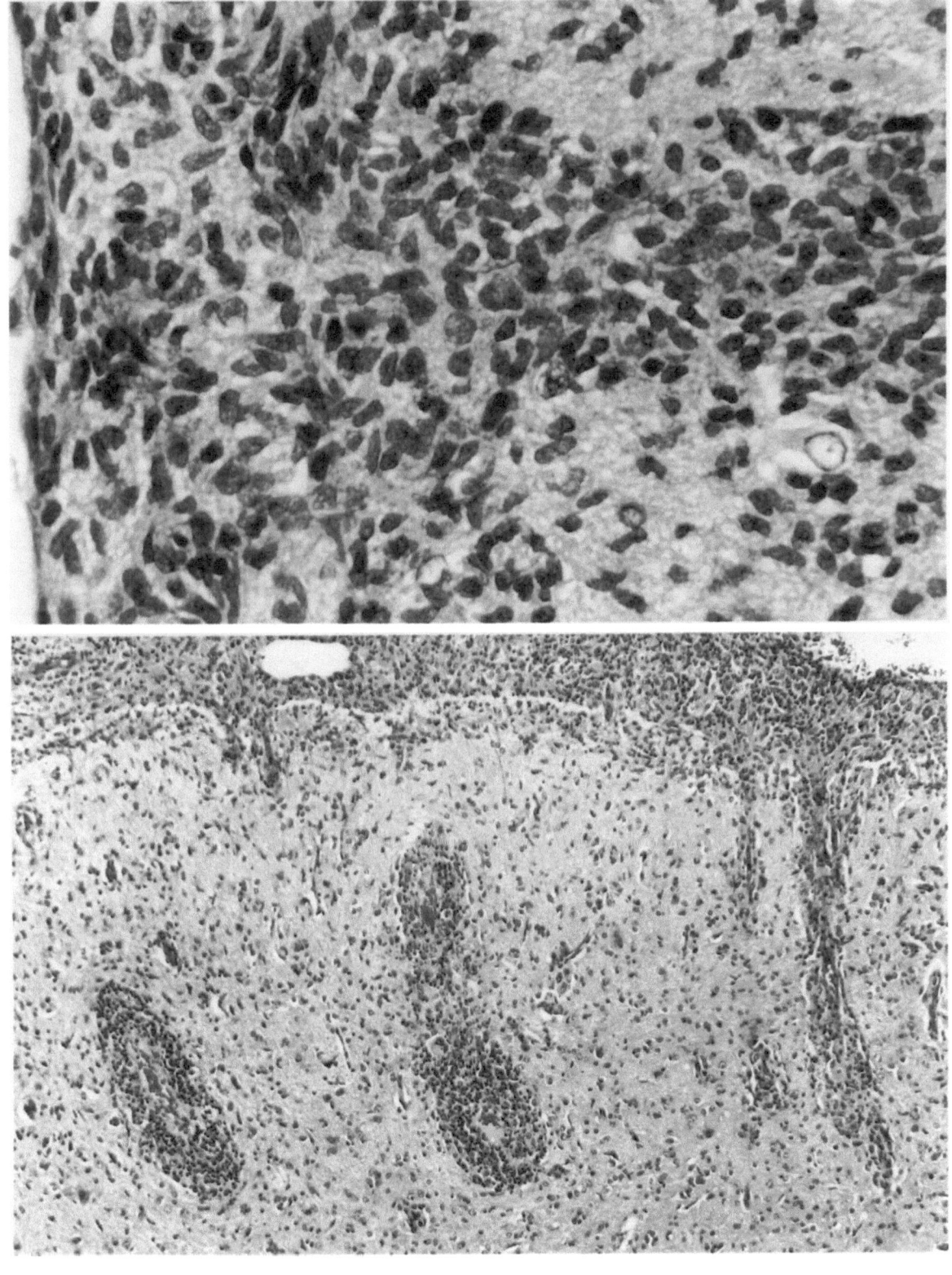

Fig. 124 *(above)*. Malignant reticulosis, cerebral cortex, rat. Infiltrated meninges *(to left)* of a second case of malignant reticulosis in a rat. Note that many of the nuclei within the meninges and Virchow-Robin space (and particularly those within the neuropil) have the elongated irregular shape characteristically associated with the microglial cell. Case 2, H and E, ×520

Fig. 125 *(below)*. Third case of malignant reticulosis in a rat, involving the surface, perivascular spaces and neuropil of the mesencephalon. Even at this magnification, this tumor may be seen to be more pleomorphic than the first two cases. Case 3, H and E, ×80

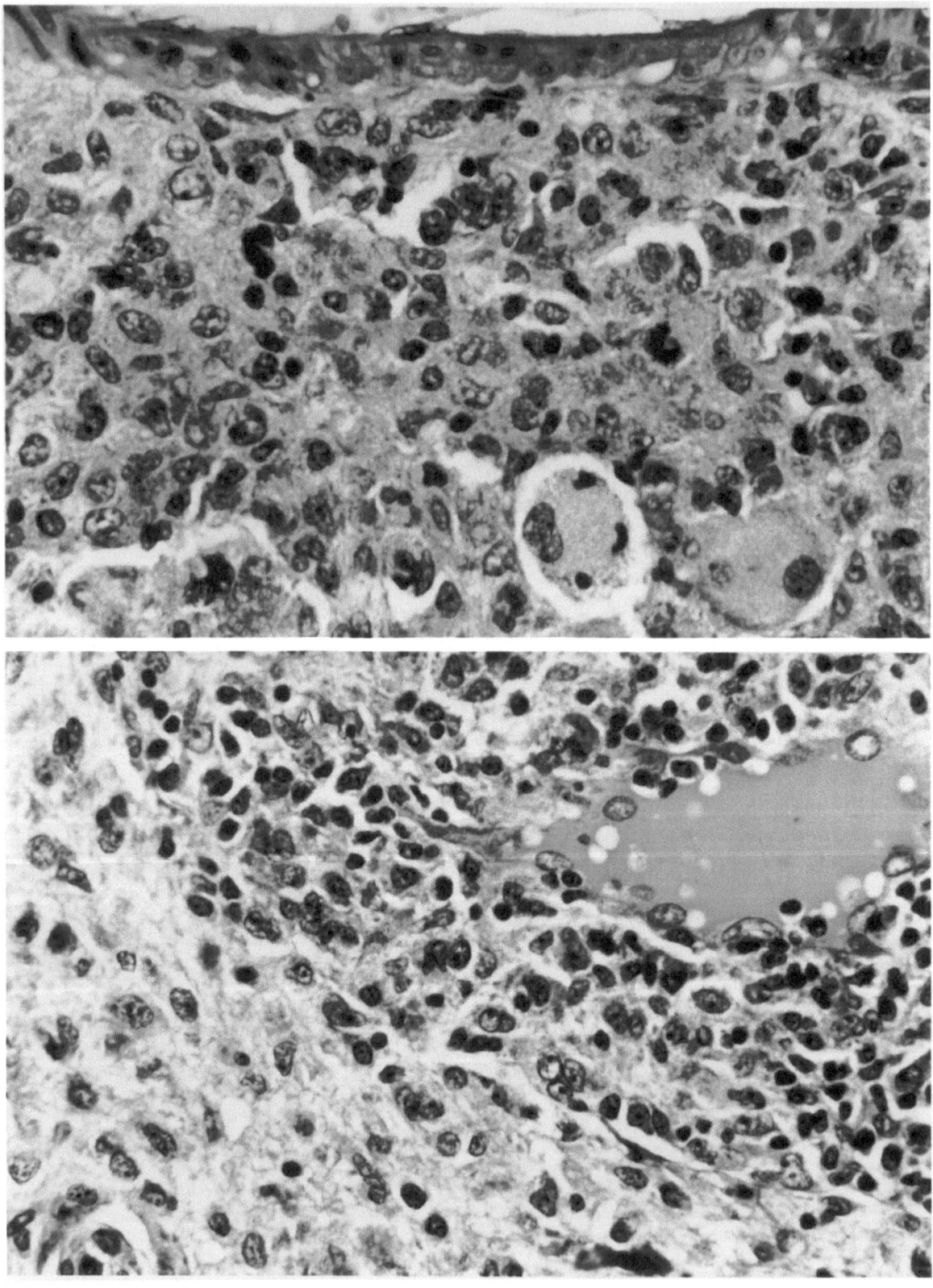

Fig. 126 *(above).* Perivascular infiltrate in case 3. Note the variability in cell size and the presence of small multinucleated giant cells. Case 3, H and E, ×520

Fig. 127 *(below).* Malignant reticulosis, cerebrum, rat. Perivascular infiltrate at a point distant to the area of major tumor involvement. Here, the infiltrate is comprised of a mixture of neoplastic cells and small- to medium-sized lymphocytes. Case 3, H and E, ×520

Fig. 128 *(above)*. Malignant reticulosis, rat. Positive reticulum stain of meningeal infiltrate in case 3. Note the intimate association of the reticulin fibers with the neoplastic cells, the latter often being circumscribed by individual fibers. Case 3, Wilder's reticulum, × 520

Fig. 129 *(below)*. Malignant reticulosis, rat. Negative or equivocal reticulum stain of meningeal infiltrate in case 2. Although reticulin fibers are present, they are not intimately associated with individual tumor cells as in Fig. 128. The neoplastic cells are not thought to be the source of the reticulin in this case. Case 2, Wilder's reticulum, × 520

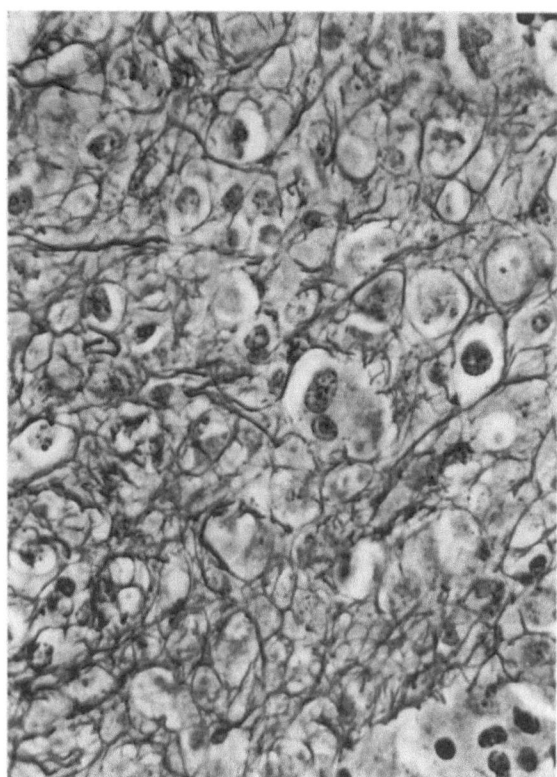

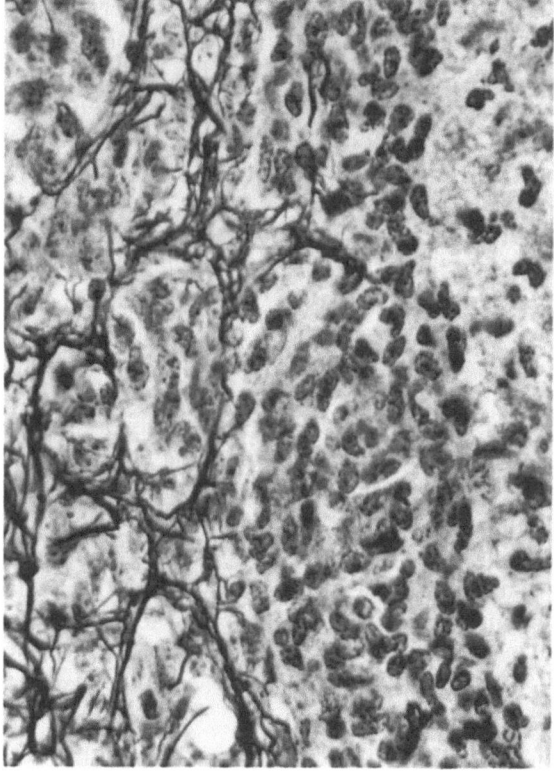

tion of the neoplasm (Fig. 127). Increased amounts of reticulin are usually associated with malignant reticulosis, particularly in perivascular locations and, to a lesser extent, within the meninges, but this should not necessarily be taken as evidence that the neoplastic cells manufacture this material. In some cases, the reticulin fibers are intimately associated with the neoplastic cells (Fig. 128). More commonly, the neoplastic cells infiltrate between the reticulin fibers but do not appear to be producing them (Fig. 129).

It has been suggested that the reticulin network is produced by nonneoplastic cells (possibly pericytes or astrocytes) as an attempt to restrict the spread of the neoplastic cells (Kalimo et al. 1985).

Because the constituent neoplastic cells are highly infiltrative, bilaterality and widespread involvement of the brain are usually seen in rats dying of malignant reticulosis.

Involvement of the cerebral cortices with infiltration of the underlying white matter, corpus callosum, and deeper structures, including the hippocampus and diencephalon, is often present. In the largest series (19 cases) reported in the literature, subcortical involvement was most commonly seen (Krinke et al. 1985).

Ultrastructure

There are no reports in the literature describing the ultrastructural appearance of this neoplasm in the rat.

Differential Diagnosis

Malignant reticulosis may be differentiated from inflammatory reticulosis by the marked degree of infiltration of the neuropil which is seen in the former. Although malignant glial cell neoplasms in the rat may demonstrate a moderate degree of perivascular infiltration and may occasionally be characterized by meningeal involvement, these features are not as pronounced as they are in malignant reticulosis. Before a diagnosis of malignant reticulosis is made, a complete microscopic examination must be performed on all available tissues to exclude the possibility of generalized lymphosarcoma with central nervous system involvement.

Biologic Features

Because of its rarity, a comprehensive understanding of the natural history of malignant reticulosis in the rat is not available. Only one publication (Krinke et al. 1985) reports a sizable number of tumors (19 neoplastic reticuloses out of a total of 89 primary brain tumors seen in a population of 4480 male and 4480 female Sprague-Dawley-derived rats). Nine of the affected rats were males, and ten were females. Sixteen of the affected rats were greater than 600 days of age. Only seven other cases of malignant reticulosis in the rat are reported in the literature. For three of these (Luginbühl 1963; Luginbühl et al. 1968), the strain was not stated. Two were reported in Sprague-Dawley-derived rats (Mawdesley-Thomas and Newman 1974; Newman and Mawdesley-Thomas 1974) and two in the Fischer 344 strain (Garman et al. 1985, 1986). In addition, three cases of "polymorphic cell sarcoma" have been reported in the rat spinal cord, one each in a Long-Evans (Innes and Borner 1961), Wistar-derived (Mawdesley-Thomas 1967) and Sprague-Dawley-derived (Mawdesley-Thomas and Newman 1974) rat. I have encountered malignant reticulosis only three times in a population of 3703 treated and control Fischer 344 rats aged 18 months or older. This same population had a total of 55 brain tumors (i.e., a frequency of 1.5% for all brain neoplasms and 0.08% for malignant reticulosis). Two of the rats with malignant reticulosis were males, and one was a female.

Malignant reticulosis in man is now generally considered to represent primary non-Hodgkin's lymphoma of the central nervous system (Casadei and Gambacorta 1985). Immunohistologic evaluations of these tumors for cell-associated immunoglobulin indicate that most are of B cell origin (Houthoff et al. 1978; Taylor et al. 1978). Isolation of Epstein-Barr virus DNA from a human central nervous system lymphoma (but not from adjacent normal brain tissue) has suggested a possible etiologic role for this virus (Hochberg et al. 1983). An association between primary cerebral lymphoma and immunosuppression is also recognized (Kay 1983). Whether immunosuppression plays a role in the development of malignant reticulosis in the rat is not known.

Comparison with Other Species

Malignant reticulosis in the rat is histologically similar to the comparable entity (i.e., primary lymphoma of the central nervous system) in man, but a series of rat neoplasms has yet to be evaluated for the presence of cell-associated immunoglobulins. Approximately 5% of human primary brain tumors are reported to be lymphomas, with half of these lymphomas being confined to the brain (Zimmerman 1984). The relative frequency of malignant reticulosis in our own series of Fischer 344 rats was similar (i.e., 5.4% of primary brain tumors). Primary reticulosis of the central nervous system has been reported in the dog (e.g., Koestner and Zeman 1962; Vandevelde et al. 1976), and lymphosarcomas represent a significant proportion of primary central nervous system neoplasms in the cat (Zaki and Hurvitz 1976). These neoplasms have been reported less frequently in the horse and cow (Luginbühl 1963; Luginbühl et al. 1968).

References

Casadei GP, Gambacorta M (1985) A clinicopathological study of seven cases of primary high-grade malignant non-Hodgkin's lymphoma of the central nervous system. Tumori 71: 501-507

Garman RH, Snellings WM, Maronpot RR (1985) Brain tumors in F344 rats associated with chronic inhalation exposure to ethylene oxide. Neurotoxicology 6: 117-137

Garman RH, Snellings WM, Maronpot RR (1986) Frequency, size and location of brain tumors in F-344 rats chronically exposed to ethylene oxide. Food Chem Toxicol 24: 145-153

Hochberg FH, Miller G, Schooley RT, Hirsch MS, Feorino P, Henle W (1983) Central nervous system lymphoma related to Epstein-Barr virus. N Engl J Med 309: 745-748

Houthoff HJ, Poppema S, Ebels EJ, Elema JD (1978) Intracranial malignant lymphomas: a morphologic and immunocytologic study of twenty cases. Acta Neuropathol (Berl) 44: 203-210

Innes JRM, Borner G (1961) Tumors of the central nervous system of rats: with report of two tumors of the spinal cord and comments on posterior paralysis. JNCI 26: 7719-735

Kalimo H, Lehto M, Nänto-Salonen K, Jalkanen M, Risteli L, Risteli J, Narva EV (1985) Characterization of the perivascular reticulin network in a case of primary brain lymphoma. Immunohistological demonstration of collagen types I, III, IV, V; laminin; and fibronectin. Acto Neuropathol (Berl) 66: 299-305

Kay HEM (1983) Immunosuppression and the risk of brain lymphoma. N Engl J Med 308: 1099-1100

Koestner A, Zeman W (1962) Primary reticuloses of the central nervous system in dogs. Am J Vet Res 23: 381-393

Krinke G, Naylor DC, Schmid S, Fröhlich E, Schnider K (1985) The incidence of naturally-occurring primary brain tumours in the laboratory rat. J Comp Pathol 95: 175-192

Luginbühl H (1963) Comparative aspects of tumors of the nervous system. Ann NY Acad Sci 108: 702-721

Luginbühl H, Fankhauser R, McGrath JT (1968) Spontaneous neoplasms of the nervous system in animals. Prog Neurol Surg 2: 85-164

Mawdesley-Thomas LE (1967) A polymorphic-cell sarcoma of the rat spinal cord. Lab Anim 1: 31-34

Mawdesley-Thomas LE, Newman AJ (1974) Some observations on spontaneously occurring tumours of the central nervous system of Sprague-Dawley derived rats. J Pathol 112: 107-116

Newman AJ, Mawdesley-Thomas LE (1974) Spontaneous tumours of the central nervous system of laboratory rats. J Comp Path 84: 39-50

Taylor CR, Russell R, Lukes RJ, Davis RL (1978) An immunohistological study of immunoglobulin content of primary central nervous system lymphomas. Cancer 41: 2197-2205

Vandevelde M, Higgins RJ, Greene CE (1976) Neoplasms of mesenchymal origin in the spinal cord and nerve roots of three dogs. Vet Pathol 13: 47-58

Zimmerman HM (1984) The pathology of primary brain tumors. Semin Roentgenol 19: 129-138

Zaki FA, Hurvitz AI (1976) Spontaneous neoplasms of the central nervous system of the cat. J Small Anim Pract 17: 773-782

Gliomas, Mouse

Kevin T. Morgan and Roger H. Alison

Synonyms. Oligodendroglioma, astrocytoma, oligoastrocytoma, mixed glioma, mixed oligoastroblastoma, glioblastoma, astroblastoma, spongioblastoma, ganglioglioma.

Gross Appearance

The mouse brain is small and requires careful examination if neoplasms are to be detected grossly. Large glial tumors may be evident on the exterior or cut surface of the brain during necropsy or tissue trimming. These neoplasms may occur as soft masses associated with the meninges or in the substance of the brain and they may be associated with areas of discoloration, cysts, or cavitation. Gliomas are whitish gray, but may contain zones of reddish or brownish discoloration due to the presence of erythrocytes or blood pigments.

Microscopic Features

Glial cell tumors vary in morphologic appearance and may be subclassified on the basis of histologic features according to a number of simple (Ward and Rice 1982) or complex (Zimmerman and Innes 1979; Morgan et al. 1984) classification schemes. The majority of these neoplasms are comprised of well-differentiated oligodendrocytes (Fig. 130), astrocytes (Fig. 131), or a mixture of these cells (Fig. 132). Nuclear morphology is a useful diagnostic feature, with oligodendrocytes having round-to-oval, darkly staining nuclei, while astrocyte nuclei are oval and contain little chromatin. However, in routine histologic preparations, it may be difficult to distinguish these cell types from each other or from poorly differentiated neoplastic cells of nonglial origin. Special stains (Zimmerman and Innes 1979), electron microscopy (Zülch 1981), and immunocytochemistry (Schneider et al. 1986) may be of value if the tissue is appropriately fixed.

Gliomas Derived from Oligodendroglia. These neoplasms are generally present in the cerebrum and/or diencephalon, especially involving the thalamus, hypothalamus, and amygdala (Morgan et al. 1984). Oligodendrogliomas are generally poorly circumscribed and may involve the overlying meninges (Fig. 133). The histologic pattern

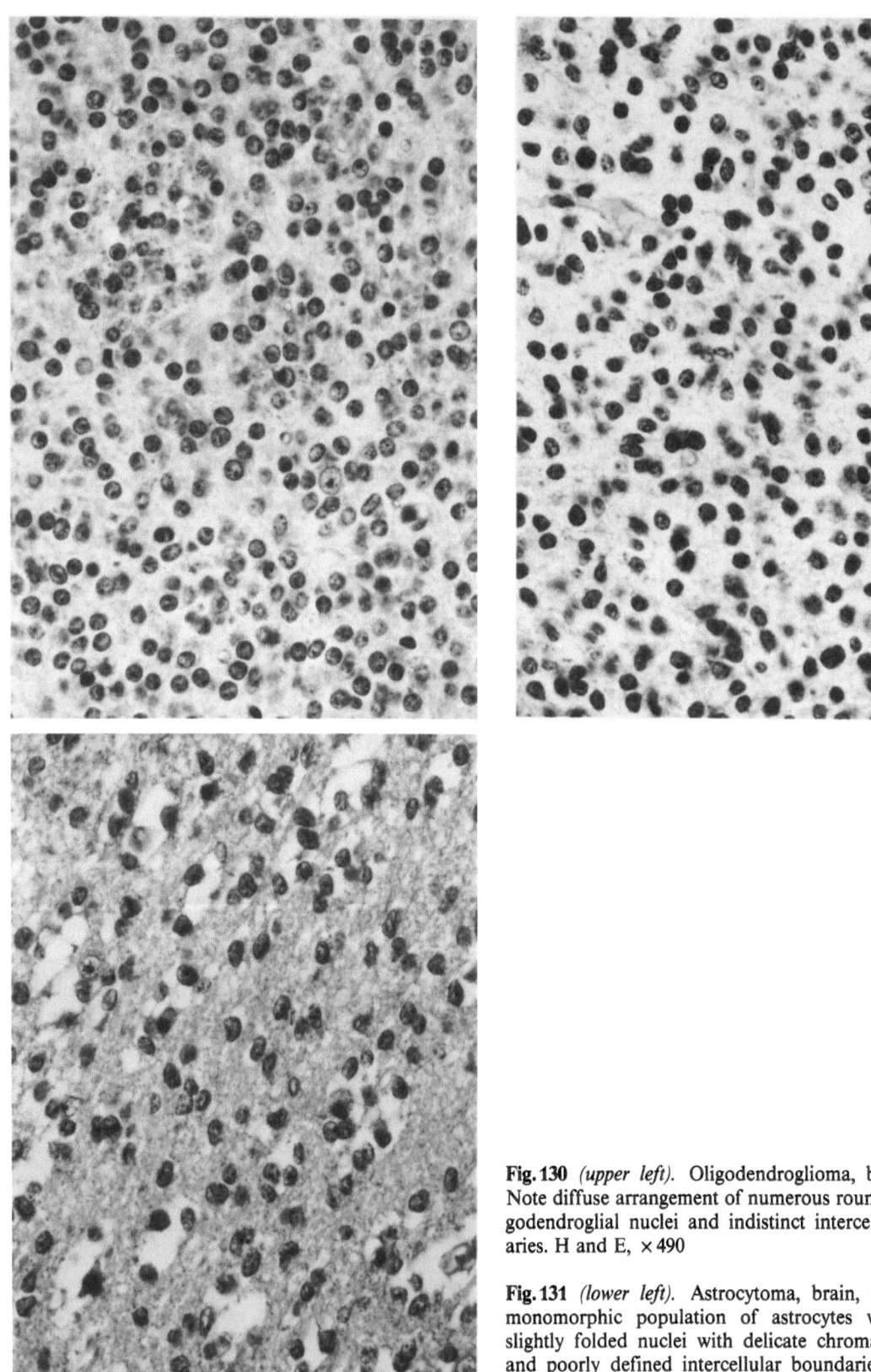

Fig. 130 *(upper left)*. Oligodendroglioma, brain, mouse. Note diffuse arrangement of numerous round-to-oval oligodendroglial nuclei and indistinct intercellular boundaries. H and E, × 490

Fig. 131 *(lower left)*. Astrocytoma, brain, mouse. Note monomorphic population of astrocytes with oval or slightly folded nuclei with delicate chromatin stippling and poorly defined intercellular boundaries. H and E, × 490

Fig. 132 *(upper right)*. Mixed glioma, brain, mouse. Note glial cell nuclei with both oligodendroglial and astroglial characteristics. H and E, × 490

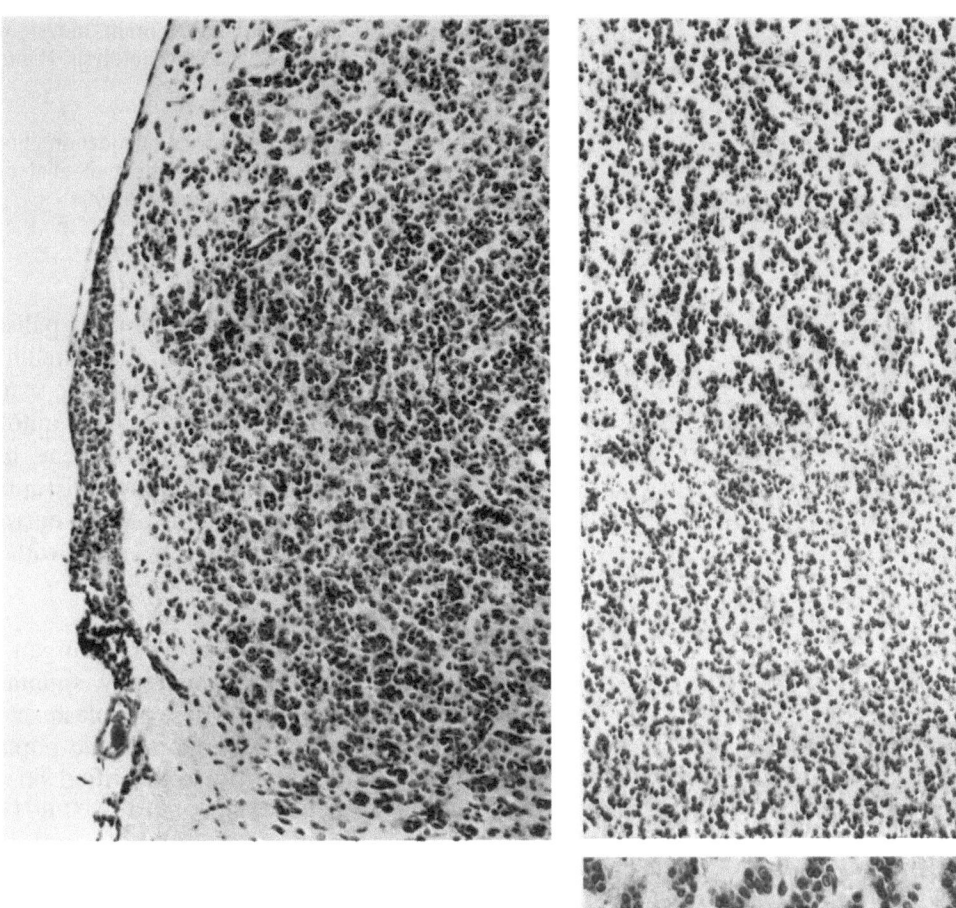

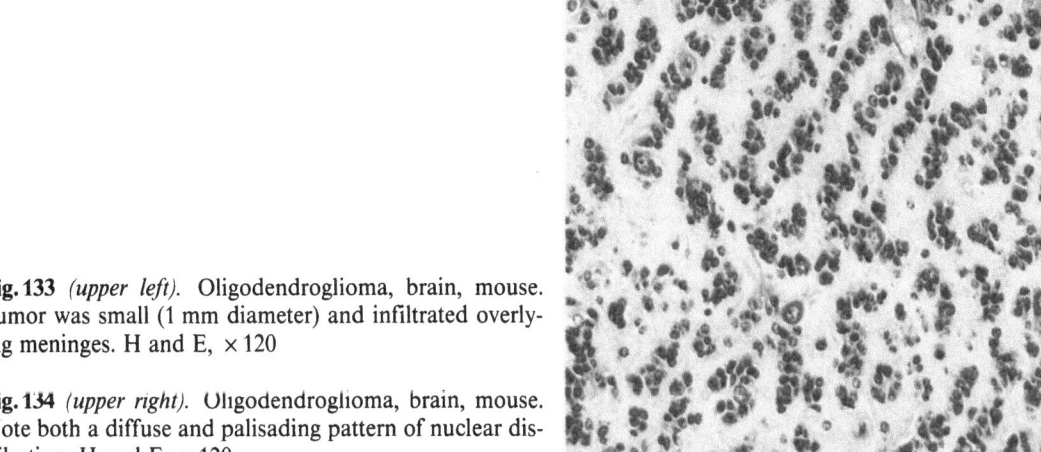

Fig. 133 *(upper left)*. Oligodendroglioma, brain, mouse. Tumor was small (1 mm diameter) and infiltrated overlying meninges. H and E, × 120

Fig. 134 *(upper right)*. Oligodendroglioma, brain, mouse. Note both a diffuse and palisading pattern of nuclear distribution. H and E, × 120

Fig. 135 *(lower right)*. Oligodendroglioma, brain mouse, with nuclear palisading and neuronal satellitosis. H and E, × 245

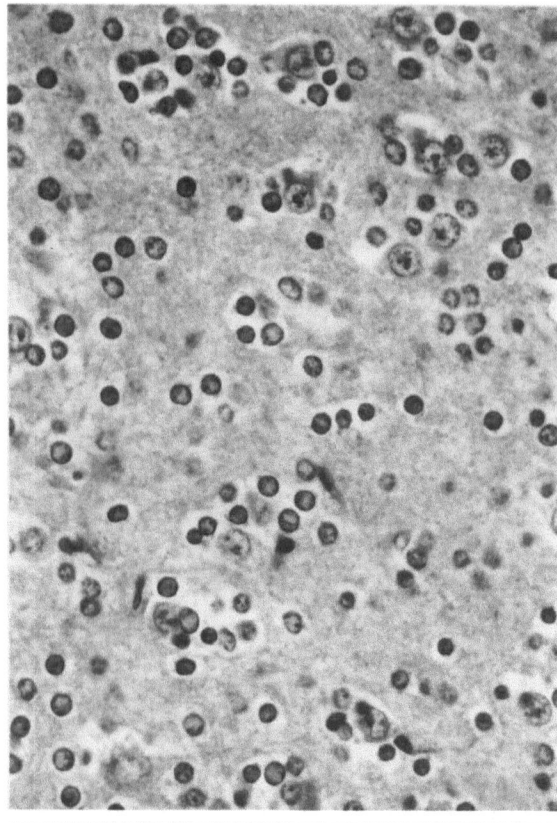

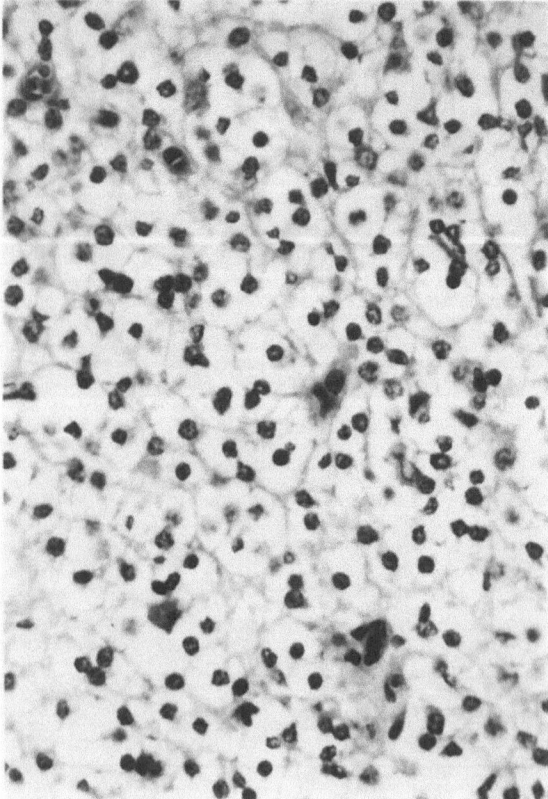

◀ **Fig. 136** *(above)*. Oligodendroglioma, brain, mouse, with perinuclear halos associated with early autolysis. H and E, × 490

Fig. 137 *(below)*. Glioma, probably an oligodendroglioma, brain, mouse. Note severe clear swelling of glial cytoplasm as a result of autolysis. H and E, × 490

is often diffuse (Fig. 134), while nuclear palisading (Figs. 134 and 135) and neuronal satellitosis may be present. The neoplastic cells have scanty, indistinct cytoplasm which may undergo autolytic distension resulting in a perinuclear halo (Fig. 136) or severe edematous disruption (Fig. 137). Mitotic figures are rare, while necrosis and hemorrhage may be present along with an associated inflammatory response.

Gliomas Derived from Astrocytes. Morgan et al. (1984) described four, apparently spontaneous, astrocytomas in mice. These neoplasms were composed of a generally monomorphic population of astrocytes which were identified on the basis of their nuclear characteristics (Fig. 131). These astrocytomas were present in the ventrolateral cerebrum and were comprised of cells with indistinct cytoplasmic boundaries and large, oval or slightly folded nuclei with very delicate chromatin stippling. The neoplasms had indistinct margins and contained areas of edema and hemorrhage. Variable numbers of oligodendroglia were also present as a minor component. Astrocytic tumors with necrosis, anaplasia, and giant cell formation may be further classified as "glioblastoma multiforme" (Morgan et al. 1984). With the present small number of reported murine gliomas the value of such subclassification remains speculative. Astrocytomas occur with fairly high frequency on BRVR and VM mice, in the forebrain (Figs. 138 and 139), mid- and hindbrain, or the spinal cord. These neoplasms consist of undifferentiated astrocytes which infiltrate but do not distort the brain (Fraser 1986).

Gliomas of Mixed or Intermediate Cell Types. Tumors with morphologic characteristics intermediate between astrocytes and oligodendrocytes, or in which neoplastic cells derived from both of these cell types contribute significantly to the neoplastic process (Fig. 132), may be classified as "mixed gliomas."

Other Glial Neoplasms. Neoplasms with histologic features of other glial tumors of humans, such as

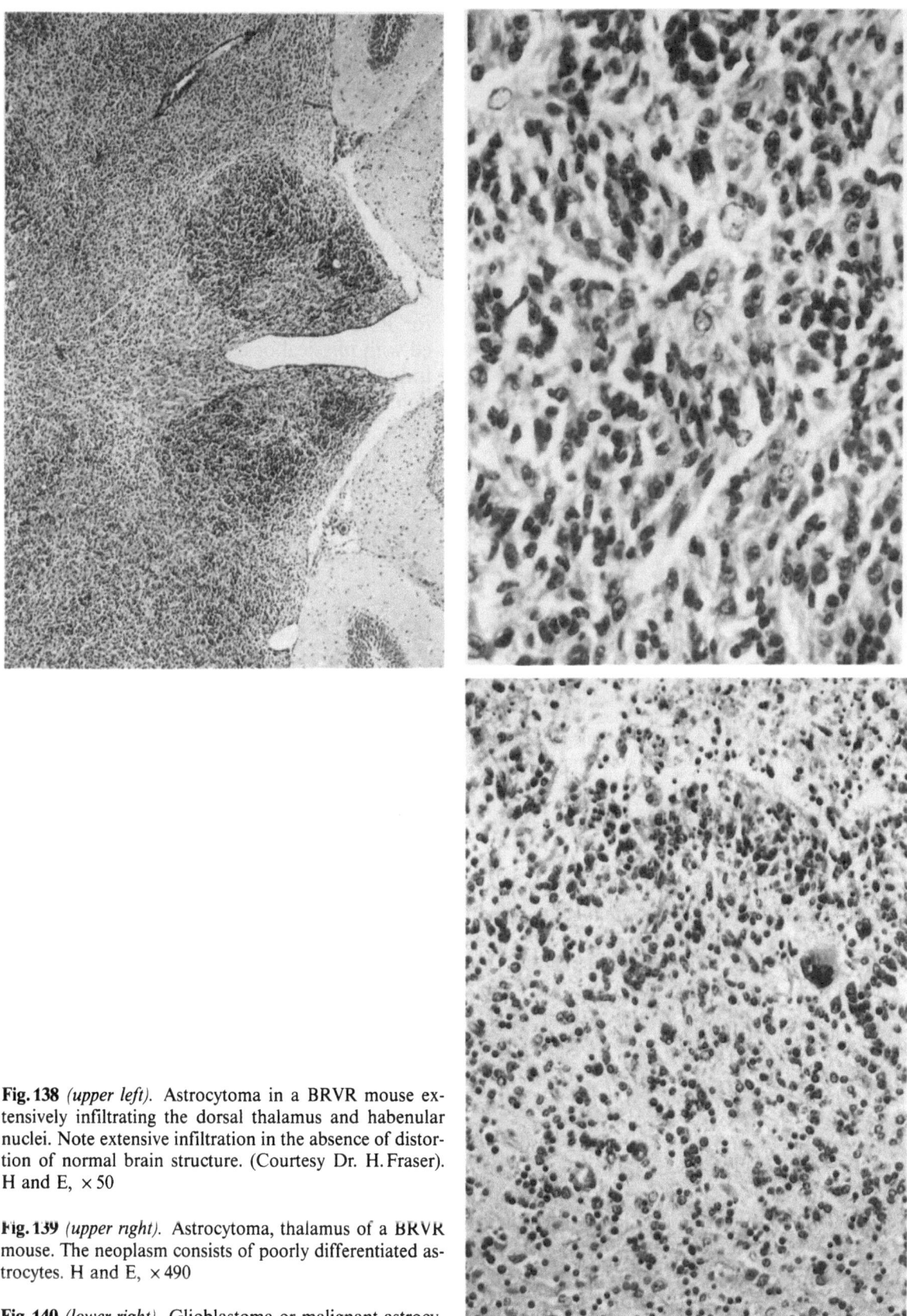

Fig. 138 *(upper left).* Astrocytoma in a BRVR mouse extensively infiltrating the dorsal thalamus and habenular nuclei. Note extensive infiltration in the absence of distortion of normal brain structure. (Courtesy Dr. H. Fraser). H and E, × 50

Fig. 139 *(upper right).* Astrocytoma, thalamus of a BRVR mouse. The neoplasm consists of poorly differentiated astrocytes. H and E, × 490

Fig. 140 *(lower right).* Glioblastoma or malignant astrocytoma, brain, mouse, with pleomorphic neoplastic astrocytes, giant cells, and an area of necrosis with pseudopalisading. H and E, × 245

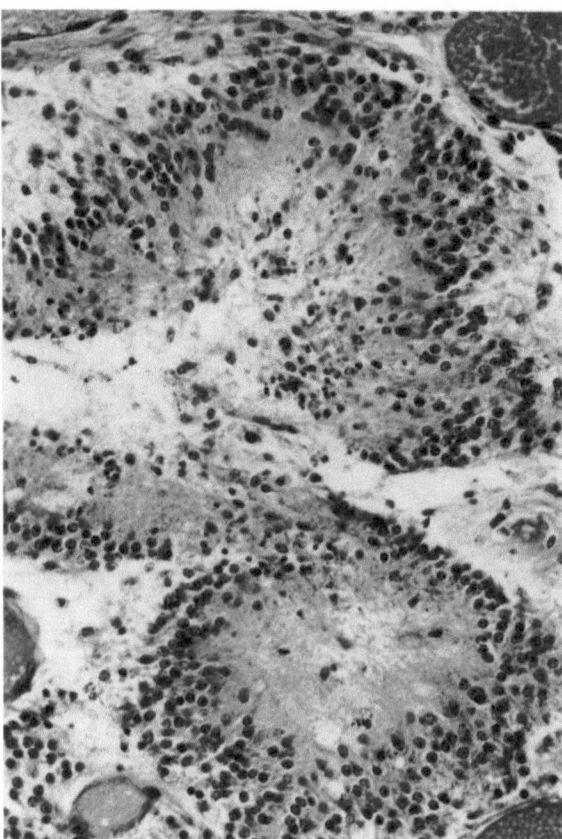

Fig. 141. Glioma of uncertain type (possibly glioblastoma or astroblastoma) with a distinctive cellular arrangement. Note small, densely basophilic nuclei arranged adjacent to connective tissue containing blood vessels, and small foci of necrotic tumor cells. H and E, × 245

glioblastoma (Figs. 140 and 141), glioblastoma multiforme, monstrocellular glioma, and spongioblastoma have been reported in mice (Zimmerman and Innes 1979; Morgan et al. 1984) and should be considered during diagnosis. Ependymomas, tumors of the ependyma, are also considered to be derived from glial cells (Rubinstein 1972) and are classified with the gliomas and have been reported to occur in mice (Zimmerman and Innes 1979).

Ultrastructure

Electron microscopy might be of diagnostic value by permitting the idenfication of cell-specific organelles, such as glial fibrils. This technique is, however, becoming superseded by more specific immunocytochemical methods which may be applied directly to tissue sections.

Differential Diagnosis

Lack of familiarity with the normal mouse brain may result in misdiagnoses. Structures which may be mistaken for glial tumors include the subcommissural and subfornical organs (Zimmerman and Innes 1979) and the pineal body. Adequate examination of brains from control animals, the use of carefully prepared transverse sections which display the bilateral symmetry of normal brain structures, and reference to texts of rodent neuroanatomy should prevent such an error. Rare brain malformations or gliosis associated with physical or chemical damage to the central nervous systems may result in glial proliferation resembling a neoplastic process. Metastases from lymphomas and other neoplasms comprised of small rounded cells can mimic gliomas, particularly when autolyzed. The perivascular location of tumor metastases and identification of the primary neoplasm should help one to make a correct diagnosis.

Biologic Features

Gliomas of the brain and spinal cord originate from cells of the glial stroma, oligodendrocytes, astrocytes, and ependymal cells, while the other basic glial cell type, microglia, appear not to produce neoplasms (Zimmerman and Innes 1979). There has been much debate concerning the classification of glial tumors in humans, for which there is a fairly large data base with considerable information on the associated clinical course (Rubinstein 1972). This debate has been complicated by the fact that many, if not all, gliomas contain a mixture of different glial types (Zimmerman and Innes 1979). In mice, with the exception of certain strains, spontaneous glial tumors are extremely rare (Zimmerman and Innes 1979; Morgan et al. 1984); Solleveld et al. 1986). Thus, in spite of the morphologic similarity between murine and human gliomas, little information is available concerning the biology and significance of histologic patterns with respect to malignant potential of glial tumors in mice. During examination of brain tumors it is worth noting that all central nervous system neoplasms may be considered malignant due to the harmful effects of a space occupying lesion within the rigidly enclosed cranial space (Cordy 1978). In mice, glial cell tumors may be associated with clinical signs of nervous system disturbance (Zimmerman and Innes 1979; Morgan et al. 1984), and these tumors can spread via the meninges or the cerebrospinal fluid, but rarely metastasize to remote sites (Cordy 1978).

The unusually high incidence of astrocytomas found by Fraser (1971) in VM and BRVR mice permitted immunocytochemical demonstration of their astrocytic nature and determation of biologic features including growth characteristics following transplantation into different strains of mice (Fraser 1986). Furthermore, a transplantable astrocytoma was derived from a spontaneous neoplasm which arose in a VM female, and from this tumor cell lines have been propogated in extraneural locations and in tissue culture (Fraser 1986).

Etiology and Frequency. Little is known of the etiology of spontaneous gliomas in mice, but they generally arise in older animals (Morgan et al. 1984). The high incidence of astrocytomas in VM and BRVR mice, and the higher frequency of these neoplasms in males, suggests possible genetic influence, but this association is apparently independent of the histocompatibility of the strains concerned (Fraser 1986). Unidentified environmental factors may also play a role in the induction of 'spontaneous' murine glial tumors. Gliomas have been induced experimentally in many species, including mice, by a wide range of procedures, including exposure to radiation, certain viral agents, and intracerebral injections of chemicals such as methylcholanthrene and benzpyrene. These procedures and the numerous results achieved have been reviewed extensively (Jänisch and Schreiber 1977a, b; Zimmerman and Innes 1979; Swenberg 1982).

Spontaneous tumors of the central nervous system of mice are very rare (Zimmerman and Innes 1979; Morgan et al. 1984). Excluding certain strains of mice with an unusually high incidence of brain tumors, the overall incidence was reported to be less than 0.1%, with a range of 0.01%–0.07% for strains of mice in which more than 2000 brains had been examined (Swenberg 1982). Morgan et al. (1984) reported an incidence of 0.54%, of which the majority were considered to be spontaneous, in a population of 77.410 mice. Only 17 gliomas (0.022%) were present in this study, the majority of which occurred in BALB/c mice and were classified as oligodendrogliomas. Thus apart from VM and BRVR mice (Fraser 1986), with a 1% incidence of astrocytomas, spontaneous gliomas are rare in mice.

Comparison with Other Species

Tumors of the central nervous system in mice bear a striking morphologic resemblance to their human equivalents (Zimmerman and Innes 1979). It remains to be determinend whether rodent brain tumors have similar biologic behavior to their human counterparts (Morgan et al. 1984). Spontaneous gliomas generally occur much less frequently in mice than in humans. The increased frequency of astrocytomas in male VM and BRVR mice parallels the sex relationship for human brain tumor incidence (Fraser 1986). Tumors of the central nervous system have been reported in many domestic species and have been most extensively investigated in the dog (Cordy 1978). Gliomas are more common in brachycephalic dogs, especially boxers, and as in mice, brain tumors in dogs are age associated (Cordy 1978).

References

Cordy DR (1978) Tumors of the nervous system and eye. In: Moulton JE (ed) Tumors in domestic animals. University of California Press, Berkeley, CA, pp 430-455

Fraser H (1971) Astrocytomas in an inbred mouse strain. J Pathol 103: 266-270

Fraser H (1986) Brain tumours in mice, with particular reference to astrocytoma. Food Chem Toxicol 24: 105-111

Jänisch W, Schreiber D (1977a) Spontaneous CNS tumors in animals. In: DD Bigner, JA Swenberg (eds) Experimental tumors of the central nervous system. Upjohn, Kalamazoo, Michigan, pp 81-82

Jänisch W, Schreiber D (1977b) Methods of inducing experimental CNS tumors. In: DD Bigner, JA Swenberg (eds) Experimental tumors of the central nervous system. Upjohn, Kalamazoo, Michigan, pp 83-99

Morgan KT, Frith CH, Swenberg JA, McGrath JT, Zulch KJ, Crowder DM (1984) A morphologic classification of brain tumors found in several strains of mice. JNCI 72: 151-160

Rubinstein LJ (1972) Tumors of mesodermal tissues. In: Atlas of tumor pathology. Tumors of the central nervous system. Second Series, Fascicle 6. AFIP, Washington, DC

Schneider SL, Sasaki F, Zeltzer PM (1986) Normal and malignant neural cells: a comprehensive survey of human and murine nervous system markers. CRC Crit Rev Oncol Hematol 5: 199-234

Solleveld HA, Bigner DD, Averill DR Jr, Bigner SH, Boorman GA, Burger PC, Gillespie Y, Hubbard GB, Laerum OD, McComb RD, McGrath JT, Morgan KT, Peters A, Rubinstein LJ, Schoenberg BS, Schold SC, Swenberg JA, Thompson MB, Vandevelde M, Vinores SA (1986) Brain tumors in man and animals: report of a workshop. Environ Health Persp 68: 155-173

Swenberg JA (1982) Neoplasms of the nervous system. In: Foster HL, Small JD, Fox JG (eds) The mouse in biomedial research, vol IV. Academic, New York, pp 529–537

Ward JM, Rice JM (1982) Naturally occurring and chemically induced brain tumors of rats and mice in carcinogenesis bioassays. Ann NY Acad Sci 381: 304–319

Zimmermam HM, Innes JRM (1979) Tumours of the central and peripheral nervous systems. In: Turusov VS (ed) Tumours of the mouse. IARC, Lyon, pp 629–654 (Pathology of tumours in laboratory animals, vol II)

Zülch KJ (1981) Problems of the classification of tumors of the nervous system and the significance of electron microscopy. Folia Histochem Cytochem 19: 171–178

Lipoma, Brain, Mouse

Kevin T. Morgan and Winslow G. Sheldon

Synonyms. Intracranial "lipoma," lipomatous hamartoma, lipomatous choristoma.

Gross Appearance

Lipomas in the brains of mice are generally small and are unlikely to be observed during gross examination. Only one of 15 lipomas in one series was detected grossly. It formed a small whitish mass in the cerebellar meninges (Morgan et al. 1984).

Microscopic Features

These tumors consist of small, well-demarcated foci or masses of cells which contain abundant stored fat and resemble fat cells of adipose tissue (Morgan et al. 1984). Lipomas may be present as single (Figs. 142 and 143) or multiple (Figs. 144 and 145) small clusters of adipocytes, each cell generally containing a single large fat droplet (Figs. 143 and 146).

These fatty nodules may be found in the connective tissue between the corpus callosum and the roof of the third ventricle (Fig. 142), in the choroidal interstitium (Figs. 145 and 146), or in the meninges of the median longitudinal fissure adjacent to the cingulate cortex (Fig. 144). They have also been reported in the choroid plexus of the lateral ventricles and fourth ventricle, and in the cerebellar meninges (Morgan et al. 1984).

Cartilage-like material and tissue resembling bone marrow devoid of hematopoietic elements have been reported within these neoplasms (Morgan et al. 1984). Intracranial lipomas of mice may be associated with dysgenesis of the corpus callosum (Figs. 144, 145 and 147) and lateral displacement of adjacent blood vessels (Fig. 148).

Ultrastructure

No information was found on the ultrastructure of murine intracranial lipomas.

Differential Diagnosis

These masses of mature adipocytes have a characteristic appearance and are unlikely to be misdiagnosed. Teratomas of the third ventricle may contain adipose tissue and thus might be confused with lipomas if other structures represent a minimal component of the tumor. Displacement of soft tissues from the skin and adnexa could re-

Fig. 142 *(upper left).* Lipoma adjacent to the roof of the ▶ third ventricle, brain, mouse. H and E, × 120

Fig. 143 *(lower left).* Higher magnification of lipoma shown in Fig. 142. The mass is composed of well-differentiated adipocytes resembling those seen in adipose tissue, the majority having a single, large fat vacuole. H and E, × 490

Fig. 144 *(upper right).* Brain, mouse. Three small lipomas in the choroid plexus and meninges of the median fissure. These may represent three parts of a single mass. Note abnormal constriction of the corpus callosum at the midline. H and E, × 50

Fig. 145 *(lower right).* Brain, mouse. Higher magnification of Fig. 144. Bilateral clusters of adipocytes in the choroid plexus of the third ventricle, midline constriction of the corpus callosum, and excessive connective tissue in the midline. H and E, × 120

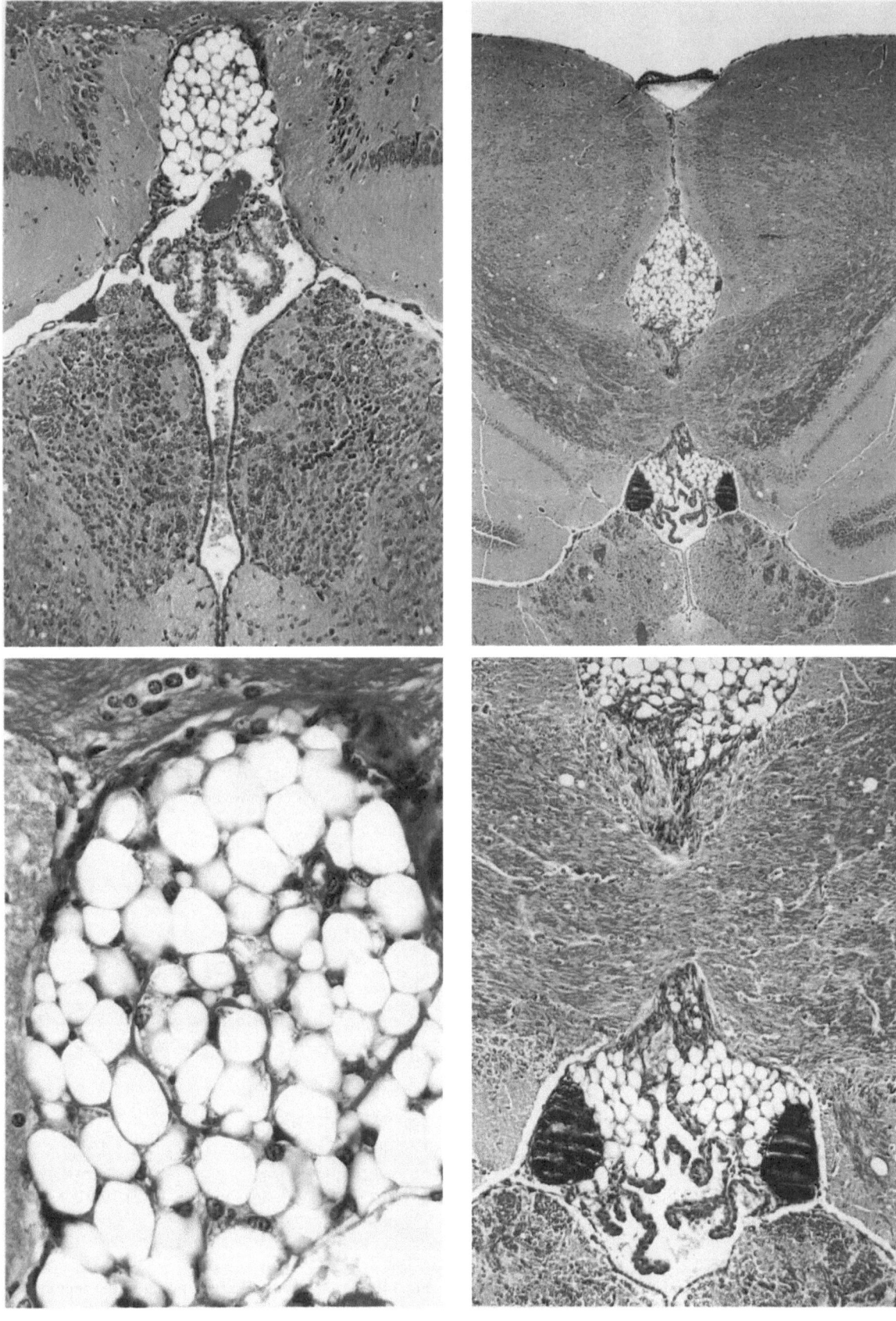

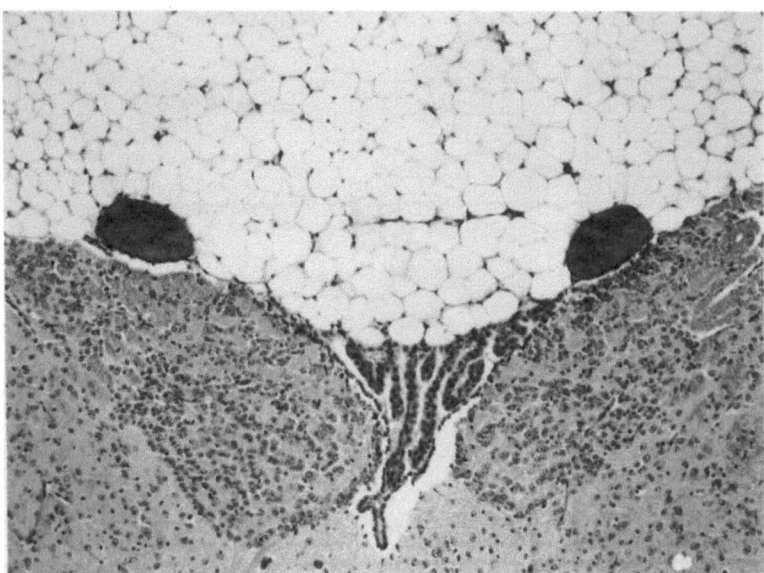

Fig. 146. Brain, mouse. Small lipoma in the interstitium of the choroid plexus of the third ventricle. H and E, × 120

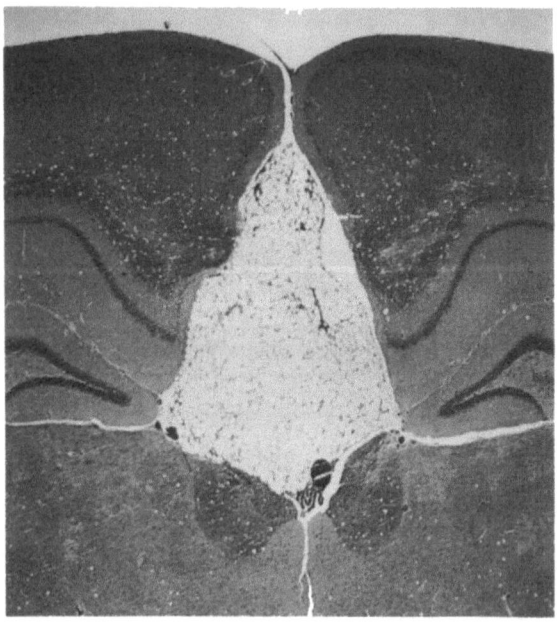

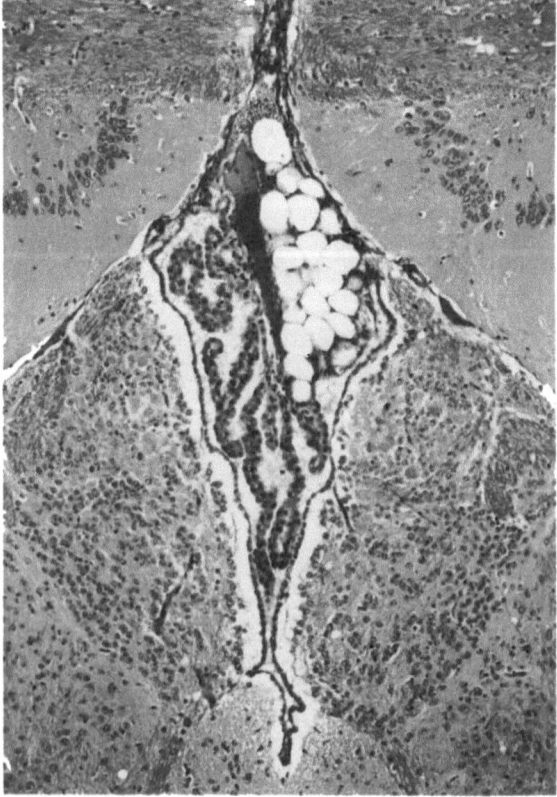

Fig. 147. Brain, mouse. Lipoma in region of the third ventricle and median fissure. Corpus callosum and other midline structures replaced by the mass of adipocytes; other structures, including the habenular nuclei are displaced ventro-laterally. H and E, × 25

Fig. 148. Brain, mouse. Large lipoma in the region of the roof of the third ventricle, associated with distortion and lateral displacement of the habenular nuclei and adjacent blood vessels. H and E, × 120

sult in the artifactual transfer of adipocytes to the brain (Zimmerman and Innes 1979). Evidence of tissue damage and the presence of hairs or other adnexal structures would prevent such misinterpretation.

Biologic Features

Intracranial "lipomas" in mice are probably not true neoplasms (Morgan et al. 1984; Fraser 1986) and, as in man, they may represent a consequence of a neural tube closure defect during embryogenesis (Soeur et al. 1979). Intracranial lipomas in mice are generally close to the midline (Fraser 1986; Morgan et al. 1984), but they occur in a number of sites, suggesting that the defect may arise at different stages during neural tube closure. These lipomas may be associated with defective formation of structures adjacent to the roof of the third ventricle, including the corpus callosum (Figs. 144 and 147). The term "lipomatous hamartoma" may be more appropriate for these lesions (Budka 1974); however, numerous reports of human examples use the term "lipoma." Until the pathogenesis of this lesion is finally clarified, toxicologic pathologists might be best advised to continue with this practice. It is important to provide a clear indication to nonpathologists that this lesion is not neoplastic in nature. Intracranial lipomas have been reported in a number of strains of mice, including C57BL, BRVR, VM, and VM crosses (Fraser 1971, 1986), BALB/c (Morgan et al. 1984), and B6C3F$_1$ (Solleveld et al. 1986), in both males and females.

Etiology and Frequency. The cause of intracranial lipomas in mice is at present unknown. Similar lesions in humans have been classified with other midline anomalies of the brain, for which the exact causes also remain unknown (Fitz 1982). Intracranial lipomas are rare in mice, having an incidence of 0.019% in one study in which 77.410 mice were examined (Morgan et al. 1984). Most murine intracranial lipomas are small, and cases may have been missed during section preparation, resulting in underestimation of their true incidence. No reports were found on experimental induction of intracranial lipomas in mice.

Comparison with Other Species

Intracranial lipomas in mice show remarkable resemblance in sites of occurrence and morphology to lipomas reported in the brains of humans. In humans, as in mice, intracranial lipomas are rare, with only about 100 cases having been reported since their first description in 1856 (Fujii et al. 1982). Human intracranial lipomas are frequently associated with agenesis of the corpus callosum (Fitz 1982), dysraphism, frontal bone defects (Zee et al. 1981), and vascular abnormalities (Eldevik and Gabrielsen 1975). During examination of slides for the present article, similar lesions to those reported in man were found in association with lipomas in BALB/c mice from the National Center for Toxicological Research. These abnormalities included dysgenesis of the corpus callosum and displacement of associated blood vessels. These lesions in mice closely parallel cases reported in man, providing a potentially useful model for a condition which may be associated with severe nervous system disturbance in humans (Fujii et al. 1982). The authors located only two reports of intracranial lipomas in other species. One was associated with a meningocele in bovine calf (Gopal and Leipold 1979), and the other was found in the brain of a humpback whale (Pilleri 1966).

References

Budka H (1974) Intracranial lipomatous hamartomas (intracranial "lipomas"). A study of 13 cases including combinations with medulloblastoma, colloid and epidermoid cysts, angiomatosis and other malformations. Acta Neuropathol (Berl) 28: 205–222

Eldevik OP, Gabrielsen TO (1975) Fusiform aneurysmal dilatation of pericallosal artery: a sign of lipoma of corpus callosum. Acta Radiol [Suppl] (Stockh) 347: 71–76

Fitz CR (1982) Midline anomalies of the brain and spine. Radiol Clin North Am 20: 95–104

Fraser H (1971) Astrocytomas in an inbred mouse strain. J Pathol 103: 266–270

Fraser H (1986) Brain tumours in mice, with particular reference to astrocytoma. Food Chem Toxicol 24: 105–111

Fujii T, Takao T, Ito M, Konishi Y, Okuno T, Suzuki J (1982) Lipoma of the corpus callosum: a case report with a review. Comput Radiol 6: 301–304

Gopal T, Leipold HW (1979) Lipomeningocele in a calf. Vet Pathol 16: 610–612

Morgan KT, Frith CH, Swenberg JA, McGrath JT, Zulch KJ, Crowder DM (1984) A morphologic classification of brain tumors found in several strains of mice. JNCI 72: 151–160

Pilleri G (1966) Brain lipoma in the humpback whale, *Megaptera novaeangliae* (in German). Pathol Vet 3: 341–349

Soeur M, Monseu G, Ketelbant P, Flament-Durand J (1979) Intramedullary ependymoma producing collagen. A clinical and pathological study. Acta Neuropathol (Berl) 47: 159-160

Solleveld HA, Bigner DD, Averill DR Jr, Bigner SH, Boorman GA, Burger PC, Gillespie Y, Hubbard GB, Laerum OD, McComb RD, McGrath JT, Morgan KT, Peters A, Rubinstein LJ, Schoenberg BS, Schold SC, Swenberg JA, Thompson MB, Vandevelde M, Vinores SA (1986) Brain tumors in man and animals: reports of a workshop. Environ Health Persp 68: 155-173

Zee C-S, McComb JG, Segall HD, Tsai FY, Stanley P (1981) Lipomas of the corpus callosum associated with frontal dysraphism. J Comput Assist Tomogr 5: 201-205

Zimmerman HM, Innes JRM (1979) Tumours of the central and peripheral nervous systems: in: Turusov VS (ed) Tumours of the mouse. IARC, Lyon, pp 629-654 (Pathology of tumours in laboratory animals, vol II)

Gliomas, Rat

Vernon E. Walker and James A. Swenberg

Synonyms. Astrocytoma; astrocytic glioma; oligodendroglioma; oligodendrocytoma; mixed glioma; oligo-astrocytoma; glioblastoma; spongioblastoma; ependymoma.

Gross Appearance

Gliomas may range in size from microscopic foci to masses 10 mm or more in diameter, but less than half are visible grossly. In a recent review of brain tumors in untreated control rats only five of the 18 astrocytomas in females (28%) and 12 of the 28 astrocytomas in males (43%) were macroscopically detectable at necropsy (Gopinath 1986).

Astrocytomas are reported to occur throughout the brain in F344 rats (Ward and Rice 1982) and predominately in the cerebrum in Sprague-Dawley rats (Newman and Mawdesley-Thomas 1974; Gopinath 1986). They may be apparent on the surface of the brain as symmetrical or asymmetrical swellings, areas of varying discoloration, grayish masses, or surface depressions. On the cut surface, astrocytomas generally appear as poorly circumscribed, spherical, soft to moderately firm, smooth, gray-white to tan masses. Occasional areas of hemorrhage and necrosis may make the tissue mottled and friable, and cysts are sometimes present. Tumor margins usually blend into the surrounding parenchyma.

Oligodendrogliomas have been found chiefly in the cerebral hemispheres, basal ganglia, and corpus callosum (Ward and Rice 1982). Small tumors are generally well-defined masses which otherwise resemble astrocytomas grossly. Larger neoplasms frequently have less discrete borders and friable, discolored foci of hemorrhage and necrosis.

Mixed gliomas commonly have the topographic distribution and gross appearance of oligodendrogliomas except that they are usually poorly demarcated. Large neoplasms are frequently cystic.

Microscopic Appearance

Astrocytomas vary considerably in their architecture and degree of differentiation. They have nondiscrete borders and are composed of sheets of moderately to densely packed cells in a fine vascular stroma (Fig. 149). Less frequently, cells occur in loosely scattered whorls and clusters (Fig. 150) or interlacing bundles (Fig. 151). Cell morphology may vary slightly depending upon the anatomic location of the neoplasm, but areas of fibrous astrocytes are usually present. Individual cells are generally fusiform to round with indistinct cell borders, moderate amounts of homogeneous to fibrillar eosinophilic cytoplasm, and spindle-shaped to round euchromatic or hyperchromatic nuclei. Nuclear chromatin is evenly distributed to marginated, and nucleoli range from distinct to indistinct. A rate tumor may have bizarre and/or multinucleated giant cells. Normal and abnormal mitotic figures range in occurrence from rare to frequent. Tumor margins frequently exhibit diffusely infiltrative growth with neoplastic astrocytes surrounding neurons (neuronal satellitosis) (Fig. 152) and blood vessels (Fig. 153). Invasion along blood vessels may be seen considerable distances from the main tumor mass. Meningeal, ependymal, and ventricular in-

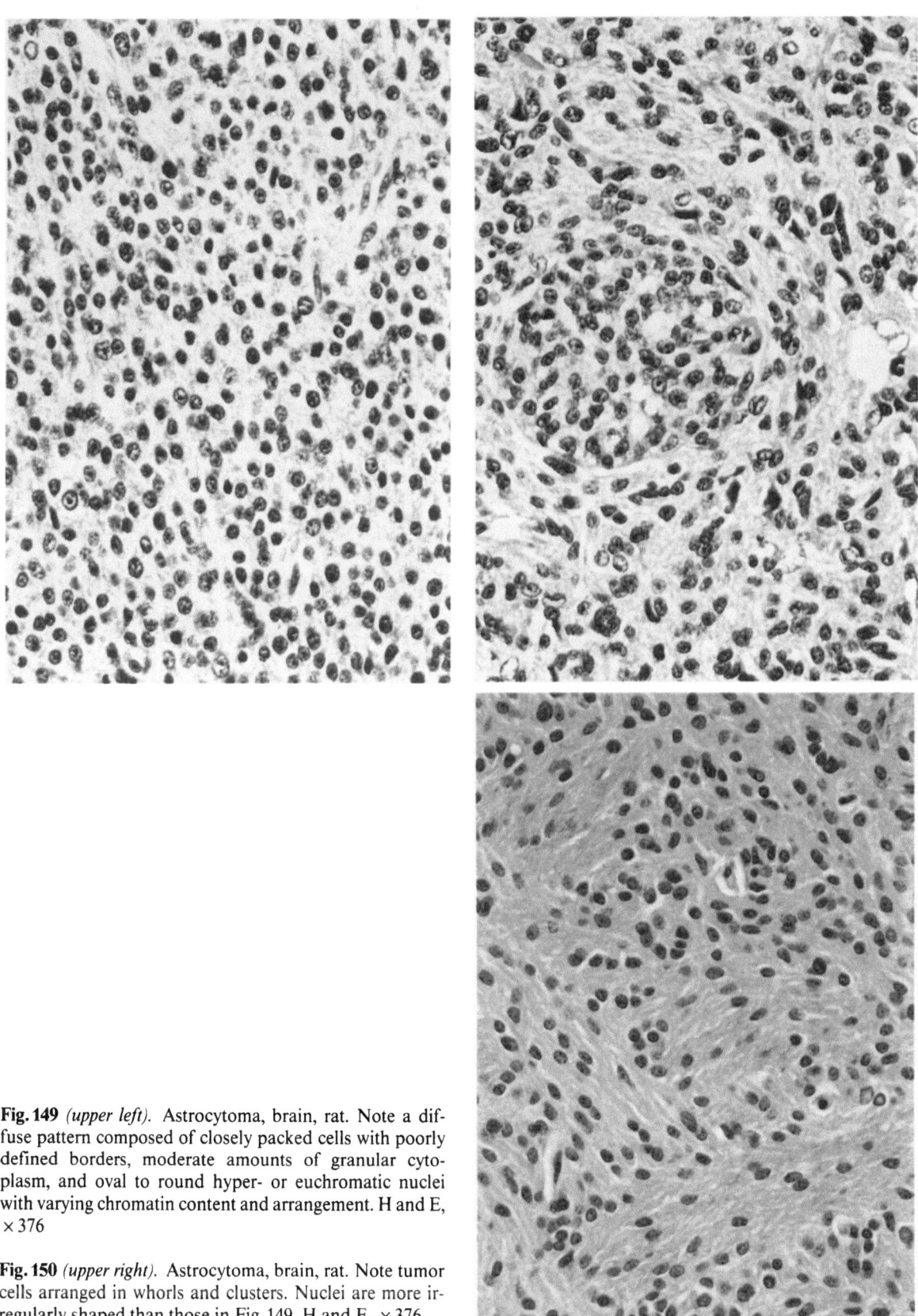

Fig. 149 *(upper left).* Astrocytoma, brain, rat. Note a diffuse pattern composed of closely packed cells with poorly defined borders, moderate amounts of granular cytoplasm, and oval to round hyper- or euchromatic nuclei with varying chromatin content and arrangement. H and E, ×376

Fig. 150 *(upper right).* Astrocytoma, brain, rat. Note tumor cells arranged in whorls and clusters. Nuclei are more irregularly shaped than those in Fig. 149. H and E, ×376

Fig. 151 *(lower right).* Astrocytoma, brain, rat. Note interlacing bundles of spindle-shaped cells with fibrillar cytoplasm. H and E, ×310

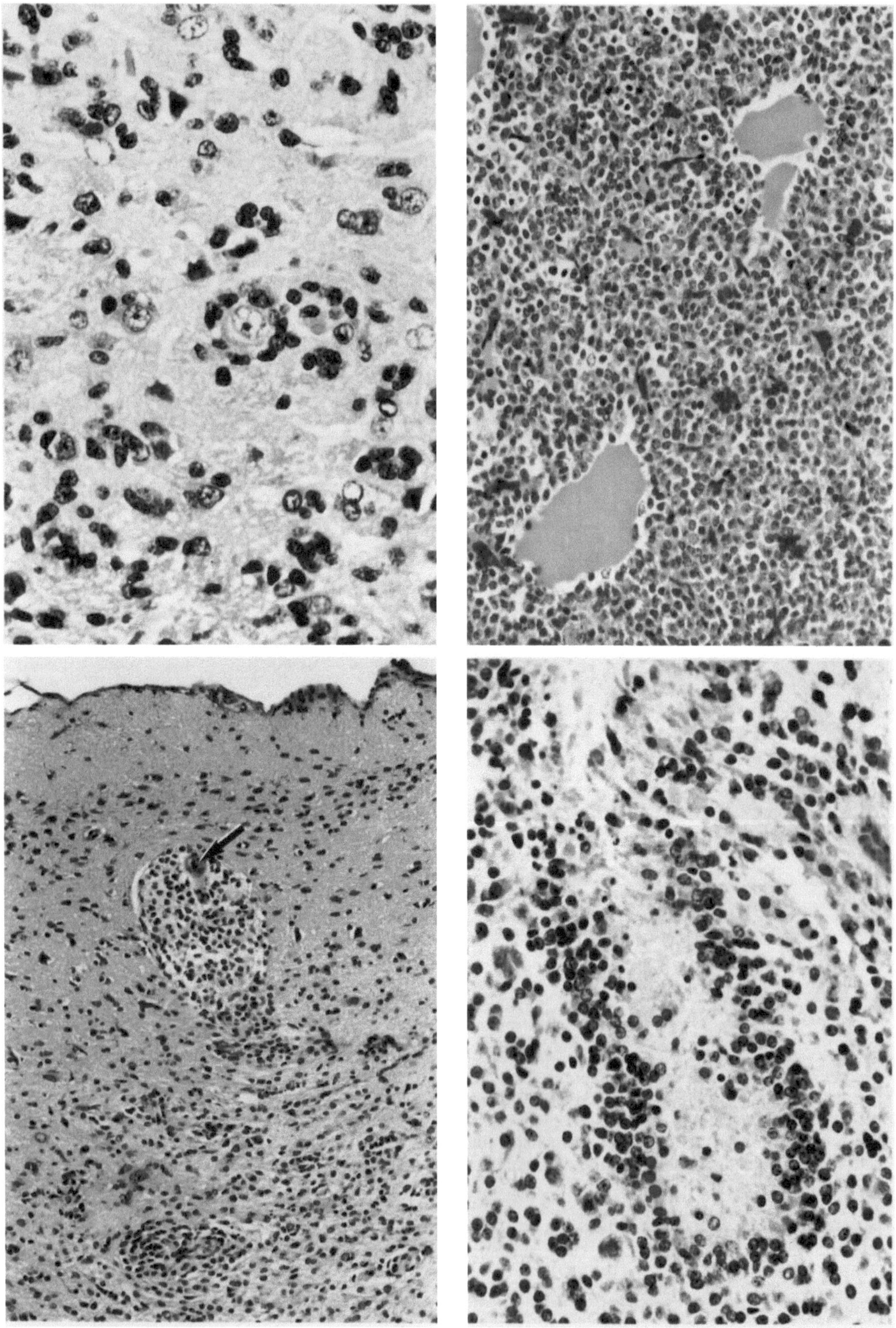

vasions are common. Cystic changes (Fig. 154) and pseudopalisading of tumor cells around foci of hemorrhage or necrosis (Fig. 155) occur infrequently and are usually associated with anaplastic astrocytomas. Most astrocytomas contain small numbers of oligodendroglial elements.

Oligodendrogliomas are generally well-differentiated and well-demarcated, expansile masses composed of sheets of uniform cells in a fine vascular stroma (Fig. 156). Individual cells usually have delicate cell membranes and finely granular to clear cytoplasm enveloping small round, moderately to densely staining nuclei. Autolytic distension of the cytoplasm may result in perinuclear halos and impart a honeycomb appearance to the tumor (Fig. 157). In well-fixed material, clusters of cells have indistinct cell borders, moderate amounts of pale pink, finely granular cytoplasm and lack perinuclear halos (Fig. 158). Mitoses are infrequent. Vascular endothelial hypertrophy and hyperplasia are frequently observed (Fig. 159), often at tumor margins. Larger oligodendrogliomas tend to be less discrete and more anaplastic. Focal areas of tumor cells may be arranged in clusters or cords and palisades or rows. Tumor cells may form pseudorosettes or be oriented around blood vessels or neurons. Necrotic and hemorrhagic foci are commonly seen, and areas of mineralization are occasionally observed. Most oligodendrogliomas contain minor

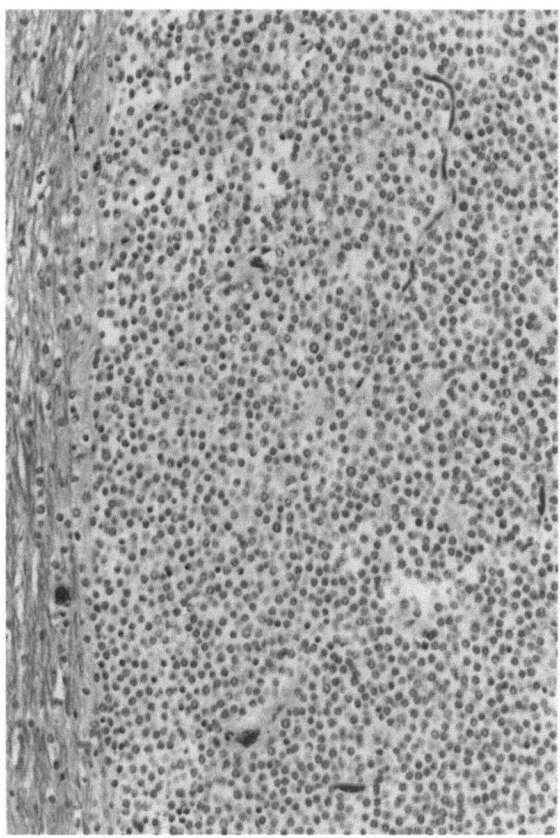

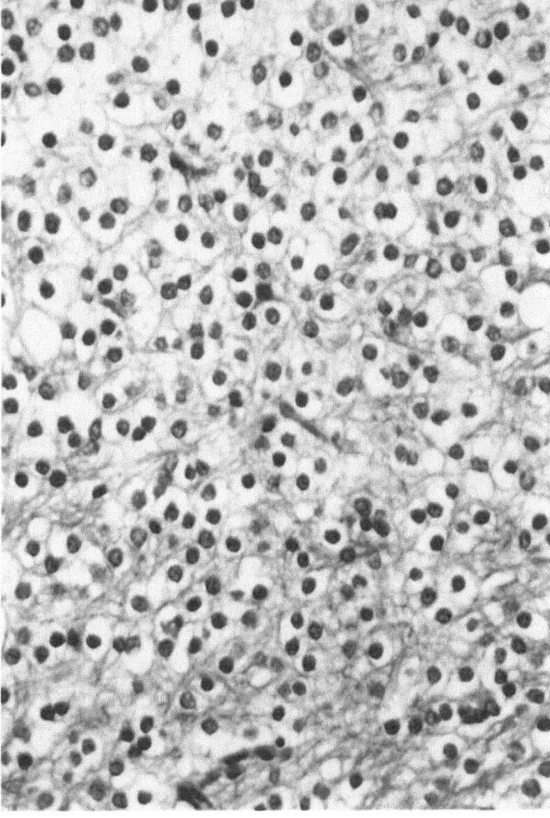

◄ **Fig. 152** *(upper left).* Astrocytoma, brain, rat. Note orientation of neoplastic astrocytes around neurons (neuronal satellitosis). H and E, ×410

Fig. 153 *(lower left).* Astrocytoma, brain, rat. Perivascular orientation of tumor cells and diffusely infiltrative growth at the margins. Note that one blood vessel *(arrow)* is encircled by neoplastic astrocytes within the Virchow-Robbin space. H and E, ×130

Fig. 154 *(upper right).* Anaplastic astrocytoma, brain, rat. Note cystic areas filled with proteinaceous material. H and E, ×300

Fig. 155 *(lower right).* Glioma, brain, rat. Note pseudopalisading of tumor cells around a focus of necrosis. H and E, ×300

Fig. 156 *(above).* Oligodendroglioma, brain, rat. Well-demarcated margins and diffuse sheets of uniform tumor cells. H and E, ×118 ▶

Fig. 157 *(below).* Oligodendroglioma, brain, rat. Tumor cells with moderate to densely staining nuclei, delicate cell membranes, and artifactual perinuclear halos associated with early autolysis. H and E, ×310

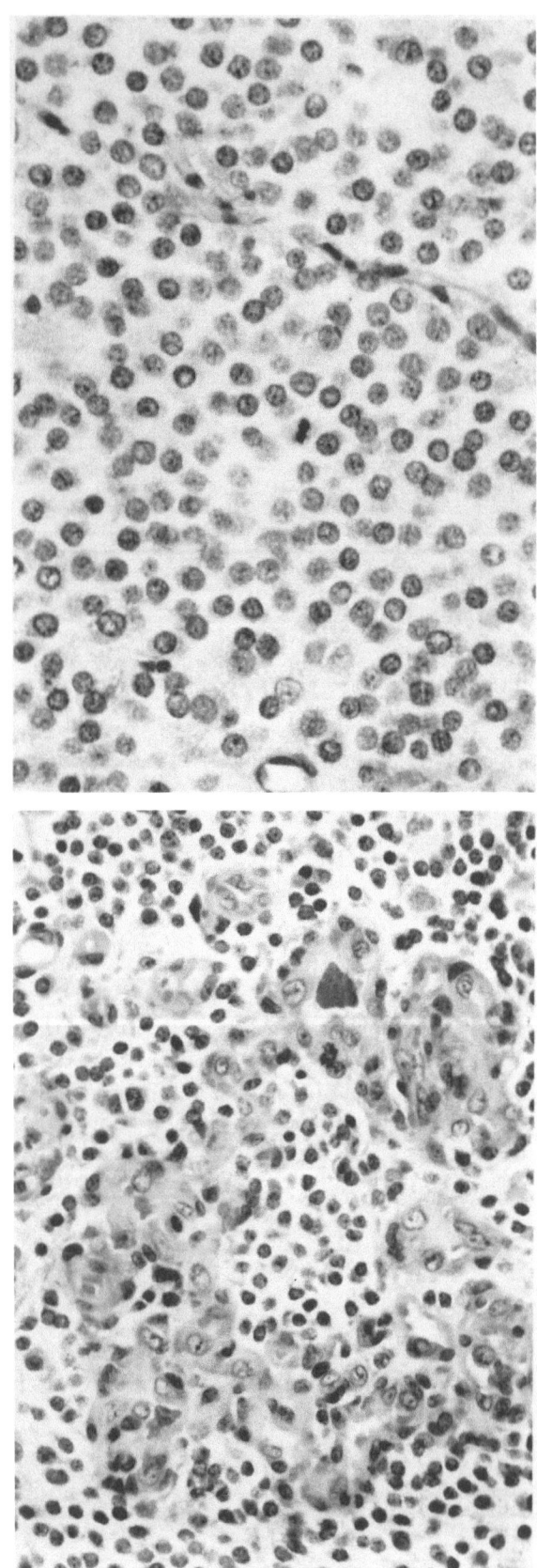

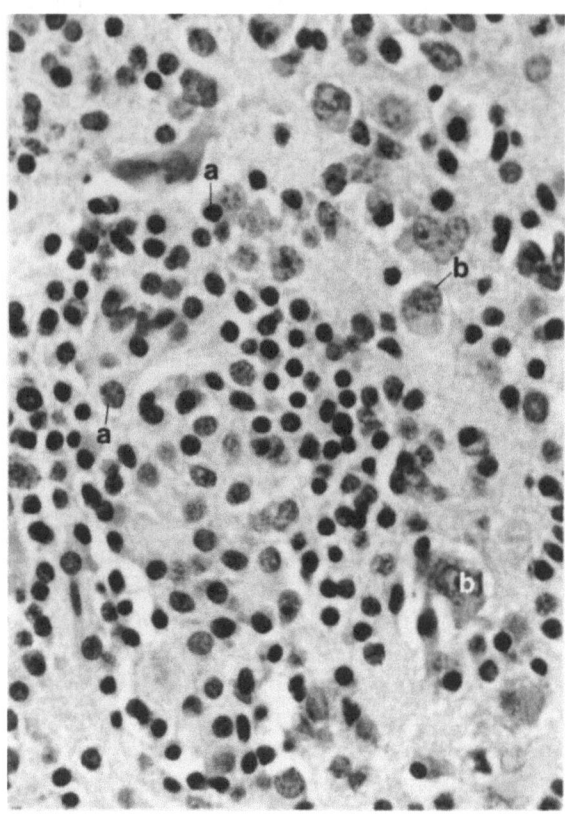

Fig. 158 *(upper left).* Oligodendroglioma, brain, rat. Note the monomorphic population of tumor cells with indistinct cell borders, moderate amounts of granular cytoplasm, and euchromatic nuclei. A well-fixed specimen. Note the absence of artifactual perinuclear halos. H and E, ×376

Fig. 159 *(lower left).* Oligodendroglioma, brain, rat. Vascular endothelial hypertrophy and hyperplasia. H and E, ×300

Fig. 160 *(upper right).* Mixed glioma, brain, rat. Admixture of two neoplastic cell types: oligodendrocytes with scant cytoplasm and small hyperchromatic nuclei *(a)* and astrocytes with moderate amounts of cytoplasm and larger euchromatic nuclei with stippled chromatin *(b).* H and E, ×436

amounts of astroglial elements, including reactive astrocytes.

Mixed gliomas range from well-differentiated to anaplastic masses with varying proportions of neoplastic astrocytes and oligodendroglia (Fig. 160). They frequently have an oligodendroglial pattern with vascular proliferation and perivascular extension of astrocytic elements beyond poorly circumscribed margins. Larger tumors tend to be anaplastic and commonly have cystic changes, areas of necrosis and pseudopalisading, frequent mitoses, occasional giant cells, and occasional areas of microcalcificiation.

Ultrastructure

Transmission electron microscopy of spontaneous gliomas of the rat has not been reported.

Differential Diagnosis

Differential diagnoses for astrocytomas include several neoplastic and nonneoplastic lesions. Astrocytomas can be difficult to distinguish from the controversial diagnostic entity, malignant reticuloses (reticulum cell sarcoma, neoplastic reticulosis, microgliomatosis, cerebral lymphoma) (Garman et al. 1985, 1986). Malignant reticulosis are composed of cells resembling lymphocytes, pleomorphic microglia, and fibroblastic astrocytes. Features common to both astrocytomas and malignant reticuloses include a solidly cellular central region and a more dispersed periphery with neuronal satellitosis, perivascular invasion, and frequent infiltration of the meninges and ventricular spaces. Malignant reticulosis may be more nodular in appearance and exhibit greater peripheral involvement. Special stains sometimes assist in differentiating these lesions. Astrocytomas will frequently stain with phosphotungstic acid hematoxylin (PTAH), while malignant reticuloses usually stain positive for reticulin fibers.

A pleomorphic astrocytoma that has invaded the ventricular system or meninges may be mistaken for an inflammatory process due to the presence of such misleading changes as glial proliferation, congestion, and necrosis. For example, Mawdesley-Thomas (1968) reported an ependymitis which was later reclassified as an astrocytoma (Mawdesley-Thomas and Newman 1974).

Marked hyperplasia of reactive astrocytes may occasionally mimic tumor formation in response to infiltrating sarcomas or meningiomas and must be distinguished from astrocytomas.

Astrocytomas composed of sheets of small cells with delicate processes may resemble oligodendrogliomas in cell pattern and morphology. These may be differentiated with stains for neuroglial fibers.

Differential diagnoses for oligodendrogliomas include several primary brain tumors in addition to astrocytomas. Glial tumors with vascular proliferation and cells arranged in rows and pseudorosettes are often diagnosed as ependymomas based merely on these features. However, this pattern is seen in some spontaneous and experimentally induced oliodendrogliomas and should not be attributed to ependymomas alone (Schreiber et al. 1977; Solleveld et al. 1987). Cerebellar oligodendrogliomas with small, uniform, dark-staining cells with little or no evidence of perinuclear halos can resemble medulloblastomas; while subpial oligodendrogliomas may invade the meninges and induce a fibrous reaction mimicking an endotheliomatous meningioma.

Astrocytomas and oligodendrogliomas are the primary differential diagnoses for mixed gliomas, especially when the neoplasms are poorly differentiated. Unfortunately there is no universally accepted criterion setting the proportions of the two neoplastic cell populations for distinguishing astrocytomas, oligodendrogliomas, and mixed gliomas (Solleveld et al. 1986). Other differential diagnoses for mixed gliomas include those listed for astrocytomas and oligodendrogliomas.

Anaplastic gliomas must be differentiated from glioblastoma multiforme (cellular glioblastoma; spongioblastoma multiforme; glioblastoma). In man, glioblastoma multiforme is considered to be an extreme manifestation of anaplasia and dedifferentiation on the part of mature glial tumors, which are mostly astrocytic (Rubinstein 1972). However, the morphologic pattern as it occurs in man has not been recognized in recent reviews of spontaneous brain tumors of the rat (Gopinath 1986; Solleveld et al. 1986, 1987). Copeland et al. (1976) suggested that the nosologic criteria developed for human brain tumors permits the use of the term "glioblastoma multiforme" only when unequivocal endothelial proliferation is present. Vascular endothelial proliferation and areas of spongioblastic astrocytes were not observed in the above series of rat brain tumors (Gopsinath 1986; Solleveld et al. 1986, 1987), nor were these features described or shown in the few published descriptions and photographs of glioblastoma multiforme in the rat (Mawdesley-Thomas and

Newman 1974; Newman and Mawdesley-Thomas 1974; Burek 1978). Thus, true spontaneous glioblastomas must be exceedingly rare in the rat, if they occur at all. Furthermore, glioblastoma multiforme and glioblastoma are not included in the most recent classification schemes for spontaneous brain tumors of the rat (Dagle et al. 1979; Ward and Rice 1982; Solleveld et al. 1987).

Proper classification of brain tumors and determination of which classifications should be combined for statistical evaluation is a continuing problem in evaluations of chemical safety (Swenberg 1986). There is little difficulty if all of the tumors are well-differentiated gliomas since it seems reasonable to group such tumors for statistical interpretation. Problems arise when the neoplasms are unusual in morphology or poorly differentiated so that astrocytomas cannot be confidently distinguished from reticuloses or sarcomas, and oligodendrogliomas cannot be separated from ependymomas or sarcomas. Under these circumstances, considerations such as dose-response relationships, tumor latency, tumor size and progression, and a shift to more anaplasia and invasion in larger tumors must provide the weight of evidence that is used to establish a causal relationship between the chemical and brain tumors (Koestner 1986; Swenberg 1986).

Biologic Features

Gliomas grow by expansion and have compressive space-occupying effects. Many are also destructive, infiltrating tumors. Metastasis through the cerebrospinal spaces may occur (Newman and Mawdesley-Thomas 1974), but extraneural metastasis appears to be exceedingly rare. A small proportion of tumor-bearing animals exhibit signs of neurologic dysfunction such as abnormal gait, head tilt, torticollis, loss of balance, loss of grip reflex, and/or posterior paralysis. The observed signs tend to reflect the anatomic location and size of the neoplasm, rather than tumor type.

Pathogenesis. It has not been established whether spontaneous glial tumors arise from the neoplastic transformation of glial cell precursors or from the dedifferentiation of differentiated glial elements. Investigations in chemical and viral neurooncogenesis have shown that during the late stage of neuroepithelial development, migrating cells of the subependymal plate are highly susceptible to neoplastic transformation (Copeland and Bigner 1977; Lantos and Pilkington 1977). These periventricular cells are glial cell precursors which migrate in the nearly mature fetal and neonatal brain to later differentiate into astrocytes and oligodendroglia. Sequential morphologic studies have demonstrated a progession from preneoplastic or early neoplastic glial proliferations to microtumors, and finally to lethal gross tumors (Swenberg et al. 1972; Schiffer et al. 1978). These early lesions are not randomly distributed, but occur in areas in which tumors later develop. Since the location of precursor cells responsive to experimental carcinogens overlaps with the predilection sites for spontaneous gliomas, similarities in the origin of spontaneous and experimentally induced gliomas may exist (Dagle et al. 1979).

Etiology. Glial neoplasms have been induced in rats by intracerebral injection of chemicals or viruses, or by transplacental, parenteral, oral, or topical exposure to chemical carcinogens. Models of experimental induction of brain tumors with chemicals (Kleihues et al. 1976; Swenberg 1976; Janisch and Schriber 1977) and viruses (Bigner and Pegram 1976; Janisch and Schriber 1977; Walker and Bigner 1985) have been comprehensively reviewed. Chemical agents capable of inducing glial neoplasms range from large polycyclic hydrocarbons to small alkylating agents. In routine bioassays, however, we know of only two chemicals which induced brain tumors in experimental animals: acrylonitrile and ethylene oxide. Exposure of rats to acrylonitrile produced brain tumors tentatively classified as "anaplastic astrocytomas" (Bigner et al. 1986), whereas ethylene oxide induced glial tumors of various types (Snellings et al. 1984; Lynch et al. 1984; Garman et al. 1985, 1986).

Frequency. Relative to other organ systems, tumors of the central nervous system are rare in the laboratory rat. The incidence of brain tumors in general averaged 1%–3% in untreated control rats, depending upon the strain, sex, and age (Table 9). The Sprague-Dawley rat appears to have a more variable incidence than the F344 strain (Ward and Rice 1982; Solleveld et al. 1984; Koestner 1986; Swenberg 1986). Brain tumors usually occur more frequently in males and increase in incidence with advancing age (Solleveld et al. 1984; Gopinath 1986). For example, a recent comparison of astrocytomas in F344 rats demonstrated an average incidence of 0.4% in

Table 9. Brain tumors in aged rats[a]

Strain	Sex	Age (months)	Incidence (D)	(%)	Most common tumor type	Reference
SD	F	24/ >24	29/2765	1.0	Astrocytoma	Gopinath
SD	M	24/ >24	59/2630	2.2	Astrocytoma	(1986)
TIF:RAI	F	24/ >24	39/4480	0.9	Granular cell tumor	Krinke
TIF:RAI	M	24/ >24	51/4480	1.1	Granular cell tumor	et al. (1985)
F344/DuCrj	F	24	3/ 346	0.9	Astrocytoma	Maekawa
F344/DuCrj	M	24	5/ 346	1.5	Astrocytoma	et al. (1984)
F344/N	F	24	20/2370	0.8	Astrocytoma	Solleveld
F344/N	M	24	27/2320	1.2	Astrocytoma	et al. (1984)
F344/N	F	>24	12/ 529	2.2	Astrocytoma	Solleveld
F344/N	M	>24	15/ 529	2.9	Astrocytoma	et al. (1984)
SD	F/M	24	5/ 234	2.1	Astrocytoma	Koestner (1984)
SD	F	>24	9/ 465	1.9	Astrocytoma	Dagle
Wistar	F	>24	3/ 250	1.2	Astrocytoma	et al. (1979)[b]
OM	F	>24	20/1572	1.3	Ependymoma	
WAG/RIJ	F	>24	4/ 101	3.9	Astrocytoma	Burek (1978)
WAG/RIJ	M	>24	3/ 124	2.4	Astrocytoma	
BN/BI	F	>24	14/ 236	5.9	Granular cell tumor	Burek (1978)
BN/BI	M	>24	2/ 74	2.7	Granular cell tumor	
AF/Han-EMD	F	24	1/ 32	3.1	Pleomorphic glioma	Sumi
AF/Han-EMD	M	24	0/ 33	0		et al. (1976)
AF/Han-EMD	F	>24	7/ 128	5.5	Meningioma	Sumi
AF/Han-EMD	M	>24	10/ 149	6.7	Meningioma	et al. (1976)

[a] Data from selected long-term (24 months) or life span (>24 months) studies.
[b] Histologic examination restricted to animals with neurologic signs or gross brain lesions.

males and 0.5% in females from 2-year bioassays (26 months), whereas the incidence was 2.7% in males and 1.5% in females allowed to live out their lifespan (up to 34 months) (Solleveld et al. 1984).

Astrocytoma is typically reported as the most common brain tumor of control rats (Table 9). In a review of the natural occurrence of brain tumors in the F344 rats (Ward and Rice 1982), glial tumors represented 83% of the neoplasms with astrocytomas (54%) being the most common tumor type followed by oligodendrogliomas (19%) and mixed gliomas (10%). In contrast, an analysis of 1731 nervous system neoplasms induced by ethylnitrosourea and other alkylating agents demonstrated the most common chemically induced brain tumor type to be mixed glioma followed, in order, by ependymoma, oligodendroglioma, and astrocytoma (Mennel and Zülch 1976).

Comparison with Other Species

The incidence of brain tumors in untreated control rats is relatively high compared with that in other species (Koestner 1986). Solleveld et al. (1986) recently compared the incidence and morphology and classification of brain tumors in man, domestic animals, and laboratory animals.

In man, age-associated increases in the incidence of brain tumors occur in childhood and between the ages of 60 and 80 (Rubinstein 1972; Solleveld et al. 1986). Astrocytoma and glioblastoma multiforme rank second and third in frequency among children. In adults, glioblastoma multiforme accounts for more than half of the intracranial tumors, whereas astrocytoma ranks third in occurrence. While the characteristic patterns of human glioblastoma multiforme may not occur in the rat, comparisons reveal that astrocytic tumors of the rat are more atypical and less differentiated than those in man (Gopinath 1986; Solleveld et al. 1986). Furthermore, examinations of rat glial tumors for cellular markers such as glial fibrillary acidic protein (GFAP) and S-100 protein have not compared well with human studies. GFAP and S-100 protein are useful in the characterization of brain tumors in man, but spontaneous glial tumors in the rat have been uniformly negative for both markers (Krinke et al. 1985; Solleveld et

al. 1986, 1987). While putative neoplastic astrocytes failed to show GFAP expression, reactive
astrocytes around and within lesions stained
strongly positive. As a consequence, the view that
spontaneous astrocytomas of the rat arise from
astrocytes is debatable.

Tumors of the central nervous system occur in all
the domestic species and have been most carefully studied in the dog (Luginbühl et al. 1968;
Fankhauser et al. 1974; Cordy 1978; Solleveld et
al. 1986). Brachycephalic breeds of dogs, especially boxers, have a high incidence of brain tumors, particularly gliomas. As in the rat, gliomas
of the dog occur more frequently in males (Solleveld et al. 1986) and are age associated (Cordy
1978). In contrast to the rat, GFAP has proved
useful in the characterization of some gliomas in
the dog (Solleveld et al. 1986).

Spontaneously arising neoplasia of the central
nervous system is extremely rare in mice, with
the exception of two strains and their crosses
(Swenberg 1982; Morgan et al. 1984; Morgan
and Alison this volume, p. 123). VM and BRVR
mice have respective brain tumor incidences of
1.6% and 1.1%, with astrocytomas representing
nearly 100% of the brain tumors (Fraser 1971,
1986).

References

Bigner DD, Pegram CN (1976) Virus-induced experimental brain tumors and of the putative association of
viruses with human brain tumors: a review. Adv Neurol
13: 57–83

Bigner DD, Bigner SH, Burger PC, Shelburne JD, Fried-
man HS (1986) Primary brain tumours in Fischer 344
rats chronically exposed to acrylonitrile in their drink-
ing-water. Food Chem Toxicol 24: 129–137

Burek JD (1978) Pathology of aging rats. CRC, West
Palm Beach, pp 148–150

Copeland DD, Bigner DD (1977) The role of the subependymal plate in avian sarcoma virus brain tumor induction: comparison of incipient tumors in neonatal
and adult rats. Acta Neuropathol (Berl) 38: 1–6

Copeland DD, Talley FA, Bigner DD (1976) The fine
structure of intracranial neoplasms induced by the inoculation of avian sarcoma virus in neonatal and adult
rats. Am J Pathol 83: 149–176

Cordy DR (1978) Tumors of the nervous system and eye.
In: Moulton JE (ed) Tumors in domestic animals. University of California Press, Berkeley, CA, pp 430–455

Dagle GE, Zwicker GM, Renne RA (1979) Morphology
of spontaneous brain tumors in the rat. Vet Pathol 16:
318–324

Fankhauser R, Luginbühl H, McGrath JT (1974) Tumours
of the nervous system. Bull WHO 50: 53–69

Fraser H (1971) Astrocytomas in an inbred mouse strain.
J Pathol 103: 266–270

Fraser H (1986) Brain tumors in mice, with particular reference to astrocytoma. Food Chem Toxicol 24:
105–111

Garman RH, Snellings WM, Maronpot RR (1985) Brain
tumors in F344 rats associated with chronic inhalation
exposure to ethylene oxide. Neurotoxicology 6:
117–137

Garman RH, Snellings WM, Maronpot RR (1986) Frequency, size and location of brain tumors in F344 rats
chronically exposed to ethylene oxide. Food Chem
Toxicol 24: 145–153

Gopinath C (1986) Spontaneous brain tumors in Sprague-
Dawley rats. Food Chem Toxicol 24: 113–120

Jänisch W, Schreiber D (1977) Experimental tumors of
the central nervous system. Upjohn, Kalamazoo, Michigan

Kleihues P, Lantos PL, Magee PN (1976) Chemical carcinogenesis in the nervous system. Int Rev Exp Pathol
15: 153–232

Koestner A (1984) Aspartame and brain tumors: pathology issues. In: Stegink LD, Filer LJ Jr (eds) Aspartame:
physiology and biochemistry. Dekker, New York,
pp 447–457 (Food Science and Technology, vol 12)

Koestner A (1986) The brain tumour issue in long-term
toxicity studies in rats. Food Chem Toxicol 24: 139–143

Krinke G, Naylor DC, Schmid S, Fröhlich E, Schnider K
(1985) The incidence of naturally-occurring primary
brain tumours in the laboratory rat. J Comp Pathol 95:
175–192

Lantos PL, Pilkington GJ (1977) Neuroblasts in cerebral
tumor induced by ethylnitrosourea in rats. A fine structural study. Virchows Arch [B] 25: 243–259

Luginbühl M, Frankhauser R, McGrath JT (1968) Spontaneous neoplasms of the nervous system in animals.
In: Krayenbuhl H, Maspes PE, Sweet WH (eds) Progress in neurological surgery, vol 2. Yearbook Medical
Publishers, Chicago, pp 85–164

Lynch DW, Lewis TR, Moorman WJ, Burg JR, Groth
DH, Khan A, Ackerman LJ, Cockrell BY (1984) Carcinogenic and toxicologic effects of inhaled ethylene
oxide and propylene oxide in F344 rats. Toxicol Appl
Pharmacol 76: 69–84

Maekawa A, Onodera H, Tanigawa H, Furuta K, Takahashi M, Kurokawa Y, Kokubo T, Ogiu T, Uchida O,
Kobayashi K, Hayashi Y (1984) Spontaneous tumors
of the nervous system and associated organs and/or tissues in rats. Jpn J Cancer Res 75: 784–791

Mawdesley-Thomas LE (1968) Ependymitis in a rat. J Pathol Bacteriol 95: 317–319

Mawdesley-Thomas LE, Newman AJ (1974) Some observations on spontaneously occurring tumours of the central nervous system of Sprague-Dawley derived rats. J
Pathol 112: 107–116

Mennel HD, Zülch E (1976) Tumours of the central and
peripheral nervous systems. In: Turusov VS (ed) Tumours of the rat. Part 2. IARC Scientific Publ no 6.
IARC, Lyon, pp 295–311 (Pathology of tumours in laboratory animals, vol 1)

Morgan KT, Frith CH, Swenberg JA, McGrath JT, Zülch
KJ, Crowder DM (1984) A morphologic classification
of brain tumors found in several strains of mice. JNCI
72: 151–160

Newman AJ, Mawdesley-Thomas LE (1974) Spontaneous
tumours of the central nervous system of laboratory
rats. J Comp Pathol 84: 39–50

Rubinstein LJ (1972) Tumors of central neurogenic origin. Classification and grading. In: Tumors of the central nervous system. Atlas of tumor pathology, second series, fascicle 6. AFIP, Washington, pp 7-17

Schiffer D, Giordana MT, Pezzotta S, Lechner C, Paoletti P (1978) Cerebral tumors induced by transplacental ENU: study of the different tumoral stages, particularly of early proliferations. Acta Neuropathol (Berl) 41: 27-31

Schreiber D, Jänisch W, Rath F (1977) Zur Klassifikation experimenteller Hirntumorem. Exp Pathol 13: 3-10

Snellings WM, Weil CS, Maronpot RR (1984) A two-year inhalation study of the carcinogenic potential of ethylene oxide in Fischer 344 rats. Toxicol Appl Pharmacol 75: 105-117

Solleveld HA, Haseman JK, McConnell EE (1984) Natural history of body weight gain, survival, and neoplasia in the F344 rat. JNCI 72: 929-940

Solleveld HA, Bigner DD, Averill DR Jr, Bigner SH, Boorman GA, Burger PC, Gillespie Y, Hubbard GB, Laerum OD, McComb RD, McGrath JT, Morgan KT, Peters A, Rubinstein LJ, Schoenberg BS, Schold SC, Swenberg JA, Thompson MB, Vandevelde M, Vinores SA (1986) Brain tumors in man and animals: report of a workshop. Environ Health Perspect 68: 155-173

Solleveld HA, Bigner SH, Boorman G, Bigner DD (1987) Neoplasms of the central nervous system. In: Atlas of tumor pathology in the Fischer rat. CRC, Boca Raton (in press)

Sumi N, Stavrou D, Frohberg H, Jochmann G (1976) The incidence of spontaneous tumors of the central nervous system of Wistar rats. Arch Toxicol 35: 1-13

Swenberg JA (1976) Chemical induction of brain tumors. In: Thompson RA, Green JR (eds) Neoplasia in the central nervous system. Raven, New York, pp 85-99 (Advances in neurology, vol 15)

Swenberg JA (1982) Neoplasms of the nervous system. In: Foster HL, Small JD, Fox JG (eds) The mouse in biomedical research, vol IV. Academic, New York, pp 529-537

Swenberg JA (1986) Brain tumours-problems and perspectives. Food Chem Toxicol 24: 155-158

Swenberg JA, Koestner A, Wechsler W (1972) The induction of tumors of the nervous system with intravenous methylnitrosourea. Lab Invest 26: 74-85

Walker JS, Bigner DD (1985) Virus induced brain tumors. In: Wilkins RM, Rengachary SS (eds) Neurosurgery. McGraw-Hill, New York, pp 522-525

Ward JM, Rice JM (1982) Naturally occurring and chemically induced brain tumors in rats and mice in carcinogenesis bioassays. Ann NY Acad Sci 381: 304-319

Peripheral Nerve Sheath Tumors, Rat

Dale M. Walker, Vernon E. Walker, Jerry F. Hardisty, Kevin T. Morgan, and James A. Swenberg

Synonyms. Neurofibroma, neurofibrosarcoma; schwannoma, malignant schwannoma; neurilemoma, malignant neurilemoma; neurilemmoma, malignant neurilemmoma; neurinoma, malignant neurinoma; Schwann-cell tumor; fibroma, fibrosarcoma; fibroblastoma.

Gross Appearance

Peripheral nerve sheath tumors are round to oval, soft to firm, discrete, unencapsulated masses which range up to 10 cm along the longest axis. The cut surface is usually smooth, shiny, and translucent or white. Subcutaneous tumors may have an ulcerated surface.

In the cases reviewed for this manuscript, a few tumors diagnosed as neurofibromas were described as fibrous and tan, pink, or purple on the cut surface. A few reported neurofibrosarcomas were described as lobular or pitted and mottled tan to red on the cut surface. One tumor had a necrotic center. A reported schwannoma was described as soft and fluctuant. One tumor diagnosed as a malignant schwannoma had a central blood-filled cyst.

The majority of peripheral nerve sheath tumors of the rat occur in subcutaneous tissues (Figs. 161-164), especially of the ear, neck, head, and shoulder (Table 10) (Schardein et al. 1968; Goodman et al. 1979, 1980; Solleveld et al. 1984). A neurofibroma has also been reported in the adrenal capsule, and neurofibrosarcomas have been reported in the retroperitoneal space and in the parotid salivary gland (Schardein et al. 1968; Anver et al. 1982). Benign and malignant schwannomas have been described in association with spinal nerve roots, in the eye, and in the uterus and adjacent tissues (Abbott 1982; Solleveld et al. 1984; Gough et al. 1986).

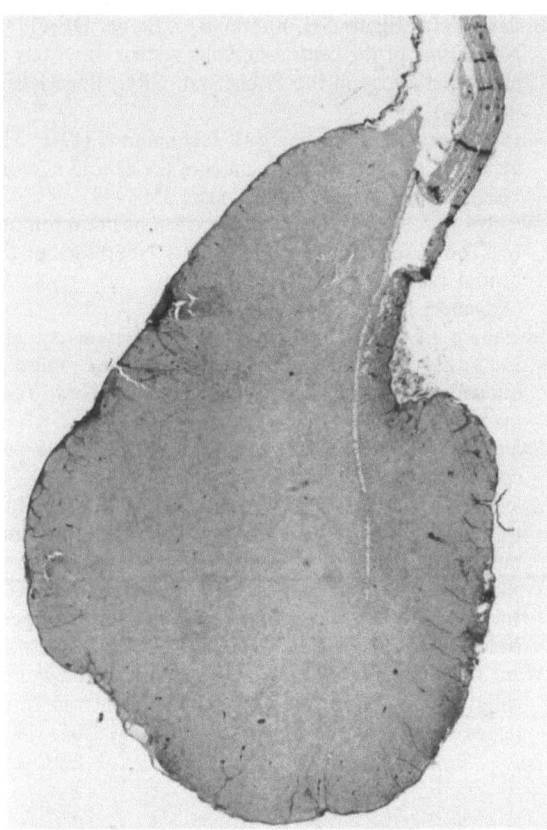

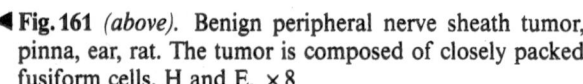

◀ **Fig. 161** *(above)*. Benign peripheral nerve sheath tumor, pinna, ear, rat. The tumor is composed of closely packed fusiform cells. H and E, × 8

Fig. 162 *(below)*. Higher magnification of tumor in Fig. 161. Note closely packed fusiform cells forming bundles which intersect at right angles. H and E, × 410

Fig. 163 *(upper left)*. Benign peripheral nerve sheath tumor, subcutis, rat. The tumor is oval and discrete. H and E, × 10 ▶

Fig. 164 *(lower left)*. Higher magnification of tumor in Fig. 163. Compressed tumor cells at the margins and artificial separation create the appearance of a thin capsule. H and E, × 330

Fig. 165 *(upper right)*. Benign peripheral nerve sheath tumor, subcutis, rat. Note loosely arranged fusiform cells in interlacing bundles. The tumor is infiltrated by two mast cells. H and E, × 200

Fig. 166 *(lower left)*. Benign peripheral nerve sheath tumor, subcutis, rat. Bundles of tumor cells intersect at right angles. Tumor cells are nondiscrete and the cytoplasm blends with the stroma. H and E, × 240

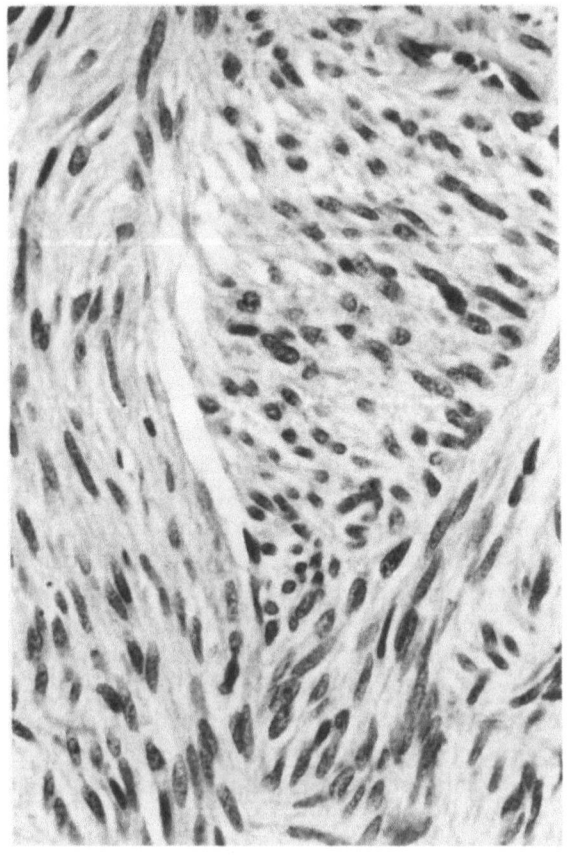

Table 10. Distribution of peripheral nerve sheath tumors[a]

Reported tumor type	Number reviewed	Tumors (Location)	(D)
Neurofibroma	10	Subcutis of pinna	9
		Subcutis-other	1
Neurofibrosarcoma	23	Subcutis of pinna	3
		Subcutis-other	14
		Salivary gland	1
		Pituitary gland	1
		Stomach	1
		Body cavity	1
		Thorax	1
		Spinal cord and surrounding musculature	1
Schwannoma	12	Subcutis of pinna	5
		Subcutis-other	5
		Salivary gland	2
Malignant schwannoma	7	Subcutis of pinna	2
		Subcutis-other	3
		Salivary gland	1
		Uterus	1

[a] Based upon a review of records of control rats used in 63 bioassays conducted by the National Toxicology Program.

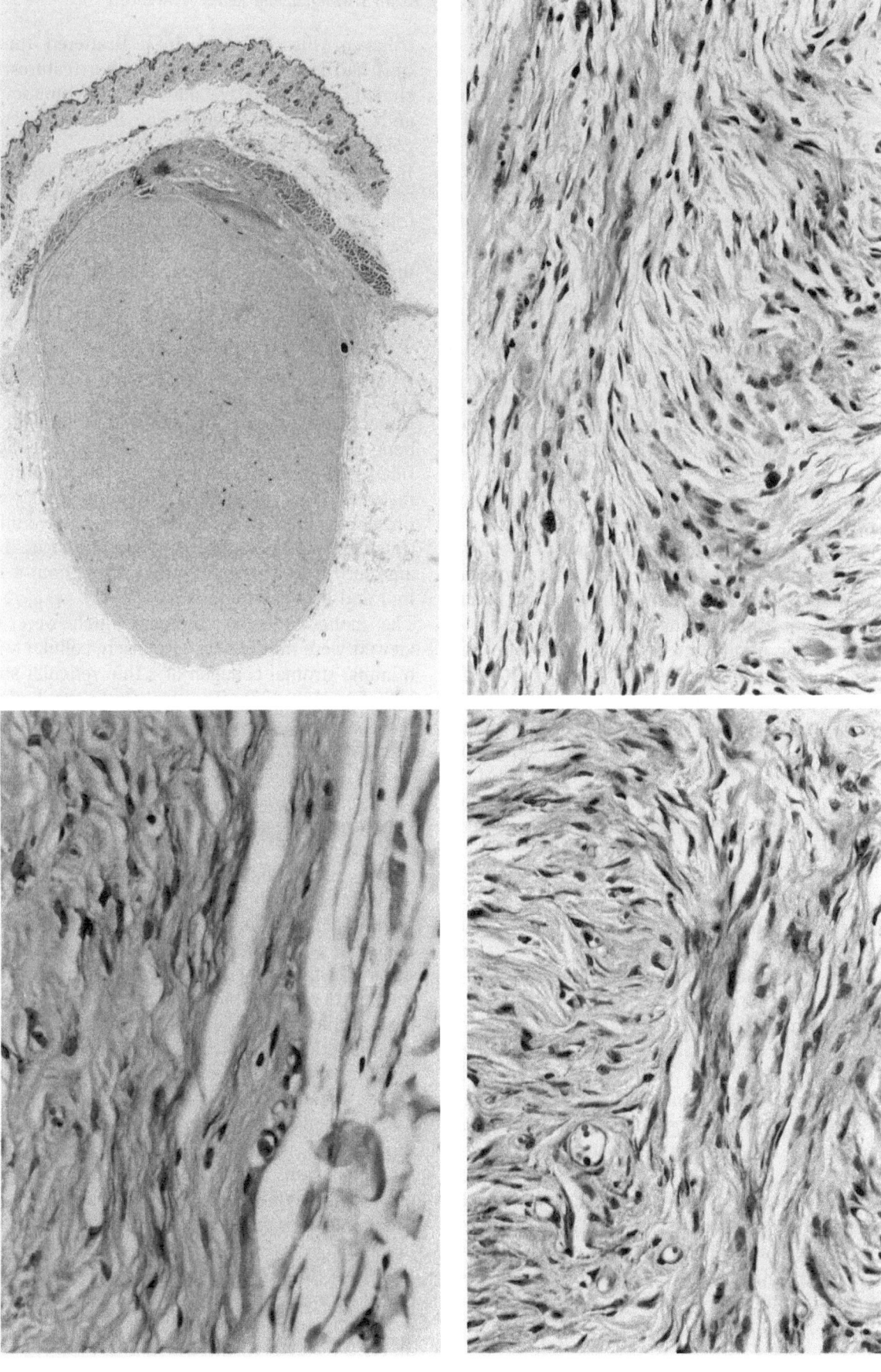

Microscopic Features

Benign peripheral nerve sheath tumors are round to oval, expansile, rarely encapsulated masses which are composed of fusiform cells arranged in interlacing bundles, cords, sheets, and occasional whorls in a loose to moderately compact, fibrillar, collagenous stroma (Figs. 161–166). Bundles may intersect at right angles in focal areas (Figs. 162, 165, 166). Compressed cells at the margins of some tumors may create the appearance of a capsule (Fig. 164). Individual tumor cells are nondiscrete and have variable amounts of eosinophilic fibrillar cytoplasm that blends with the stroma (Figs. 162, 165, 166). Nuclei are single, oval and have moderate to abundant fine granular or reticular chromatin. Nucleoli are rare. Mitotic figures are uncommon (less than one per five high-power fields in the tumors reviewed). Nerve fibers may be present within or near the periphery of the tumor mass.

Malignant peripheral nerve sheath tumors are similar to their benign counterparts with several exceptions. The margins may be moderately well defined or nondiscrete with invasion of tumor cells into surrounding tissues (Figs. 167–169). Tumors are moderately to densely cellular with varying amounts of stromal collagen (Figs. 167–170). Moderate to marked cellular and nuclear pleomorphism (Fig. 168), and foci of necrosis, suppuration, hemorrhage, or ulceration may also be present. In the malignant nerve sheath tumors reviewed, mitotic figures ranged up to six per high-power field. Bizarre mitotic figures may be present, but are uncommon.

The reported neurofibromas which were reviewed were composed of loosely arranged fusiform cells in an abundant compact fibrillar to collagenous stroma (Figs. 164–166). Tumor cells were arranged in bundles, cords, and sheets; the proportions of each arrangement varied between and within individual tumors. Scattered individual tumor cells had uni- or bipolar cytoplasmic processes and/or large hyperchromatic nuclei with abundant chromatin. A few cells had two to three nuclei. Rarely, cells had a single small basophilic nucleolus. Tumors in the subcutis occasionally involved the dermis and were frequently (in more than 50% of the cases surveyed) infiltrated by mast cells (Figs. 165, 171) and fewer small round cells resembling lymphocytes. Focal areas of collagen degradation were present in a few tumors.

The reported neurofibrosarcomas reviewed were moderately to densely cellular with little stromal collagen (Figs. 167 and 168). Scattered tumor cells had large bizarre nuclei. Other features included infiltration by mast cells, lymphocytes and/or round cells containing intracytoplasmic golden-brown pigment.

In the cases reviewed, tumors diagnosed as schwannomas frequently had one or more of the following patterns. In focal areas, tumor cells were densely packed with areas of palisading of tumor cells along their long axes (Antoni type A pattern). Cells palisaded or whorled around vessels in a few tumors. In other foci, tumor cells were loosely arranged in an abundant, loose, pale pink, reticular stroma (Antoni type B pattern). In a few tumors, nuclei palisaded at the periphery of aggregates of parallel eosinophilic fibers (Verocay body) (Fig. 171). Cystic spaces filled with erythrocytes or eosinophilic granular material (Fig. 170) and lined by tumor cells were present in a few cases. Rarely, tumors were infiltrated by small nests of foamy macrophages. The amount of each pattern varied throughout a tumor and between tumors.

The malignant schwannomas which were reviewed were moderately to densely cellular with minimal stromal collagen or a thin reticular stroma (Figs. 169–172). The features described in schwannomas were present in a few focal areas or were absent.

Ultrastructure

Gough et al. (1986) described the ultrastructural features of two benign nerve sheath tumors of Wistar rats. Tumor cells ranged from round to oval with numerous interwoven cytoplasmic processes. Intercellular junctions were moderately frequent and resembled tight junctions or hemidesmosomes. Individual cells were surrounded by a basal lamina which ranged from continuous to discontinuous. The extracellular organelles included mitochondria, rough endoplasmic reticulum, ribosomes and fewer lysozomes. In one tumor, Gough et al. (1986) described loosely scattered inclusions composed of multiple concentric osmiophilic lamellae with a periodicity of approximately 15 nm (resembling myelin membranes).

No description of the ultrastructural characteristics of spontaneous neurofibromas and neurofibrosarcomas of the rat is available. Denlinger et al. (1973) described the electron-microscopic appearance of a neurofibrosarcoma induced in a CDF rat by intravenous injection of methylni-

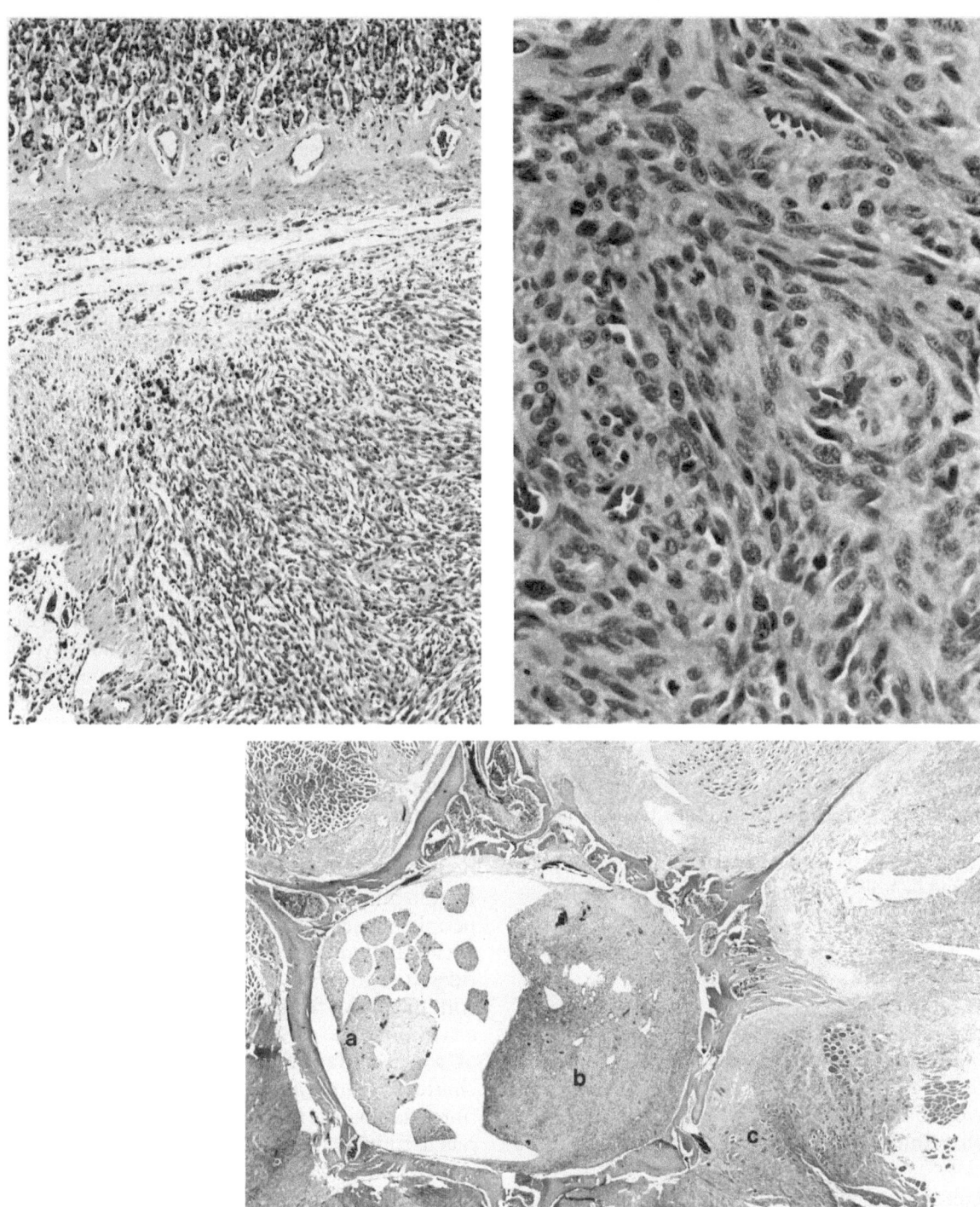

Fig. 167 *(upper left).* Malignant peripheral nerve sheath tumor, muscular layer, stomach, rat. Tumor cells have invaded and replaced smooth muscle. H and E, ×66

Fig. 168 *(upper right).* Higher magnification of the tumor in Fig. 167. Note the dense cellularity and absence of stromal collagen. H and E, ×300

Fig. 169 *(below).* Malignant peripheral nerve sheath tumor, spinal nerve root, rat. Tumor cells have invaded and partially replaced the spinal cord and paravertebral musculature *(a).* The masses *(b)* on the right and above the spinal canal consists of tumor cells. The fragmented tissue *(c)* on the left of the spinal canal consists of spinal cord partially replaced by tumor cells. The location and cellular morphology of this tumor closely resembles peripheral nerve sheath tumors induced by ethylnitrosourea. H and E, ×12

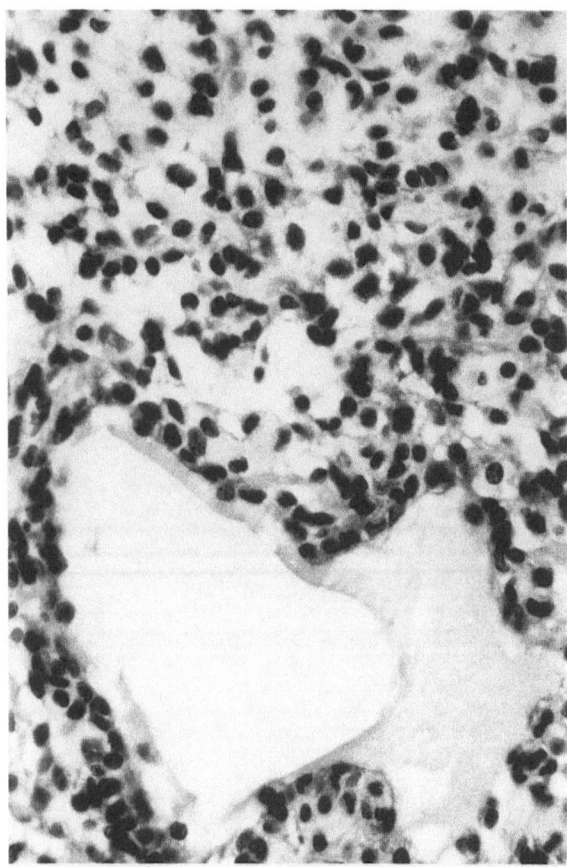

Fig. 170. Higher magnification of the tumor in Fig. 169. Note fluid-filled cystic space, the dense cellularity, the absence of stromal collagen, and the nuclear pleomorphism. H and E, × 400

trosourea. The tumor consisted of interlacing bundles of Schwann's cells admixed with fusiform fibroblasts with oval vesicular nuclei. An abundant amount of collagen was present. Tumor cells invaded the perineurium focally.

Laber-Laird and Jokinen (personal communication) noted a schwannoma in a F344 rat. The ultrastructural morphology of the neoplastic cells was similar to that described above. In addition, some tumor cells contained pinocytotic vesicles.

Differential Diagnosis

Peripheral nerve sheath tumors may be difficult to distinguish from any spindle cell tumor including leiomyoma, leiomyosarcoma, fibroma,

fibrosarcoma, hemangioma, hemangiosarcoma, malignant fibrous histiocytoma, and undifferentiated sarcoma. Electron-microscopic and immunohistochemical studies may be useful in distinguishing these tumors (Weiss et al. 1983). However, poorly differentiated tumors may lack distinguishing features.

Neurofibromas and neurofibrosarcomas are difficult to distinguish from benign and malignant schannomas, respectively. Neurofibromas or neurofibrosarcomas typically have a collagenous stroma and lack Verocay bodies and Antoni type A and type B tissue. These features are not adequate, however, for differentiation. Peripheral nerve sheath tumors are composed of spindle cells with varying amounts of collagen. The amount of collagen decreases as tumor cells are more densely packed and in malignant tumors of both types. Antoni type A and B tissues may be present in less than 10% of a mass, and absence from one cut surface does not preclude their presence elsewhere in the tumor. Foci of loosely arranged tumor cells resembling Antoni type B tissue may be scattered throughout neurofibromas and neurofibrosarcomas. Densely cellular foci in neurofibromas/neurofibrosarcomas may resemble Antoni type A tissue. Some Verocay bodies resemble areas of palisading seen in neurofibromas and neurofibrosarcomas. Many tumors diagnosed as schwannomas lack Verocay bodies.

Harkin and Reed (1969) suggested that in human peripheral nerve sheath tumors the presence of encapsulation and few acid mucopolysaccharides stained by Alcian blue may be used, along with the above features, as definitive evidence of a schwannoma, either benign or malignant. Lack of a capsule and abundant acid mucopolysaccharides are indicative of a neurofibroma/neurofibrosarcoma. In the data collected from control rats used in the National Toxicology Program no association between the presence or absence of a capsule and tumor type was noted. One mass diagnosed as a neurofibrosarcoma had a capsule which had been invaded by tumor cells. One tumor diagnosed as a neurofibroma had a thin fibrous capsule. No other evidence of encapsulation was present in the tumors surveyed. In several reported neurofibromas and schwannomas, compressed cells near the margins of the mass resembled a capsule. No information is available concerning staining characteristics of rat nerve sheath tumors using Alcian blue stain. Harkin and Reed (1969) noted that, in man, staining patterns vary between individual tumors and are not definitive for one tumor type in the absence of other diagnostic features.

The electron-microscopic features described above may aid in distinguishing peripheral nerve sheath tumors from other spindle cell tumors, but are not diagnostic for any one cell type. For instance, myofibroblasts may have structures resembling desmosomes and may be surrounded by basal lamina material (Greaves and Faccini 1984). Basal lamina may be present around fibroblasts, endothelial cells, smooth muscle cells, Schwann's cells, and perineurial cells (see Pathogenesis).

Peripheral nerve sheath tumors of man have been demonstrated to contain vimentin and S-100 protein (Gould et al. 1986), and in the recent past the presence of S-100 protein was considered diagnostic of tumors of Schwann-cell origin. More recently several authors have demonstrated that tumors of man with light- and electron-microscopic evidence of Schwann's cells may show variable expression of S-100 protein (Weiss et al. 1983; Matsunou et al. 1985; Wick et al. 1987). Gough et al. (1986) and Laber-Laird and Jokinen (personal communication) described peripheral nerve sheath tumors in rats which contained S-100 protein. However, S-100 protein is more difficult to demonstrate in anaplastic or malignant peripheral nerve sheath tumors of man, and Wechsler et al. (1973) reported similar findings in methyl- and ethylnitrosourea (MNU and ENU)-induced peripheral nerve sheath tumors of rats. In addition, S-100 protein has been observed in human cases of spindle cell malignant melanoma, clear cell sarcoma, and in a few cases of leiomyosarcoma (Wick et al. 1987). Wick et al. (1987) proposed the use of multiple immunohistochemical stains in evaluating possible peripheral nerve sheath tumors.

Diagnostic Problems. For the purpose of preparing this manuscript, 52 spontaneous neoplasms, previously diagnosed as peripheral nerve sheath tumors of rats, were reviewed by the authors. Each author independently classified the tumors without reference to case history or previous diagnoses. For purposes of comparison, the original set of diagnoses was included. Complete agreement by all pathologists was not found for any tumor reviewed. Five of six pathologists agreed upon the diagnosis of one tumor, which was diagnosed as a fibroma. Four of six pathologists agreed upon the diagnoses of eight tumors; four were diagnosed as neurofibrosarcomas, three as fibromas, and one as a malignant

schwannoma. No agreement was found between the pathologists for one of the 52 tumors, and this tumor was diagnosed as a malignant schwannoma, neurofibrosarcoma, malignant fibrous histiocytoma, fibrosarcoma, anaplastic sarcoma, and malignant spindle cell tumor. The highest degree of correlation between any two pathologists was 38%. While agreement was evident concerning the light-microscopic features of these tumors, opinion varied concerning the most significant features and terminology used in classification of the tumors. The results of electron-microscopic and immunohistochemical studies were not available for the 52 tumors reviewed and are not usually available to the pathologist involved in toxicology/pathology studies.

This review emphasizes the difficulty of differentiating between benign schwannomas, malignant schannomas, neurofibromas, neurofibrosarcomas, fibromas, fibrosarcomas, and other spindle cell tumors. In contrast to the information available for nerve sheath tumors of man, no definitive information is available concerning the cell or cells of origin of rat nerve sheath tumors, and the detailed electron-microscopic and immunohistochemical studies are too few to guide evaluation of light-microscopic characteristics (see Pathogenesis).

The authors feel that the terms "benign or malignant peripheral nerve sheath tumor" should be used in classifying rat nerve sheath tumors. If the results of electron-microscopic and immunohistochemical studies are available, it may then be appropriate to subclassify tumors. The term "schwannoma" should be used to distinguish those tumors which show strong evidence of consisting primarily of Schwan's cells. Tumors composed of a mixed population of cells including Schwann's cells, perineurial cells, and/or endoneurial fibroblasts should be classified as "neurofibromas" or "neurofibrosarcomas". A tumor composed of perineurial cells has been reported in man (see Pathogenesis); this tumor may occur in the rat, but it remains to be identified.

Biologic Features

Natural History. In benign peripheral nerve sheath tumors little to no evidence of local invasion is seen. Malignant nerve sheath tumors are locally and extensively invasive but metastasize infrequently. Clinical signs associated with peripheral nerve sheath tumors reflect the tumor size and location. Some animals may die suddenly with no

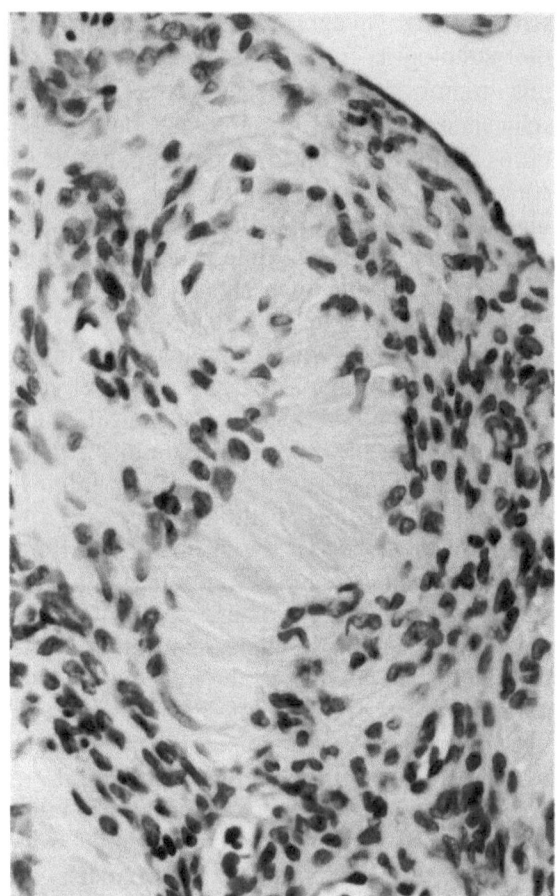

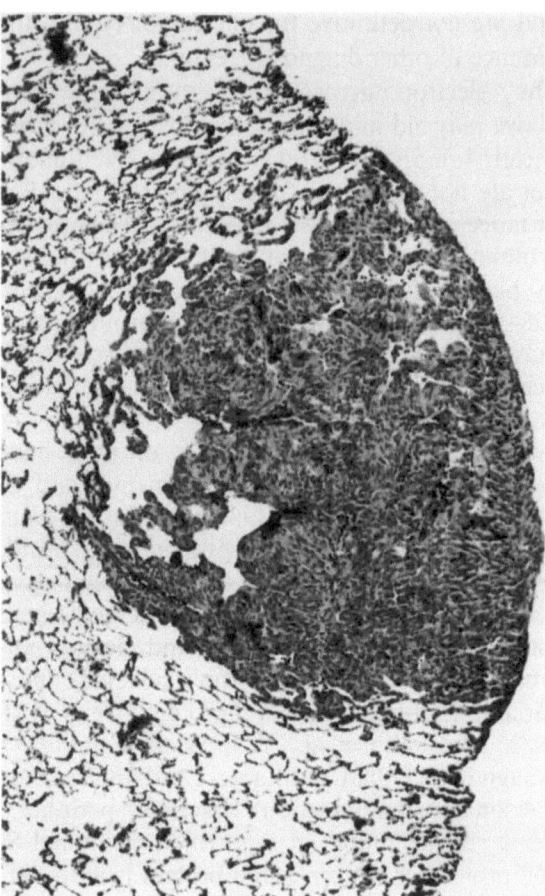

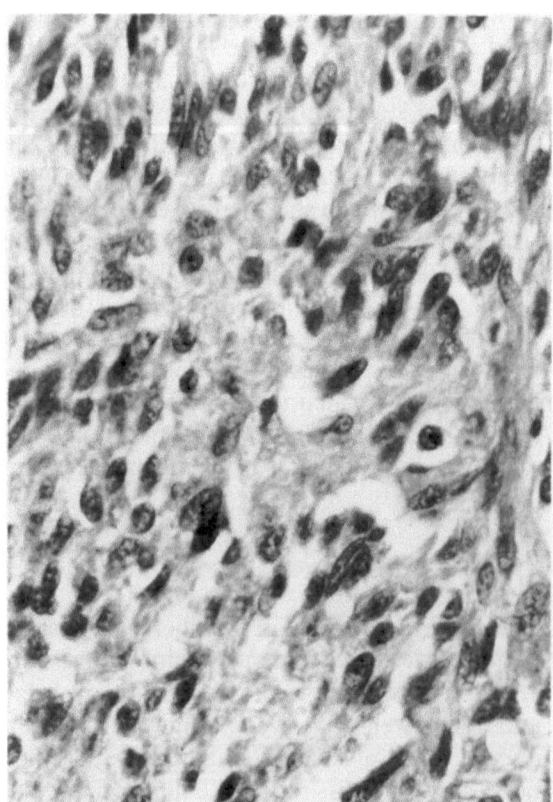

Fig. 171 *(upper left).* Malignant peripheral nerve sheath tumor within the meninges. One prominent Verocay body is present. H and E, × 400

Fig. 172 *(lower left).* Malignant peripheral nerve sheath tumor, subcutis, pinna of the ear, rat. This tumor metastasized to the lung (Fig. 173) H and E, × 410

Fig. 173 *(upper right).* One of several foci of metastasis in the lung, rat. The primary of this tumor is shown in Fig. 172. H and E, × 52

apparent clinical signs (Laber-Laird and Jokinen, personal communication). In experimentally induced tumors, gradual weight loss was evident in some animals (Denlinger et al. 1973).

Schardein et al. (1968) reported a retroperitoneal neurofibrosarcoma with metastasis to the lung in a Holtzman-source rat. In the data collected from the National Toxicology Program, seven malignant schwannomas were diagnosed. Two had metastasized to regional lymph nodes, lung (Fig. 171–173) and surrounding organs. One mass originating in the uterus had spread to the urinary bladder and colon.

Pathogenesis. The cell of origin of peripheral nerve sheath tumors has not been determined definitively. Several authors (Harkin and Reed 1968; Cordy 1978) have hypothesized that all nerve sheath tumors originate from Schwann's cells. This theory fails to explain the variations in light- and electron-microscopic and immunohistochemical characteristics noted in human and animal tumors. Other authors (Erlandson and Woodruff 1982; Ushigome et al. 1986) have hypothesized that peripheral nerve sheath tumors of man may arise from Schwann's cells, perineurial cells, and/or endoneurial fibroblasts, and that the cell of origin is reflected in subtle variations in morphology, immunohistochemical staining patterns, and biologic behavior (Chitale and Dickerson 1983).

Erlandson and Woodruff (1982) have described light- and electron-microscopic features of neurofibromas in man which aid in distinguishing them from schwannomas. Light-microscopic features include widely separated fusiform to stellate cells and "wiry cell processes" separated by individual collagen bundles. Distinguishing ultrastructural characteristics include bipolar or, rarely, tripolar, long thin cytoplasmic processes; an external lamina around approximately 50% of the cells; a fragmented or absent lamina around remaining cells; a few tight junctions; and cytoplasmic processes with prominent microfilaments, scattered microtubules, and pinocytotic vesicles in moderate to large numbers. Interdigitating or entangled cell processes are rare. The stroma consists of randomly arranged collagen fiber bundles in a fibrillar or granular matrix admixed with acellular myxoid areas. Long spacing collagen is rare. These features are consistent with those of the perineurial cell. In some tumors examined, perineurial cells were admixed with fibroblastic cells and well-differentiated Schwann's cells encircling axons. The fibroblas-

tic cells have few pinocytotic vesicles, lack a basal lamina and intercellular junctions (Weidenheim and Campbell 1986) and resemble endoneurial fibroblasts. The Schwann's cells differ from neoplastic cells in schwannomas in that neoplastic Schwann's cells rarely encircle axons.

Ushigome et al. (1986) and Weidenheim and Campbell (1986), in separate studies, concurred with Erlandson and Woodruff (1982) and suggested that peripheral nerve sheath tumors of man may fall into three categories: tumors composed primarily of Schwann's cells, tumors composed of perineurial cells, and tumors composed of both cell types with or without fibroblasts. In a survey of peripheral nerve sheath tumors of man, two tumors consisting entirely of perineurial cells were described by Ushigome et al. (1986). These tumors lacked evidence of S-100 protein and were weakly positive for blood coagulation factor XIII a, a characteristic of perineurial and endoneurial cells but not of Schwann's cells. The neurofibromas examined had varied light- and electron-microscopic appearance. Cellular features were compatible with an admixture of perineurial cells, Schwann's cells, and fibroblastic cells. Areas felt by the authors ot be composed of perineurial cells lacked evidence of S-100 protein and were weakly positive for blood coagulation factor XIII a. Other areas with microscopic features of Schwann's cells were positive for S-100 protein. Based on these findings, Ushigome et al. (1986) and Erlandson and Woodruff (1982) hypothesized that the perineurial cell is a significant component of neurofibromas and that this cell contributes to the distinctions between neurofibromas and schwannomas. The embryologic origins of perineurial cells are uncertain, but some evidence suggests that they are of modified Schwann's cells and that they originate from the neural crest (Erlandson and Woodruff 1982).

Evidence exists that peripheral nerve sheath tumors of the rat may fall into the same or similar subclassifications as those used for nerve sheath tumors of man. Gough et al. (1986) and Laber-Laird and Jokinen (personal communication) described two tumors with a random S-100-staining pattern and discontinuous basal lamina. Laber-Laird and Jokinen (personal communication) also noted pinocytotic vesicles. These features are suggestive of perineurial cells. The most detailed work using rat peripheral nerve sheath tumors has been done using neoplasms induced by ENU and MNU (Koestner et al. 1971; Swenberg et al. 1972; Denlinger et al. 1973). These tumors occur

Table 11. Incidence of peripheral nerve sheath tumors in aged rats[a]

Strain	Sex	Type of tumor								Reference
		Neurofibroma		Neurofibrosar-coma		Benign schwannoma		Malignant schwannoma		
		(n)	(%)	(n)	(%)	(n)	(%)	(n)	(%)	
F344	M	3/1794	0.2	0/1794		2/1794	0.1	0/1794		Goodman et al.
F344	F	0/1754		0/1754		0/1754		0/1754		(1979)
Osborne-Mendel	M	0/ 975		1/ 975	0.1	0/ 975		0/ 075		Goodman et al.
	F	0/ 970		0/ 970		1/ 970	0.1	0/ 970		(1980)
F344/N	M					4/2320	0.17	1/2320	<0.1	Solleveld et al.
F344/N	F					3/2370	0.13	1/2370	<0.1[b]	(1984)

[a] Data from control rats used in 2-year carcinogenicity tests.

[b] This malignant schwannoma of the uterus, with local metastasis to colon and urinary bladder, was among the tumors surveyed by the authors and was counted as one tumor for the purpose of calculating incidence.

mostly in association with the trigeminal nerve, spinal nerve roots (most frequently those of the lumbosacral plexus) and the proximal portion of peripheral nerves. MNU induces well-differentiated peripheral nerve sheath tumors; ENU induces primarily anaplastic nerve sheath tumors. The gross and light-microscopic appearance of these neoplasms resembles that of spontaneously occurring schwannomas. The electron-microscopic features of these neoplasms support the hypothesis that they are composed of Schwann's cells admixed with one or more cell types. Koestner et al. (1971) and Swenberg et al. (1972) described several features of these tumors including spindle-shaped cells with prominent convoluted cytoplasmic processes and scattered cells contained intracytoplasmic, nonmyelinated axons. Basal lamina around tumor cells ranged from absent, to discontinuous, to continuous around a few cells. Denlinger et al. (1973) reported the presence of electron-lucent fibroblasts of the perineurium scattered between Schwann's cells.

Etiology. The cause of spontaneously occurring peripheral nerve sheath tumors of rats is unknown. These tumors may be induced by alkylating agents such as nitroso compounds, triazine and related compounds administered subcutaneously, intraperitoneally, or orally (Mennel and Zülch 1976; Jänisch and Schreiber 1977). The target cell of these chemicals is unknown. The majority of these tumors have been diagnosed as benign and malignant schwannomas (Swenberg et al. 1972; Denlinger et al. 1973; Swenberg et al. 1975). Denlinger reported one neurofibrosarcoma and two perineurial fibrosarcomas in a group of rats treated with MNU intravenously. Since some ambiguity exists in the use of the terms "neurofibroma/neurofibrosarcoma" and "schwannoma," and since differentiation between these tumors is not definitive, agents capable of inducing schwannomas may also induce neurofibromas and neurofibrosarcomas. For instance, in a report on chemical induction of schwannomas using ENU and MNU (Mandybur and Brunner 1982) the morphology of metastatic foci was compatible with either a neurofibrosarcoma or a poorly differentiated malignant schwannoma.

Frequency. For this manuscript, records and tissues from 7320 F344 control rats used in chronic toxicity studies conducted in the National Toxicology Program were reviewed. A total of 52 peripheral nerve sheath tumors had been diagnosed (0.7%) (excluding cardiac neurilemmomas). Of these tumors, ten neurofibromas (0.1%), 23 neurofibrosarcomas (0.2%), 12 schwannomas (0.2%), and seven malignant schwannomas (0.1%) were described. All the reported neurofibromas (10/10) and 17 of 23 neurofibrosarcomas (82%) were in male rats. Goodman et al. (1979, 1980) reported neurofibromas and neurofibrosarcomas only in male rats (Table 11).

These data suggest that male rats may have a higher incidence of neurofibromas/neurofibrosarcomas than do female rats. In contrast, the incidence of benign and malignant schwannomas was approximately the same in male and female rats. The incidences reported here are slightly higher than those recorded in the literature (Table 11).

Comparison with Other Species

Peripheral nerve sheath tumors are rare, but have been reported in man (see Biologic Features) and all domestic species (Luginbühl et al. 1968; Fankhauser et al. 1974; Cordy 1978). Vandevelde et al. (1977) described neurofibromas in the central nervous system of two dogs. The light- and electron-microscopic descriptions of these tumors were compatible with those neurofibromas discussed by Erlandson and Woodruff (1982) and Ushigome et al. (1986). Vandevelde et al. (1977) noted that the majority of tumor cells were fibroblastic. These cells may represent endoneurial fibroblasts. Some cells were described as containing vesicles and may represent perineurial cells. Features suggestive of Schwann's cells, such as long spacing collagen and convoluted cytoplasmic processes, were described as absent. Schwannomas have been reported in a wide variety of domestic species including dogs, cats, and cattle (Luginbühl et al. 1968; Fankhauser et al. 1974; Cordy 1978). Cordy (1978) reported that schwannomas are most common in cattle, and that viral particles have been seen in tumor cells. Most common locations are the brachial plexus, intercostal nerves, and cardiac nerves. The light-microscopic appearance of these neoplasms resembles that described in rats. Patnaik et al. (1984) described schwannomas in two dogs. Both of these tumors consisted of spindle cells with light- and electron-microscopic characteristics compatible with a tumor of Schwann's cell and/ or perineurial cell origin. Scattered cells in these tumors contained melanin pigment. The production of melanin by Schwann's cells may reflect the common origin of melanocytes and Schwann's cells from neural crest cells. Production of melanin by tumor cells in schwannomas has been reported in a few tumors of man. Rothwell et al. (1986) reported a schwannoma in the testis of a dog in which tumor cells positive for S-100 protein were demonstrated. In the mouse, peripheral nerve sheath tumors are very rare in all strains with the exception of the NHO mouse. The incidence in this strain is 8.07% compared to 0.05% for all other strains (Stewart et al. 1974; Swenberg 1982). Approximately 50% of these tumors were diagnosed as schwannomas.

Acknowledgement. The information presented in this manuscript is based in part upon a review of records and tissues of control rats from 63 chronic toxicity studies conducted in the National Toxicology Program. The authors wish to acknowledge access to these files for data and tissue sections used for photomicrographs.

References

Abbott DP (1982) Malignant schwannoma of the dorsal spinal nerve root in a laboratory rat. Lab Anim 16: 265–266

Anver MR, Cohen BJ, Lattuada CP, Foster SJ (1982) Age-associated lesions in barrier-reared male Sprague-Dawley rats: a comparison between Hap: (SD) and CRL: COBS [R] (CD) [R] (SD) stocks. Exp Aging Res 8: 3–24

Chitale AR, Dickersin GR (1983) Electron microscopy in the diagnosis of malignant schwannomas: a report of six cases. Cancer 51: 1448–1461

Cordy DR (1978) Tumors of the nervous system and eye. In: Moulton JE (ed) Tumors in domestic animals. University of California Press, Berkeley, pp 430–455

Denlinger RH, Koestner A, Swenberg JA (1973) An experimental model for selective production of neoplasms of the peripheral nervous system. Acta Neuropathol (Berl) 23: 219–228

Erlandson RA, Woodruff JM (1982) Peripheral nerve sheath tumors: an electron microscopic study of 43 cases. Cancer 49: 273–287

Fankhauser R, Luginbühl M, McGrath JT (1974) Tumours of the nervous system. Bull WHO 50: 53–69

Goodman DG, Ward JM, Squire RA, Chu KC, Linehart MS (1979) Neoplastic and non-neoplastic lesions in aging F344 rats. Toxicol Appl Pharmacol 48: 237–248

Goodman DG, Ward JM, Squire RA, Paxton MB, Reichardt WD, Chu KC, Linhart MS (1980) Neoplastic and non-neoplastic lesions in aging Osborne-Mendel rats. Toxicol Appl Pharmacol 55: 433–447

Gough AW, Hanna W, Barsoum NJ, Moore J, Sturgess JM (1986) Morphologic and immunohistochemical features of two spontaneous peripheral nerve tumors in Wistar rats. Vet Pathol 23: 68–73

Gould VE, Moll R, Moll I, Inchul L, Schwechheimer K, Franke WW (1986) The intermediate filament complement of the spectrum of nerve sheath neoplasms. Lab Invest 55: 463–474

Greaves P, Faccini JM (1984) Rat histopathology: a glossary in toxicity and carcinogenicity studies. Elsevier Science, New York, pp 74–85

Harkin JC, Reed RJ (1969) Tumors of the peripheral nervous system. In: Firminger HI (ed) Atlas of tumor pathology, second series, fasc. 3. Aimed Forces Institute of Pathology, Washington, DC

Jänisch W, Schreiber D (1977) Experimental tumors of the central nervous system. Upjohn, Kalamazoo, Michigan

Koestner A, Swenberg JA, Wechsler W (1971) Transplacental production with ethylnitrosourea of neoplasms of the nervous system in Sprague-Dawley rats. Am J Pathol 63: 37–56

Luginbühl M, Fankhauser R, McGrath JT (1968) Spontaneous neoplasms of the nervous system in animals. In: Krayenbuhl H, Maspes PE, Sweet WH (eds) Progress in neurological surgery, vol. z. Karger, New York, pp 85–164

Mandybur TI, Brunner GD (1982) Experimental hematogenic metastasis of malignant schwannomas in the rat. Acta Neuropathol (Berl) 57: 151–157

Matsunou H, Shimoda T, Kakimoto S, Yamashita H, Ishikawa E, Mukai M (1985) Histopathologic and immunohistochemical study of malignant tumors of peripheral nerve sheath (malignant schwannoma). Cancer 56: 2269–2279

Mennel HD, Zülch E (1976) Tumours of the central and peripheral nervous systems. In: Turusov VS (ed) Tumours of the rat. Part 2. IARC Scientific Publ no 6. IARC Lyon, pp 295–311 (Pathology of tumours in laboratory animals, vol I)

Patnaik AK, Erlandson RA, Liebermen PH (1984) Canine malignant melanotic schwannomas: a light and electron microscopic study of two cases. Vet Pathol 21: 483–488

Rothwell TLW, Papadimitriou JM, Xu F-N, Middleton DJ (1986) Schwannoma in the testis of a dog. Vet Pathol 23: 629–631

Schardein JL, Fitzgerald JE, Kaump DH (1968) Spontaneous tumors in Holtzman-source rats of various ages. Pathol Vet 5: 238–252

Solleveld HA, Haseman JK, McConnell EE (1984) Natural history of body weight gain, survival, and neoplasia in the F344 rat. JNCI 72: 929–940

Steward HL, Deringer MK, Dunn TB, Snell KC (1974) Malignant schwannomas of nerve roots, uterus, and epididymis in mice. JNCI 53: 1749–1758

Swenberg JA, Clendenon N, Denlinger R, Gordon WA (1975) Sequential development of ethylnitrosourea-induced neurinomas: morphology, biochemistry, and transplantability. JNCI 55: 147–152

Swenberg JA, Koestner A, Wechsler W (1972) The induction of tumors of the nervous system with intravenous methylnitrosourea. Lab Invest 26: 74–85

Swenberg JA (1982) Neoplasms of the nervous system. In: Foster HL, Small JD, Fox JG (eds) The mouse in biomedical research, vol IV. Academic, New York, pp 529–537

Ushigome S, Takakuwa T, Hyuga M, Tadokoro M, Shinagawa T (1986) Perineurial cell tumor and the significance of the perineurial cells in neurofibroma. Acta Pathol Jpn 36: 973–987

Vandevelde M, Braund KG, Hoff EJ (1977) Central neurofibromas in two dogs. Vet Pathol 14: 470–478

Wechsler W, Pfeiffer SE, Swenberg JA, Koestner A (1973) S-100 protein in methyl- and ethylnitrosourea induced tumors of the rat nervous system. Acta Neuropathol (Berl) 24: 287–303

Weidenheim KM, Campbell WG jr (1986) Perineurial cell tumor: immunocytochemical and ultrastructural characterization. Relationship to other peripheral nerve tumors with a review of the literature. Virchows Arch [A] 408: 375–383

Weiss SW, Langloss JM, Enzinger FM (1983) Value of S-100 protein in the diagnosis of soft tissue tumors with particular reference to benign and malignant Schwann cell tumors. Lab Invest 49: 299–308

Wick MR, Swanson PE, Scheithauer BW, Manivel JC (1987) Malignant peripheral nerve sheath tumor: an immunohistochemical study of 62 cases. Am J Clin Pathol 87: 425–433

Schwannomas (Induced), Cranial, Spinal, and Peripheral Nerves, Rat

Jerry M. Rice and Jerrold M. Ward

Synonyms. Malignant neurinoma; malignant neurilem(m)oma; neurogenic sarcoma.

Gross Appearance

Schwannomas found early in their development are seen as inconspicuous, swollen segments of the nerve of origin. Larger neoplasms are soft, grayish-white, often cystic and sometimes hemorrhagic masses, are frequently invasive but rarely metastasize. There is no capsule. Intracranial tumors most ferquently occur ventral to the overlying brain and may adhere firmly to the brain or to the floor of the cranial vault. They often spread diffusely over the meninges and may extend through foramina and sutures of the skull to invade the soft tissues of the head, causing bizarre, asymmetrical distortions of the face. Tumors that arise from spinal ganglia commonly spread within the spinal canal, compressing the cord and causing paresis that progresses to paralysis distal to the mass. These tumors frequently also extend to the adjacent paravertebral musculature where they are seen as mediastinal, retroperitoneal, or pelvic masses that contrast sharply in color and consistency with the invaded muscle. Schwannomas may also originate demonstrably from the larger peripheral nerves, such as the sciatic; from the brachial or lumbosacral plexuses; from a myenteric plexus of the intestine; or in soft tissues, where they may bear no obvious anatomic relationship to the nerve of origin. such tumors may be grossly indistingushable from soft tissue neoplasms of mesenchymal origin, such as lipomas or soft fibromas, unless they are markedly cystic. Even small schwannomas may contain multiple, often contiguous cysts

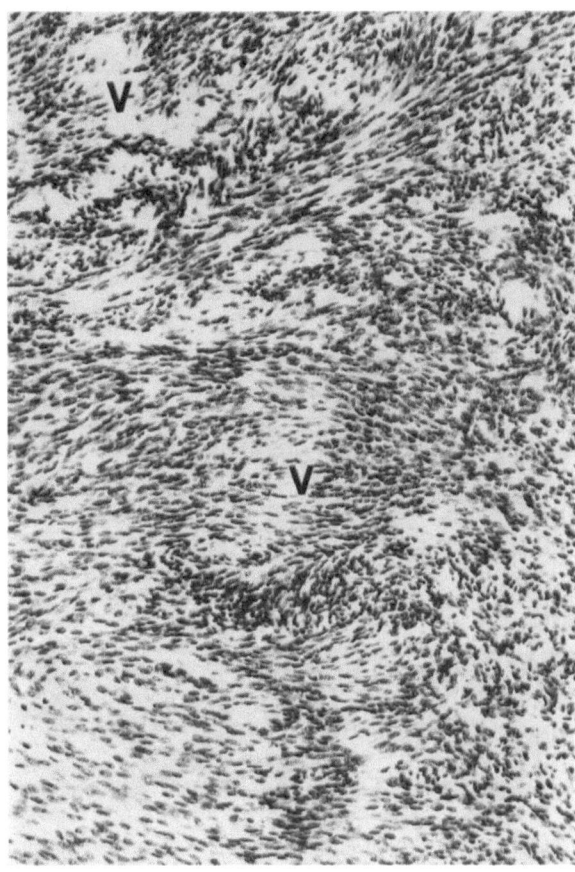

Fig. 174. Intra-abdominal schwannoma, rat, composed of Antoni type A tissue with Verocay bodies *(V)*. H and E, × 100

that contain clear or blood-tinged serous fluid, and this feature, when present, is virtually diagnostic. Schwannomas may attain maximum dimensions of several centimeters, but when much smaller often cause death by compromising the brain or cord. Photographs of careful dissections of the nervous system, showing schwannomas in relation to the brain, spinal cord, and major nerves have been published (Ivankovic and Druckrey 1968; Wechsler et al. 1969; Ivankovic 1979).

Microscopic Features

The histologic, ultrastructural, and biochemical characteristics of rat schwannomas are consistent with their origin from Schwann's cells, the myelin-forming cells of the peripheral nervous system. Differentiated schwannomas consist of both Antoni type A and type B tissue in variable proportions. Antoni type A tissue (Fig. 174) is dense-ly cellular and consists of small fusiform cells with oval nuclei that stain intensely and evenly. Cytoplasm is rather abundant and eosinophilic, but cell margins are indistinct. The cells tend to be aligned in parallel arrays. These may generate a sinusoidal pattern strongly reminiscent of that of a nerve sectioned longitudinally. In other areas they may have a whorling pattern. Nuclei of adjacent cells may lie in rows, creating palisades. Palisades of nuclei may occur at both ends of an elongated bundle of parallel cell processes that is devoid of nuclei and thus uniformly eosinophilic. Such formations are called "Verocay bodies" (Fig. 174). It must be emphasized, however, that Verocay body formation is not found in all schwannomas, and in fact this feature is more common in tumors of smooth muscle. Individual cells in Antoni type A tissue are enveloped by abundant, fine reticulin fibers (Fig. 175). Schwann's cells, unlike other neuroectodermally derived cells such as glia, are able to form collagen. Mitoses are easily found.

Antoni type B tissue is less cellular and appears myxoid in sections stained with hematoxylin and eosin (Fig. 176). The cells have less cytoplasm and cell processes often project in serveral directions so that some cells appear stellate rather than spindle shaped and are widely separated by a nonstaining matrix. The cysts that are often prominent grossly in schwannomas occur in Antoni type B tissue and appear empty in paraffin sections or contain a small quantity of cellular debris. Cysts are lined by either slightly flattened tumor cells or by a narrow zone of hypercellularity. Reticulin fibers are much less abundant in Antoni type B tissue and foci of such tissue may appear afibrillar in silver impregnations (Fig. 175).

Schwannomas that arise in or adjacent to spinal or cranial nerve ganglia frequently contain remnants of the ganglion, including large neurons and axis cylinders (Fig. 177). Organoid structures that resemble Meissner's corpuscles may occur (Fig. 178); in these, nuclei are in palisades separated by fibrillar, eosinophilic cytoplasmic processes arrayed in parallel. These corpuscles, although somewhat similar to Verocay bodies, are much smaller. Granular cell (Berman et al. 1978) and melanotic (Spence et al. 1976) variants of otherwise typical schwannomas have been described (see p. 160, this volume).

Rat schwannomas contain variable amounts of S-100 protein (Wechsler et al. 1973), which can often, but not always, be demonstrated in at least a fraction of the tumor cells by immunohisto-

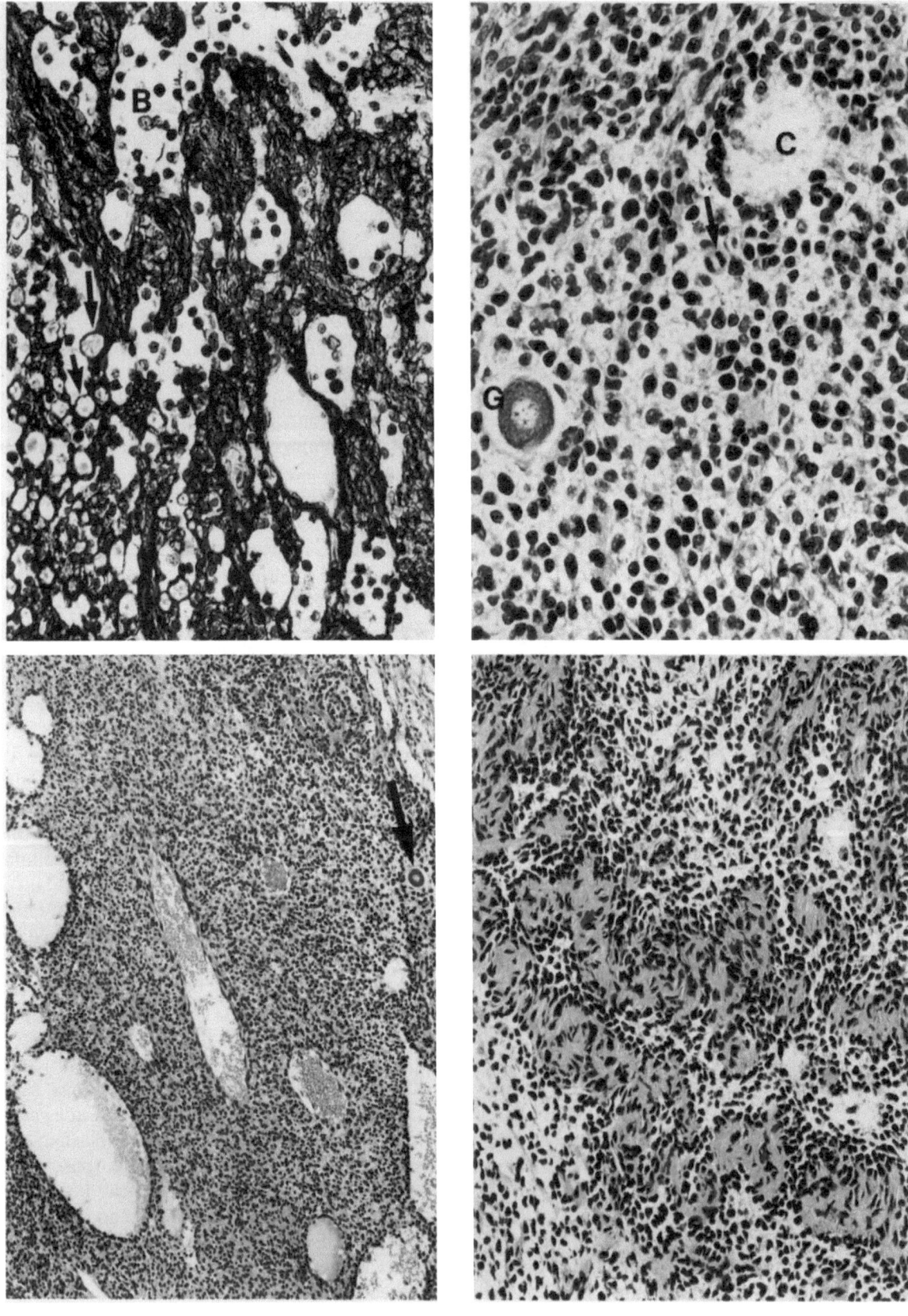

◀ **Fig. 175** *(upper left)*. Schwannoma, rat. Abundant reticulin fibers in Antoni type A tissue with apparently afibrillar foci of Antoni type B tissue *(B)*. Residual axons from the nerve of origin persist at lower left *(arrows)*. Wilder's reticulum, × 400

Fig. 176 *(lower left)*. Schwannoma, rat. Antoni type B tissue with cysts and residual ganglion cells *(arrow)*. DNA from this tumor transformed NIH 3T3 cells and contained a mutationally activated *neu* oncogene. H and E, × 100

Fig. 177 *(upper right)*. Schwannoma, rat. Higher magnification of Fig. 176 to show a ganglion cell *(G)*, a neoplastic Schwann's cell in mitosis *(arrow)* and a small cyst *(C)*. H and E, × 400

Fig. 178 *(lower right)*. Schwannoma, rat. Organoid structures resembling Meissner's tactile corpuscles within an area of Antoni type B tissue. H and E, × 250

chemistry, with predominantly nuclear localization. Although the biologic role of S-100 protein is unknown, it is a useful if nonspecific marker for neuroectodermal tumors including schwannomas (Gough et al. 1986).

Anaplastic schwannomas are more cellular and more malignant than their differentiated counterparts. They contain less reticulin, less S-100 protein, and little or no Antoni type A tissue. They may resemble hypercellular Antoni type B tissue with cysts and frequent mitoses or may contain plump, spindle-shaped cells larger than those of the Antoni type A tissue in differentiated tumors.

Schwannomas, especially anaplastic schwannomas, frequently invade skeletal muscle; intracranial tumors may invade the brain along the perivascular spaces. Anaplastic schwannomas occasionally metastasize to lung (Swenberg et al. 1972).

Ultrastructure

Neoplastic Schwann's cells that comprise differentiated schwannomas of the rat are surrounded by a single, usually interrupted layer of basal lamina (Wechsler et al. 1969; Koestner et al. 1971; Swenberg et al. 1972), like their human homologs (Harkin and Reed 1969; Henderson and Papadimitriou 1982; Dickersin 1987). This is the most important ultrastructural feature of these cells. Adjacent cells also have characteristically interdigitating plasma membranes with occasional junctional processes, and abundant collagen fibers are present in the intercellular ma-

trix. Occasionally segments of nonmyelinted axons are incorporated into the cytoplasm of the cells (Koestner et al. 1971). Melanotic schwannomas contain premelanosomes and melanosomes (Spence et al. 1976). Anaplastic schwannomas frequently contain fewer collagen fibers, and a smaller fraction of the cells have basal lamina.

Differential Diagnosis

Intracranial schwannomas that spread diffusely over the meninges may be confused with primary meningeal neoplasms of fibroblastic type. The latter usually consist of larger cells with abundant, coarse collagen fibers that are demonstrable by Masson's stain and by silver impregnations for reticulin. Meningeal tumors lack Antoni type B tissue, basal lamina, and S-100 protein. Schwannomas in the soft tissue that lack appreciable Antoni type B tissue or cystic areas may be difficult to distinguish from sarcomas; immunohistochemical staining for S-100 protein and intermediate filaments and electron microscopy may be required to establish a diagnosis with confidence. This is especially true for tumors that arise in the wall of the gastrointestinal tract and may be indistinguishable from smooth muscle tumors (which contain desmin, but not S-100 protein) by light microscopy. Anaplastic schwannomas, especially those of the intracranial segments of the trigeminal nerve, may appear as afibrillar "small blue-cell tumors" that contain residual ganglion cells and can be misinterpreted as neuroblastomas. Neuroblastoma is rare in rats and should not be diagnosed without ultrastructural confirmation that the cells are in fact neuroblasts. Intracranial schwannomas that are allowed to autolyze prior to fixation may become almost indistinguishable from oligodendrogliomas by hematoxylin and eosin staining; the reticulum often persists, however, and remains demonstrable by silver staining.

Biologic Features

Schwannomas of the rat appear biologically malignant by the criteria of local invasiveness and transplantability with local invasion and metastasis. True benign schwannomas, like the acoustic nerve tumors of man (Harkin and Reed 1969), have not been conclusively identified. Schwannomas are among those chemically induced tumors of rodents that are specifically associated

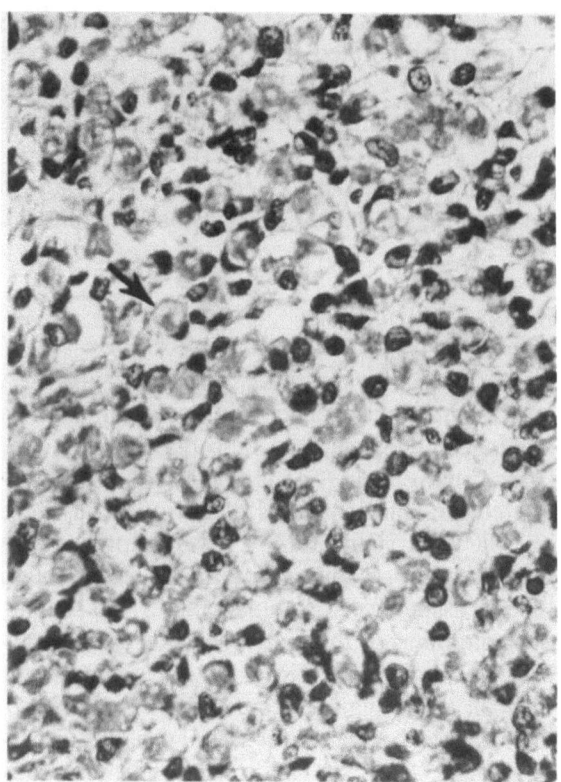

Fig. 179. Mediastinal schwannoma, invading thoracic spinal nerve, rat. Neoplastic cells surround axis cylinders *(arrow)*, reflecting the normal relationship of Schwann's cells to axons. H and E, ×630

plantation (Swenberg et al. 1975). Periaxonal orientation of the neoplastic Schwann's cells is lost as the cells proliferate to form a mass. Cysts and Antoni type B tissue are often apparent in tumors as small as 0.2 cm in diameter and are more prominent in large tumors. Most schwannomas aggressively invade adjacent tissues very early in their developement, but in the rat, metastasis from a primary schwannoma is very rare. Schwannomas grow rapidly, and signs of intracranial pressure or of posterior paresis that deepens to paralysis progress rapidly in animals that develop these tumors within the skull or spinal canal. Latency varies inversely with dose, and schwannomas that result from transplacental exposure may cause death as early as 4 months after birth, or may be found incidentally at necropsy in rats more than 2 years old, depending on the strain of rat, the dose of carcinogen, and the stage of gestation when it was administered (Ivankovic and Druckrey 1968). The tumors are readily transplantable, grow rapidly, and, from a subcutaneous transplantation site, frequently metastasize to the lungs.

with a mutationally activated oncogene. A specific thymine to adenine transversion mutation in the transmembrane region of the oncogene *neu* has been consistently found in schwannomas of cranial and spinal nerves that had been induced by *N*-nitrosoethylurea in F344 rats (Perantoni et al. 1987). This mutated oncogene was not detected in gliomas or in other neoplasms induced by chemicals in these rats.

Pathogenesis. Schwannomas begin as foci of hypercellularity within a nerve, often adjacent to or within a ganglion, that may be histologically evident as early as 20 days after exposure to carcinogen (Swenberg et al. 1975). The gassarian ganglion of the trigeminal nerve is an especially common site of origin of schwannomas induced by transplacental carcinogenesis. In the early stages, the normal relation of Schwann's cells to axons is retained, with simply a diffuse increase in the number of Schwann's cells and a resultant slight swelling of the nerve (Fig. 179). Such early lesions, when transplanted to syngeneic hosts, produce typical schwannomas at the site of im-

Etiology. Schwannomas are readily inducible in rats by a variety of chemical carciogens, and susceptibility is highest during the perinatal period, especially during the final week of intrauterine life. Although direct-acting alkylating agents (for example, *N*-nitrosoethylurea, methylmethanesulfonate) are most prominent among the transplacental carcinogens that cause schwannomas in rats after a single prenatal exposure (e.g., Druckrey et al. 1970; Ivankovic and Druckrey 1968; Koestner et al. 1971), many metabolism-dependent carcinogens including certain polynuclear aromatic hydrocarbons (e.g., 7,12-dimethylbenz[*a*]anthracene) are also effective (Rice et al. 1978). Schwannomas can also be induced selectively in young adult rats by repeated injections of *N*-nitrosomethylurea (Swenberg et al. 1972).

Frequency. Schwannomas have been reported in old, untreated control rats (Abbott 1982; Gough et al. 1986), but the incidence is so low that no accurate estimate of frequency can be made. Inbred strains of rats differ greatly in susceptibility to chemical induction of these tumors (Druckrey et al. 1970; Swenberg et al. 1972), but the pattern of inheritance is complex and more than one gene is involved (Naito et al. 1985). Males are more susceptible than females (Swenberg et al. 1972).

Comparison with Other Species

Schwannomas similar in morphology and sites of origin to those in rats have been induced by transplacental exposure to alkylating agents in the mouse (Denlinger et al. 1974; Wechsler et al. 1979), Syrian golden hamster (Cardesa et al. 1982), and rabbit (Stavrou et al. 1977). The mouse is much more resistant than the rat to carcinogensis in both the central and peripheral nervous system. Schwannomas of the mouse are generally better differentiated than those of the rat; Meissner's corpuscles are much more common in murine schwannomas. The Syrian hamster is rather susceptible to transplacental induction of schwannomas, and in the hamster tumors, Antoni type B tissue often predominantes. In addition to malignant schwannomas like those of the rat and mouse, Syrian hamsters develop a tumor that morphologically resembles the plexiform neurofibromas of man. Antoni type B tissue also frequently predominantes in rabbit schwannomas. Schwannomas have been induced in adult European hamsters by repeated subcutaneous injections of 1,1-dimethylhydrazine (Ernst et al. 1987) and in boxer dogs by repeated intravenous injections of N-nitrosomethylurea (Denlinger et al. 1978). A peculiar feature of the canine tumors is their preferential origin from the intestinal wall and frequent metastasis to the liver.

Rat schwannomas differ from those of man in that most human schwannomas are clinically benign (Harkin and Reed 1969), including the so-called cellular schwannomas (Fletcher et al. 1987) that closely resemble many rat tumors both in histologic appearance and tendency to originate from the paravertebral region of the mediastinum and retroperitoneum. Most malignant schwannomas of man occur in patients with neurofibromatosis (Recklinghausen's disease), an autosomal dominant trait due to a specific gene located in the pericentromeric region of chromosome 17 (Barker et al. 1987). The cellular schwannomas are an exception, in that most are not associated with neurofibromatosis. No comparable condition is known to exist in animals.

References

Abbott DP (1982) Malignant schwannoma of the dorsal spinal nerve root in al laboratory rat. Lab Anim 16: 265–266

Barker D, Wright E, Nguyen K, Cannon L, Fain P, Goldgar D, Bishop DT, Carey J, Baty B, Kivlin J, Willard H, Waye JS, Greig G, Leinwand L, Nakamura Y, O'Connell P, Leppert M, Lalouel J-M, White R, Skolnick M (1987) Gene for von Recklinghausen neurofibromatosis is in the pericentromeric region of chromosome 17. Sciene 236: 1100–1102

Berman JJ, Rice JM, Strandberg J (1978) Granular cell variants in a rat schwannoma. Vet Pathol 15: 725–731

Cardesa A, Rustia M, Mohr U (1982) Tumours of the nervous system. In: Turusov VS (ed) Tumours of the hamster. IARC, Lyon, pp 413–436 (Pathology of tumours in laboratory animals, vol III)

Denlinger RH, Koestner A, Wechsler W (1974) Induction of neurogenic tumors in C3HeB/FeJ mice by nitrosourea derivatives: observations by light microscopy, tissue culture, and electron microscopy. Int J Cancer 13: 559–571

Denlinger RH, Koestner A, Swenberg JA (1978) Neoplasms in purebred boxer dogs following long-term administration of N-methyl-N-nitrosourea. Cancer Res 38: 1711–1717

Dickersin GR (1987) The electron microscopic spectrum of nerve sheath tumors. Ultrasruct Pathol 11: 103–146

Druckrey H, Landschuetz C, Ivankovic S (1970) Transplacentare Erzeugung maligner Tumoren des Nervensystems. II. Aethylnitrosoharnstoff an 10 genetisch definierten Rattenstämmen. Z Krebsforsch 73: 371–386

Ernst H, Rittinghausen S, Wahnschaffe U, Mohr U (1987) Induction of malignant peripheral nerve sheath tumors in European hamsters with 1,1-dimethylhydrazine (UDMH). Cancer Lett 35: 303–311

Fletcher CDM, Davies SE, McKee PH (1987) Cellular schwannoma: a distinct pseudosarcomatous entity. Histopathology 11: 21–35

Gough AW, Hanna W, Barsoum NJ, Moore J, Sturgess JM (1986) Morphologic and immunohistochemical features of two spontaneous peripheral nerve tumors in Wistar rats. Vet Pathol 23: 68–73

Harkin JC, Reed RJ (1969) Tumors of the periphral nervous system. Atlas of tumor pathology, Secound Series, Fascicle 3. AFIP, Washington

Henderson DW, Papadimitriou JM (1982) Ultrastructural appearances of tumours. A diagnostic atlas. Churchill Livingstone, London, pp 200–207

Ivankovic LS (1979) Teratogenic and carcinogenic effects of some chemicals during prenatal life in rats, Syrian golden hamsters, and minipigs. NCI Monogr 51: 103–115

Ivankovic S, Druckrey H (1968) Transplacentare Erzeugung maligner Tumoren des Nervensystems. I. Aethylnitrosoharnstoff an BD IX Ratten. Z Krebsforsch 71: 320–360

Koestner A, Swenberg JA, Weschler W (1971) Transplacental production with ethylnitrosourea of neoplasms of the nervous system in Sprague-Dawley rats. Am J Pathol 63: 37–56

Naito M, Ito A, Aoyama H (1985) Genetics of susceptibility of rats to trigeminal schwannomas induced by neonatal administration of N-ethyl-N-nitrosourea. JNCI 74: 241–245

Perantoni AO, Rice JM, Reed CD, Watantani M, Wenk ML (1987) Activated neu oncogene sequences in primary tumors of the peripheral nervous system induced in rats by transplacental exposure to ethylnitrosourea. Proc Natl Acad Sci USA 84: 6317–6321

Rice JM, Joshi SR, Shenefelt RE, Wenk M (1978) Transplacental carcinogenic activity of 7,12-dimethylbenz[a]anthracene. In: Jones PW, Freudenthal RI (eds) Carcinogenesis: a comprehensive survey. III. Polynuclear aromatic hydrocarbons. Raven, New York

Spence AM, Rubinstein LJ, Conley FK, Herman MM (1976) Studies on experimental malignant nerve sheath tumors maintained in tissue and organ culture systems. III. Melanin pigment and melanogenesis in experimental neurogenic tumors: a reappraisal of the histogenesis of pigmented nerve sheath tumors. Acta Neuropathol (Berl) 35: 27-45

Stavrou D, Dahme E, Schroeder B (1977) Transplacentare neuroonkogene Wirkung von Äthylnitrosoharnstoff beim Kaninchen während der frühen Graviditätsphase (engl abstr). Z Krebsforsch 89: 331-339

Swenberg JA, Koestner A, Wechsler W (1972) The induction of tumors of the nervous system with intravenous methylnitrosourea. Lab Invest 26: 74-85

Swenberg JA, Clendenon N, Denlinger R, Gordon WA (1975) Sequential development of ethylnitrosourea-induced neurinomas: morphology, biochemistry, and transplantability. JNCI 55: 147-152

Wechsler W, Kleihues P, Matsumoto S, Zülch KJ, Ivankovic S, Preussmann R, Druckrey H (1969) Pathology of experimental neurogenic tumors chemically induced during prenatal and postnatal life. Ann NY Acad Sci 159: 360-408

Wechsler W, Pfeiffer SE, Swenberg JA, Koestner A (1973) S-100 protein in methyl- and ethylnitrosourea-induced tumors of the rat nervous system. Acta Neuropathol (Berl) 24: 287-303

Wechsler W, Rice JM, Vesselinovitch SD (1979) Transplacental and neonatal induction of neurogenic tumors in mice: comparison with related species and with human pediatric neoplasms. NCI Monogr 51: 219-226

Malignant Melanotic Schwannomas Induced by 1,1-Dimethylhydrazine, European Hamster

Heinrich Ernst and Ulrich Mohr

Synonyms. Malignant melanocytic schwannoma; malignant pigmented schwannoma; malignant melano(cy)tic nerve sheath tumor; malignant pigmented nerve sheath tumor; fusiform malignant melanoma.

Gross Appearance

Seventeen malignant peripheral nerve sheath tumors were induced in 29 European hamsters by weekly subcutaneous injection of 1,1-dimethylhydrazine (UDMH). Five of these tumors were classified as malignant melanotic schwannomas (Ernst et al. 1987). These tumors, which probably originated from dermal nerves, arose predominantly in the skin around the orbit as fairly firm cutaneous nodules which grew slowly but continuously up to 1 cm in diameter. As the tumors grew, the overlying epidermis became focally ulcerated (Fig. 180) and developed spots of hyperpigmentation. The cut surface of the intradermal tumor tissue was grayish-yellow with peripheral

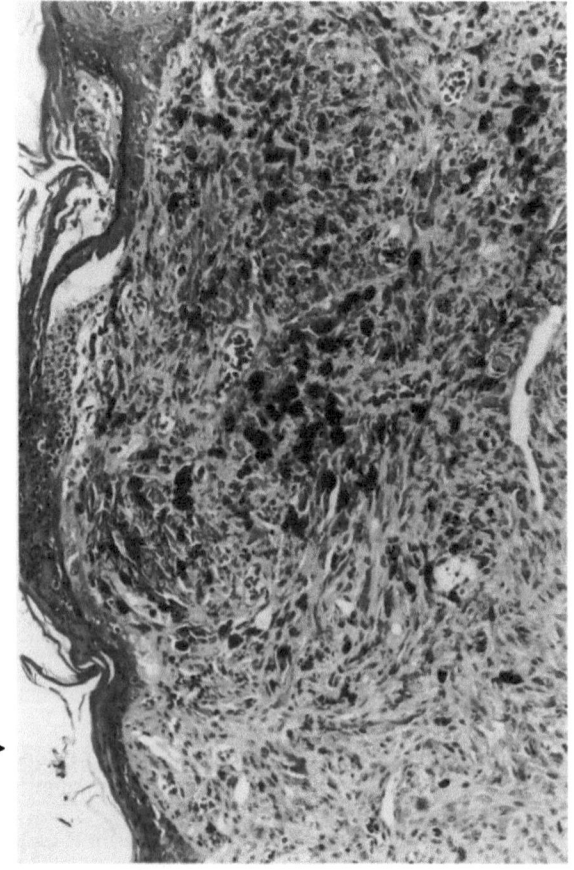

Fig. 180. Skin, European hamster, UDMH-induced malignant melanotic schwannoma of Antoni type A with ulceration of the overlying epidermis. Note clusters of heavily pigmented tumor cells and inflammatory cell infiltration within the tumor. H and E, × 120

brown to bluish-black pigmented areas. These areas varied in number, size, and degree of pigmentation from tumor to tumor, but were always located in close proximity to the epidermis. No distant metastasis was found from any of the melanotic tumors.

Microscopic Appearance

Three of the melanotic tumors were categorized as schwannomas with Antoni type A pattern, characterized by densely cellular interlacing fascicles of spindle-shaped cells with oval to elongated hyperchromatic nuclei and a moderate amount of pink cytoplasm. In some tumor areas a rhythmical nuclear palisading of the tumor cells and the formation of Verocay bodies and neuroid structures resembling tactile bodies was observed (Figs. 181, 182). The other melanotic schwannomas, with stellated and more pleomorphic tumor cells distributed in a reticular pattern and separated by interstitial edema, were classified as Antoni type B (Fig. 183). Both schwannomas types contained tumor cells with variable amounts of pigment which was positive by Fontana-Masson and negative for iron. These cells ranged from epithelial cells with coarse black pigment granules, which frequently obsured the cellular details, to bipolar and dendritic cells with fine brownish-black granular pigment dispersed in their perikarya and cytoplasmic processes (Figs. 180, 184). Melanotic tumor cells were only found in tumor fields adjacent to or within the epidermis where they formed loosely arranged aggregates (Figs. 180, 184) or densely packed cell clusters indistinguishable from true melanomas (Fig. 185). Occasionally, melanomatous nests of pigmented tumor cells appeared at the dermo-epidermal junction concomitant with irregularly scattered melanotic cells in a narrow zone of underlying schwannoma tissue (Fig. 183). Some of these junctional pigment cells were also found to have migrated across the epidermis. Since the observed melanotic schwannomas destroyed neighboring tissues by infiltrative growth and frequently elicited pronounced inflammatory reaction (Fig. 184), they were all considered to be malignant.

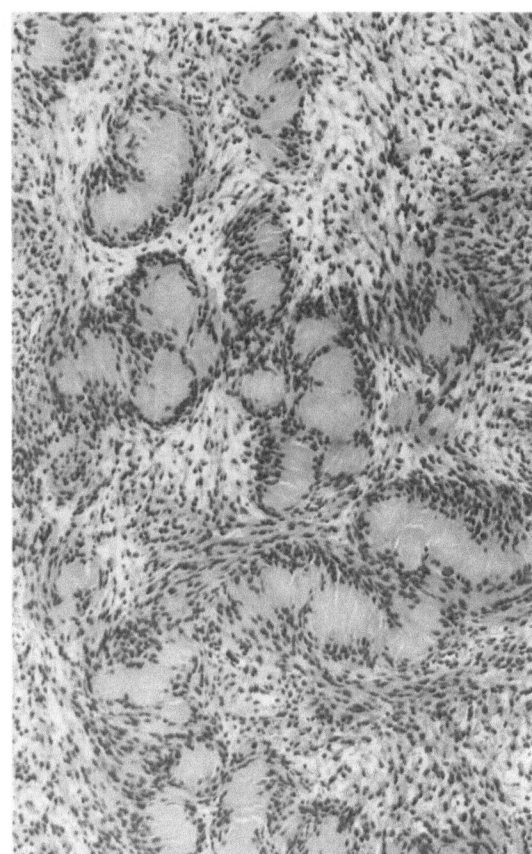

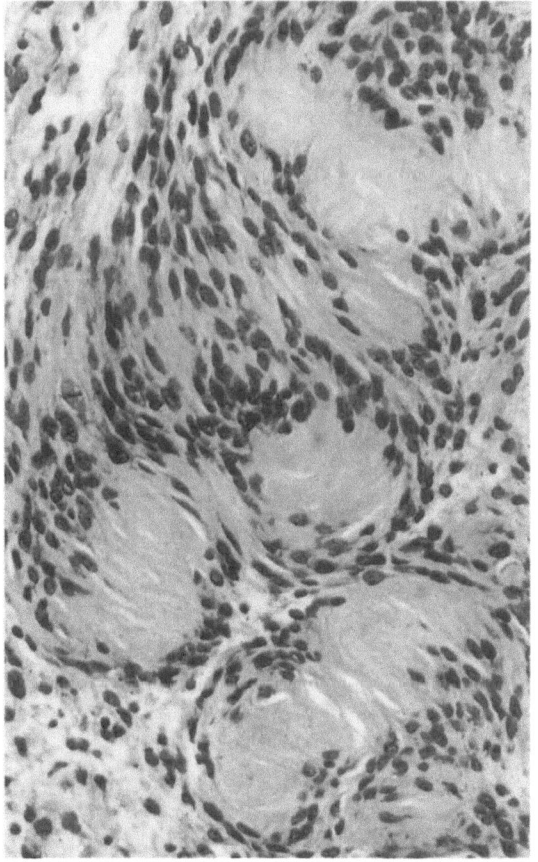

Fig. 181 *(above)*. Skin, European hamster, UDMH-induced malignant melanotic schwannoma of Antoni type A. Unpigmented tumor area with numerous Verocay (tactile) bodies. Bodian stain, × 90

Fig. 182 *(below)*. Higher magnification of Fig. 181. Bodian stain, × 300

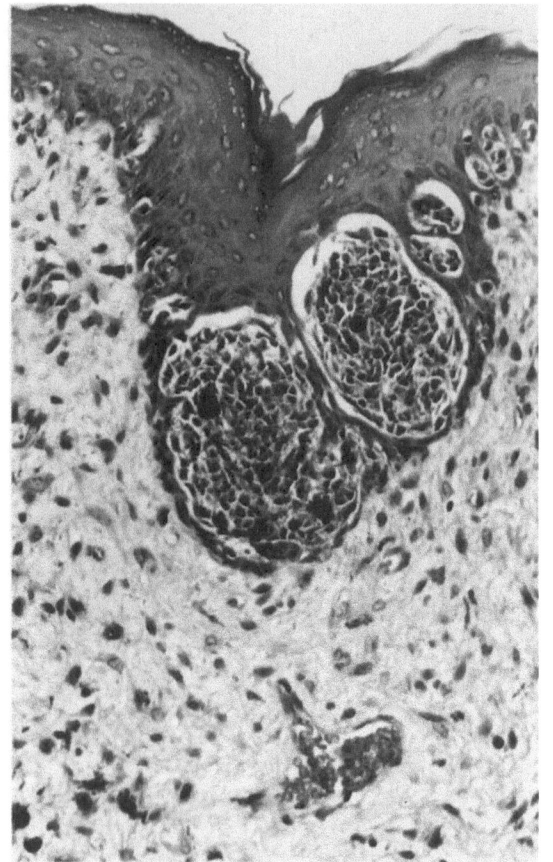

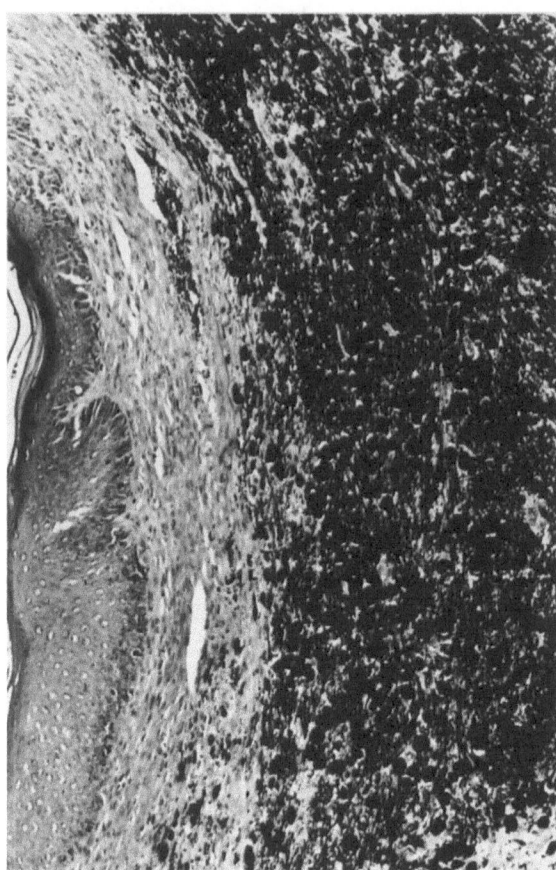

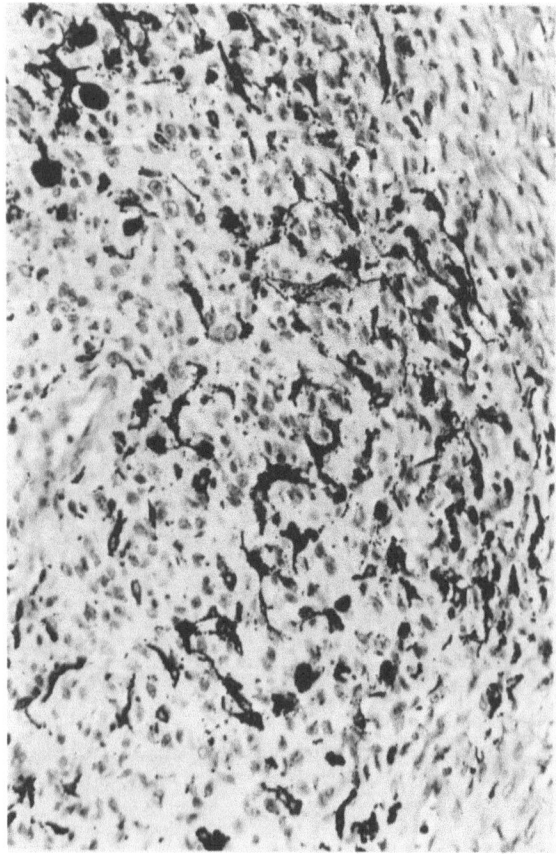

◄ **Fig. 183** *(upper left).* Skin, European hamster, UDMH-induced malignant melanotic schwannoma of Antoni type B. Clumps of pigmented tumor cells at the dermoepidermal junction concomitant with similar cells in the underlying schwannoma tissue. H and E, × 275

Fig. 184 *(lower left).* Skin, European hamster, UDMH-induced malignant melanotic schwannoma of Antoni type A. Loosely distributed epitheliod, bipolar, and dendritic tumor cells with cytoplasmic melanin granules. Fontana-Masson, × 200

Fig. 185 *(upper right).* Extensively pigmented dermal zone of the tumor shown in Figs. 181 and 182, not distinguishable from true melanoma. Fontana-Masson, × 110

Ultrastructure

Characteristic ultrastructural features of melanotic schwannomas in man (Webb 1982; Burns et al. 1983) include the presence of (a) complex laminated cytoplasmic interdigitations; (b) prominent basal laminae around the tumor cells; (c) micropinocytotic vesicles on the plasma membranes; (d) cytoplasmic premelanosomes and melanosomes in all stages of maturation; and (e) long-spacing collagen ("Luse bodies") within the interstitium.

Differential Diagnosis

Melanotic schwannomas must be differentiated from a variety of other melanin-synthesizing neoplasms and hamartomatous growths of the peripheral nervous system and the skin, the majority of which, in common with melanotic schwannomas, occur very rarely and have so far only been reported in man. Differentiation from pigmented neurofibromas (Bednar 1957; Anderson and Robertson 1979) can be made based on quantitative variation in the number of fibroblasts and collagen content. Primary malignant melanomas, which exhibit either a pseudoepitheliomatous or pseudosarcomatous histologic appearance, usually undergo no differentiation to schwannoma. Other melanogenic lesions with Schwann-cell elements, such as (cellular) blue nevi (Masson 1951; Merkow et al. 1969), pigmented hamartomas (Burkhart and Gohara 1981), pigmented ganglioneuroblastomas and neuroblastomas (Hahn et al. 1976; Mullins 1980), melanocytic tumors of the sympathetic ganglia (Fu et al. 1975), and spinal melanotic clear cell sarcomas (Parker et al. 1980), may be distinguished from melanotic schwannomas, mainly dependending on clinical and morphologic criteria.

Biologic Features

Several hypotheses have been proposed to explain the origin of melanin in melanotic schwannomas: (a) the transfer of melanin from non-neoplastic melanocytes into neoplastic Schwann's cells by a process of "cytocrine injection" (Masson 1967); (b) phagocytosis of melanin from the extracellular space by the neoplastic cells (Dastur et al. 1967); and (c) the simultaneous neoplastic proliferation of Schwann's cells and melanocytes (Hodson 1961).

However, the now most widely accepted theory is that of ectopic melanogenesis by the neoplastic Schwann's cells themselves following aberrant differentiation of metaplastic changes (Masson 1951, 1967; Hodson 1961; Mandybur 1974). This is consistent with the common ontogenetic derivation of both melanocytes and Schwann's cells from pluripotential neural crest cells. Additional evidence supporting the concept of neurogenic melanogenesis comes from reports demonstrating that both cell types have similar ultrastructural characteristics (Nakai and Rappaport 1963; Spence et al. 1976; Mennemeyer et al. 1979) and identifying melanosomes in normal human and rodent dermal Schwann's cells (Garcia and Szabo 1979).

Moreover, with regard to the striking histologic overlap between some UDMH-induced melanotic schwannomas and primary melanomas, the possibility of a complete transformation of malignant schwannoma into malignant melanoma should be considered, as has already been suggested by Krausz et al. (1984). The reverse phenomenon, the transformation of malignant melanoma to malignant schwannoma ("neurosarcoma") with loss of melanogenesis, has also been demonstrated (DiMaio et al. 1982).

The multipotentiality of neural crest cells is further illustrated by tumors composed of mixed neural crest derivatives (Karcioglu et al. 1977) and by malignant peripheral nerve sheath tumors with focal divergent differentiation to rhabdomyosarcoma, osteosarcoma, chondrosarcoma, angiosarcoma, epithelial elements, or a combination thereof (Ducatman and Scheithauer 1984).

According to Weston (1971), local environmental factors can affect the phenotypic expression of migrating neural crest cells, and the degree of dispersion of these cells determines, in part, whether they differentiate as neuronal types or pigment cells. These observations may perhaps explain why in the current study melanotic tumor areas could always be found exclusively in the epidermis-bordering periphery of the schwannomas, thus suggesting an epidermal influence on the melanomatous transformation of the neoplastic Schwann's cells.

Comparison with Other Species

Melanotic schwannomas are very rare tumors. No more than 25 cases have been reported in man, most of them biologically benign and arising from the spinal nerve roots and the soft tissues, with few tumors involving the skin, esophagus, stomach, heart, mandible, and acoustic nerve (Burns et al. 1983; Miller et al. 1986). Recently, two cases of spontaneous malignant melanotic schwannomas of the spinal cord have been described in dogs (Patnaik et al. 1984). To our knowledge, there are no further reports in the literature where spontaneously arising melanotic schwannomas have been diagnosed as such, either in domestic or laboratory animals. However, melanotic skin tumors resembling (cellular) blue nevi and melanotic schannomas were experimentally induced by means of topical application of 7,12-dimethylbenz(*a*)anthracene (DMBA) in Syrian hamsters (Nakai and Rappaport 1963). As further example of experimental oncogenesis, intracranial pigmented nerve sheath tumors developed in Long-Evans rats after transplacental exposure to ethylnitrosourea (ENU). In one of these tumors, progressive melanogenesis was seen in tissue culture; in a second one, differentiation was evident toward Schwann's cells (Spence et al. 1976).

References

Anderson B, Robertson DM (1979) Melanin-containing neurofibroma: case report with evidence of Schwann cell origin of melanin. Can J Neurol Sci 6: 139–143

Bednar B (1957) Storiform neurofibromas of the skin, pigmented and nonpigmented. Cancer 10: 368–376

Burkhart CG, Gohara A (1981) Dermal melanocyte hamartoma: a distinctive new form of dermal melanocytosis. Arch Dermatol 117: 102–104

Burns DK, Silva FG, Forde KA, Mount PM, Clark HB (1983) Primary melanocytic schwannoma of the stomach: evidence of dual melanocytic and schwannian differentiation in an extra-axial site in a patient without neurofibromatosis. Cancer 52: 1432–1441

Dastur DK, Sinh G, Pandya SK (1967) Melanotic tumor of the acoustic nerve. Case report. J Neurosurg 27: 166–170

DiMaio SM, Mackay B, Smith JL Jr, Dickersin GR (1982) Neurosarcomatous transformation in malignant melanoma: an ultrastructural study. Cancer 50: 2345–2354

Ducatman BS, Scheithauer BW (1984) Malignant peripheral nerve sheath tumors with divergent differentiation. Cancer 54: 1049–1057

Ernst H, Rittinghausen S, Wahnschaffe U, Mohr U (1987) Induction of malignant peripheral nerve sheath tumors in European hamsters with 1,1-dimethylhydrazine (UDMH). Cancer Lett 35: 303–311

Fu YS, Kaye GI, Lattes R (1975) Primary malignant melanocytic tumors of the sympathetic ganglia with an ultrastructural study of one. Cancer 36: 2029–2041

Garcia RI, Szabo G (1979) Melanosomes in dermal Schwann cells of human and rodent skin. Arch Dermatol Res 264: 83–87

Hahn JF, Netsky MG, Butler AB, Sperber EE (1976) Pigmented ganglioneuroblastoma: relation of melanin and lipofuscin to schwannomas and other tumors of neural crest origin. J Neuropathol Exp Neurol 35: 393–403

Hodson JJ (1961) An intra-osseous tumour combination of biological importance: invasion of a melanotic schwannoma by an adamantinoma. J Pathol Bacteriol 82: 257–266

Karcioglu Z, Someren A, Mathes SJ (1977) Ectomesenchymoma: a malignant tumor of migratory neural crest (ectomesenchyme) remnants showing ganglionic, schwannian, melanocytic and rhabdomyoblastic differentiation. Cancer 39: 2486–2496

Krausz T, Azzopardi JG, Pearse E (1984) Malignant melanoma of the sympathic chain: with a consideration of pigmented nerve sheath tumours. Histopathology 8: 881–894

Mandybur TI (1974) Melanotic nerve sheath tumors. J Neurosurg 41: 187–192

Masson P (1951) My conception of cellular nevi. Cancer 4: 9–38

Masson P (1967) Melanogenic system: nevi and melanomas. Pathol Annu 2: 351–397

Mennemeyer RP, Hallman KO, Hammar SP, Raisis JE, Tytus JS, Bockus D (1979) Melanotic schwannoma: clinical and ultrastructural studies of three cases with evidence of intracellular melanin synthesis. Am J Surg Pathol 3: 3–10

Merkow LP, Burt RC, Hayeslip DW, Newton FJ, Slifkin M, Pardo M (1969) A cellular and malignant blue nevus: a light and electron microscopic study. Cancer 24: 888–896

Miller RT, Sarikaya H, Sos A (1986) Melanoti schwannoma of the acoustic nerve. Arch Pathol Lab Med 110: 153–154

Mullins JD (1980) A pigmented differentiating neuroblastoma: a light and ultrastructural study. Cancer 46: 522–528

Nakai T, Rappaport H (1963) A study of the histogenesis of experimental melanotic tumors resembling cellular blue nevi: the evidence in support of their neurogenic origin. Am J Pathol 43: 175–199

Parker JB, Marcus PB, Martin JH (1980) Spinal melanotic clearcell sarcoma: a light and electron microscopic study. Cancer 46: 718–724

Patnaik AK, Erlandson RA, Lieberman PH (1984) Canine malignant melanotic schwannomas: a light and electron microscopic study of two cases. Vet Pathol 21: 483–488

Spence AM, Rubinstein LJ, Conley FK, Herman MM (1976) Studies on experimental malignant nerve sheath tumors maintained in tissue and organ culture systems. III. Melanin pigment and melanogenesis in experimental neurogenic tumors: a reappraisal of the histogenesis of pigmented nerve sheath tumors. Acta Neuropathol (Berl) 35: 27–45

Webb JN (1982) The ultrastructure of a melanotic schwannoma of the skin. J Pathol 137: 25–36

Weston JA (1971) Neural crest cell migration and differentiation. In: Pease DC (ed) UCLA forum in medical sciences, no 14. University of California Press, Berkeley, CA, pp 1–22

Cardiac Neurilemmoma, Rat

Jerry M. Rice and Jerrold M. Ward

Synonyms. Endocardial schwannoma; neurinoma; neurosarcoma; endocardial mesenchymal tumor; Anitschkow's cell sarcoma; cardiac spindle cell tumor; cardiac fibrosarcoma.

Gross Appearance

This neoplasm is often an incidental finding at necropsy and in its early stages may not be grossly evident even when the heart is cut to reveal the interiors of the chambers. The early lesion consists of a firm, white to gray coating over all or a part of the lining of one chamber, most often the left ventricle. More advanced tumors are grossly evident as firm, grayish-white masses that partially fill one or more chambers and diffusely invade the myocardium. Rarely, the tumor may grow through the myocardium and expand as an exophytic mass on the external surface of the heart. Infiltrative growth may then extend along the major blood vessels within and beyond the mediastinal cavity to involve the lungs and soft tissues of the neck and head, in some exceptional cases extending as far as the orbit. Photographs illustrating both early and advanced lesions have been published (Ivankovic 1976).

Microscopic Features

Smaller tumors consist of a very uniform, dense population of elongated fusiform cells with abundant, eosinophilic cytoplasm and inapparent cell margins that occur between the endothelial lining of the ventricles and the underlying myocardium. Nuclei are round to cigar shaped and most are hyperbasophilic. Mitotic figures are infrequent. The cells and nuclei tend to form parallel arrays, often with a pronounced serpentine pattern reminiscent of a nerve sectioned longitudinally (Fig. 186). Individual nuclei may thus appear S-shaped. This pattern is very similar to the Antoni type A tissue of a differentiated schwannoma of cranial or spinal nerves. The cells are enveloped by a dense network of fine reticulin fibers, demonstrable by silver impregnations such as Wilder's or Tibor Pap's. The serpentine pattern is accentuated by silver staining (Fig. 187).

A distinctive feature of some tumor cells is Anitschkow's nuclear pattern (Fig. 188). Anitschkow's nuclei are ellipsoidal and have distinct nuclear membranes. In sections stained with hematoxylin and eosin they are pale except for an intensely stained central bar of chromatin, usually along the major axis. This pattern has been observed in virtually every normal cell type in the heart, as well as in carcinoma cells in coronary metastases (Ragsdale 1973). It was once incorporated into an empirically descriptive, nonhistogenetic name for these tumors, "Anitschkow's cell sarcoma" (Vesselinovitch and Mihailovich 1968). Cells with Anitschkow's nuclei usually occur in small clusters and are not otherwise distinguishable from the rest of the neoplastic cell population.

Microcystic degeneration and a more myxoid pattern may be seen within larger tumors, but the multiple large cysts characteristic of Antoni type B tissue in schwannomas of cranial and spinal nerves are rarely, if ever, observed. In larger tumors with extensive invasion of the myocardium, a significant fraction of the tumor cells may be larger and sufficiently separated from one another in formalin-fixed material so that cell margins can be discerned. These plump fusiform cells are similar to those of a variety of soft tissue sarcomas and tend to predominate in portions of invasive tumors that extend beyond the heart. S-100 protein with predominantly nuclear localization can be demonstrated in a fraction of these sarcoma-like cells by ABC immunoperoxidase staining (S. Rehm et al. unpublished, Fig. 189). Staining for S-100 is more consistent and occurs in cytoplasm as well as nuclei in the more typical Antoni type A portions of these tumors.

Ultrastructure

Tumors cells often have highly convoluted cell membranes with occasional junctional complexes between cells (Berman et al. 1980). Bundles of collagen fibers are demonstrable between cells, many of which are enveloped by a single layer of basal lamina. These features are virtually identical to those of cells of schwannomas of cranial and spinal nerve roots.

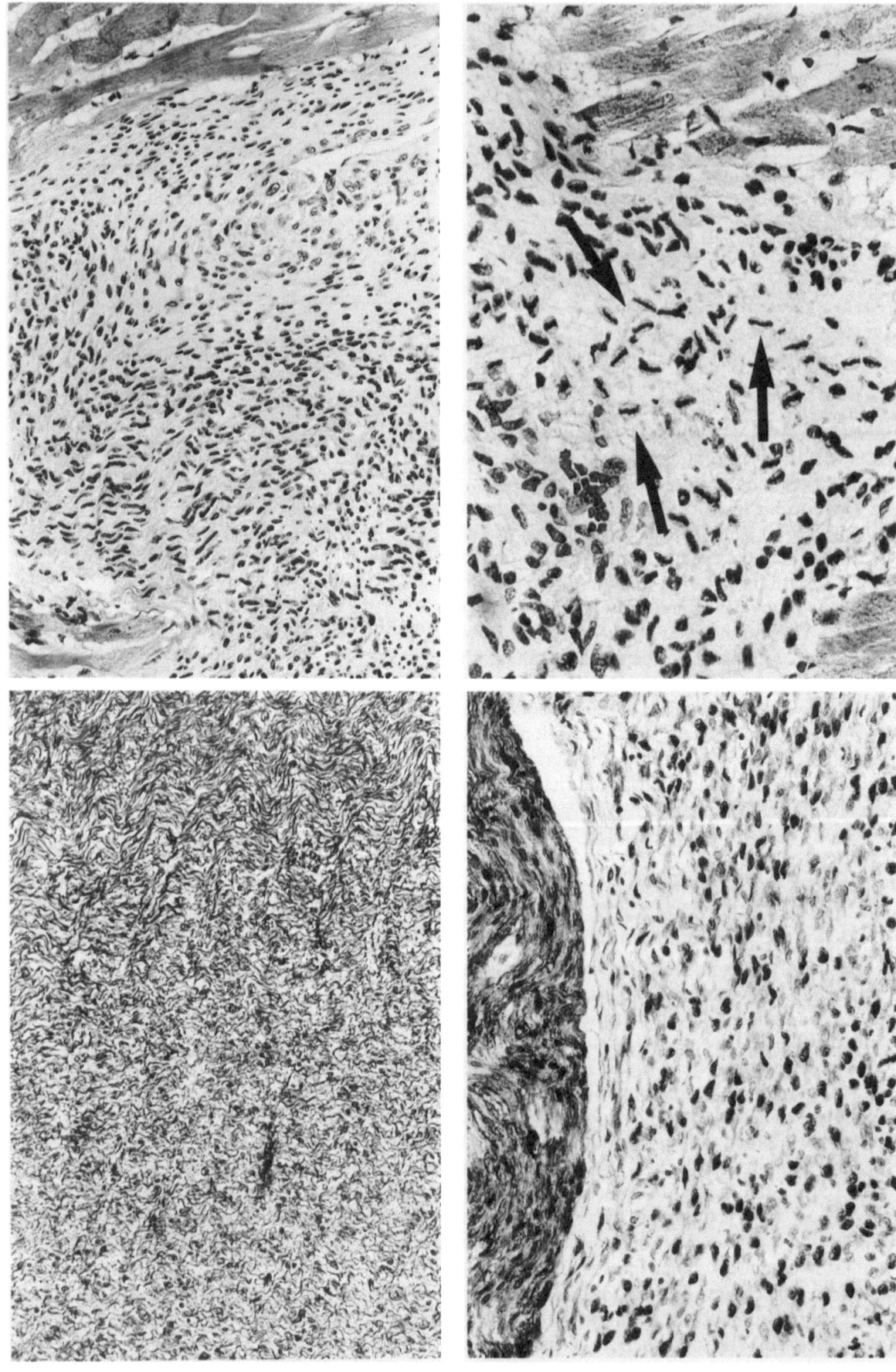

Fig. 186 *(upper left).* Endocardial neurilemmoma, rat, induced by 7,12-dimethylbenz[*a*]anthracene, confined to the lining of the left ventricle. The layer of tumor tissue was less than 1 mm thick and was only detected in histologic sections. The wavelike pattern is characteristic. H and E, ×250

Fig. 187 *(lower left).* Endocardial neurilemmoma, rat. Silver impregnation for reticulin revealing abundant fine fibers surrounding every cell. Tibor Pap, ×250

Fig. 188 *(upper right).* Endocardial neurilemmoma, rat. Anitschkow's nuclei *(arrows)* in a group of tumor cells. H and E, ×400

Fig. 189 *(lower right).* Endocardial neurilemmoma, mediastinal extension of tumor, rat. S-100 protein in nuclei of tumor cells. Approximately 50% of the tumor cell nuclei are stained, in comparison with uniform staining of both cytoplasm and nuclei within a nerve *(left)* surrounded by the tumor. ABC immunoperoxidase and hematoxylin, ×250

Differential Diagnosis

Cardiac neurilemmomas in their early stages are difficult to distinguish from endocardial proliferative lesions that are degenerative rather than neoplastic (Boorman et al. 1973; Burek 1978; Berman et al. 1980). Unfortunately, there are no unequivocal morphologic criteria that can be confidently applied to this problem using only hematoxylin and eosin staining. Myocardium-underlying non-neoplastic fibroproliferative endocardial lesions, which are not uncommon in old rats of many strains, usually show signs of degeneration including loss of cross-striations and clumping of nuclei. The fibrotic tissue itself may extend beyond the endocardial space into the myocardium, but consists of plump, fusiform, fibroblastic cells in layers only a few cells thick. It has been argued that all such lesions may represent early stages of neoplastic development (Hoch-Ligeti et al. 1986), but progressive, autonomous growth of such tissue following transplantation, or other compelling evidence for this view, has not been demonstrated. We interpret unequivocal Antoni type A tissue, like that in Fig. 186, in *any* amount to be diagnostic of neoplasia. The use of S-100 immunohistochemistry to distinguish neurogenic proliferative lesions from reactive histiocytes and fibroblasts should assist diagnosis in cases of doubt.

Masses of larger size can generally be easily distinguished from other primary tumors of the heart and from metastases or extension to the heart of tumors arising elsewhere, both of which are much less common. Primary cardiac tumors other than the endocardial neurilemmoma are extremely rare in rats and are unlikely to cause diagnostic difficulty. Atriocaval node tumor is common in rats of the NZR/Gd strain (Goodall et al. 1975), but is exceedingly uncommon in other strains (Hoch-Ligeti et al. 1986). This neoplasm is located at the atrioventricular septum, is obviously epithelial in morphology, and often metastasizes widely. Aortic body tumors (chemodectomas, paragangliomas) do occasionally occur in rats and have the morphology of tumors of the amine precursor uptake decarboxylase (APUD) cell system (Van Zwieten et al. 1979). Metastatic tumors are extremely rare in the rat heart, although cardiac metastases from osteosarcoma and from lymphomas have been observed (Wilens and Sproul 1938). Primary mediastinal neoplasms that have morphologic features similar to endocardial tumors, such as schwannomas of the thoracic spinal nerve roots, do not, in our experience, involve the heart.

The principal problem in differential diagnosis of these tumors is not so much distinguishing them from other neoplasms, but from achieving consensus on their cell of origin. Many investigators have considered them to be neurogenic on the basis of their histologic and ultrastructural similarity to schwannomas and have classified them synonymously as neurinomas (Ivankovic 1976) schwannomas (Berman et al. 1980), or neurilemmomas (Robertson et al. 1982). Others, not convinced, have argued for a mesenchymal origin (Hoch-Ligeti et al. 1983, 1986). Yet others have suggested that some were neurogenic while others were sarcomas of uncertain origin (Mennel 1971). In some descriptions the Antoni type A tissue of the early lesions has been considered a nonneoplastic lesion unrelated to the less-differentiated, sarcomatous tissue of larger tumors, even when both lesions are present and contiguous in the same heart (Burek 1978). We believe the less-differentiated unequivocally neoplastic cells are derived from the Antoni type A tissue and represent an example of loss of differentiated morphologic features in the course of tumor progression. The additional datum (Fig. 189) that the cells of both the Antoni type A tissue of early lesions and the sarcomatous tissue of large tumors contain S-100 protein strengthens the argument for a common neurogenic origin of both types of cells.

Biologic Features

Cardiac neurilemmomas behave as malignant neoplasms. Their growth is diffusely infiltrative into the myocardium from the earliest stages of tumor development and is capable of direct extension beyond the heart to involve other mediastinal structures, the lungs, and the soft tissues of the neck and head. Metastasis to the lung has also been reported (Hoch-Ligeti et al. 1983, 1986), but is uncommon. The transplantability of these neoplasms has not been established.

Pathogenesis. No systematic studies of the development of these tumors have been published. The heart is innervated by both sympathetic and parasympathetic fibers and has sensory fibers that originate from neurons in the vagal or upper cervical ganglia (Simionescu and Simionescu 1977). It has been suggested, but not demonstrated, that cardiac neurilemmomas arise from the intracardiac branches of the vagus nerve (Ivankovic 1976).

Etiology. Exposures of rats of many strains to a wide variety of direct-acting or metabolism-dependent chemical carcinogens has resulted in an increased incidence of cardiac neurilemmomas. Compounds of the metabolism-dependent 1-aryl-3,3-dialkyltriazene family have shown special selectivity for the heart (Imhof and Ivankovic 1983), but a significant incidence of cardiac neurilemmomas has also resulted from exposure to the direct-acting alkylating agents ethylmethanesulfonate (Haas et al. 1974), N-nitrosomethylurea (Schreiber et al. 1972), and N-nitrosoethylurea (Druckrey et al. 1970). Many of the agents that induce cardiac tumors, including all the agents listed above, also induce schwannomas of the cranial and spinal nerve roots. However, while susceptibility to the latter is greatest during late gestation and within the first days after birth, the highest incidences of cardiac neurilemmomas have generally been seen in rats exposed to carcinogens somewhat later in life (Imhof and Ivankovic 1983; Druckrey et al. 1970). Druckrey et al. (1970) observed four heart tumors that were the primary cause of death among 60 strain BD IX rats (7%) given a single oral dose of N-nitrosoethylurea (10–40 mg/kg) at 10 days of age. Survival of rats with heart tumors ranged from 298 to 484 days. No heart tumors were seen at higher doses; mean survival among rats given 80 mg/kg was only 215 days, with death from tumors of brain, kidney, and peripheral nerves intervening before the rats reached the age at which heart tumors might have appeared. Heart tumors also caused death in five of 64 rats (8%) treated at 30 days of age, but none were seen in rats exposed transplacentally or within 24 h after birth. However, no systematic search for microscopic lesions was performed. Similarly, no heart tumors were observed in rats of the same strain given single exposures to 1-(3-pyridyl)-3,3-dimethyltriazene transplacentally or on the 1st or 10th days after birth, but incidences of 30%, 32% and 5% were seen in rats dosed once with 50 mg/kg on days 30, 60, or 90, respectively (Imhof and Ivankovic 1983). As mean survival was significantly longer among rats treated at stages of development that yielded no heart tumors, these results strongly suggest that susceptibility to induction of these neoplasms is truly greatest in young rats between approximately 10 and 60 days of age.

Frequency. Frequency of spontaneous cardiac neurilemmomas varies widely among different strains of rats. While no such neoplasms were observed among 15 000 untreated rats of the ten inbred strains of the BD series necropsied over a period of 10 years (Druckrey 1971), in other strains the spontaneous incidence has been estimated as 0.05%–0.29% (Robertson et al. 1982), and as high as 1%–7% (Boorman et al. 1973) if all endocardial lesions are considered neoplasms (Hoch-Ligeti et al. 1986). These tumors have been observed in rats as young as 8 months (Robertson et al. 1982), but are much more frequent in older animals, especially those approaching or exceeding 2 years of age.

Comparison with Other Species

Tumors of the heart have been reported in European hamsters (Ketkar et al. 1977) and in boxer dogs (Denlinger et al. 1978) following intravenous administration of N-nitrosomethylurea. The hamster tumors resembled rat endocardial neurilemmomas histologically, but the authors used the term "fibrosarcoma" and expressed the opinion that a possible neurogenic origin could not be established without ultrastructural studies. The hamster tumors tended to originate from the atria, unlike the rat endocardial tumors. The canine tumors were diagnosed as neurinomas.

The rare cases of neurogenic tumors of the heart in man differ from the rat tumors in that they generally do not originate from the endocardium.

In some case reports, benign intramural neurilemmoma were incidental findings at autopsy (Gleason et al. 1972; Factor et al. 1976). Others were diagnosed clinically and treated (Monroe et al. 1984; Ursell et al. 1982), including one that was intracavitary in location (Betancourt et al. 1979).

References

Berman JJ, Rice JM, Reddick R (1980) Endocardial schwannomas in rats: their characterization by light and electron microscopy. Arch Pathol Lab Med 104: 187–191

Betancourt B, Defendini EA, Johnson C, De Jesus M, Pavia-Villamil A, Diaz Cruz A, Medina JC (1979) Severe right ventricular outflow tract obstruction caused by an intracavitary cardiac neurilemmoma: successful surgical removal and postoperative diagnosis. Chest 75: 522–524

Boorman GA, Zurcher C, Hollander CF, Feron VJ (1973) Naturally occurring endocardial disease in the rat. Arch Pathol 96: 39–45

Burek JD (1978) Pathology of aging rats. CRC, West Palm Beach, pp 75–86

Denlinger RH, Koestner A, Swenberg JA (1978) Neoplasms in purebred boxer dogs following long-term administration of N-methyl-N-nitrosourea. Cancer Res 38: 1711–1717

Druckrey H (1971) Genotypes and phenotypes of ten inbred strains of BD rats. Arzneimittelforschung 21: 1274–1278

Druckrey H, Schagen B, Ivankovic S (1970) Erzeugung neurogener Malignome durch einmalige Gabe von Aethylnitrosoharnstoff (ANH) an neugeborene und junge BD IX Ratten. Z Krebsforsch 74: 141–161

Factor S, Turi G, Biempica L (1976) Primary cardiac neurilemmoma. Cancer 37: 883–890

Gleason TH, Dillard DH, Gould VE (1972) Cardiac neurilemmoma. NY State J Med 72: 2435–2436

Goodall CM, Christie GS, Hurley JV (1975) Primary epithelial tumour in the right atrium of the heart and inferior vena cava in NZR/Gd inbred rats; pathology of 18 cases. J Pathol 116: 239–251

Haas J, Hilfrich J, Mohr U (1974) Induction of heart tumors in Wistar rats after a single application of ethyl methanesulphonate and dimethylnitrosamine. Z Krebsforsch 81: 225–228

Hoch-Ligeti C, Harris PN, Stewart HL (1983) Endocardial tumors induced by carbamate or fluorenylacetamide derivatives in rats. JNCI 71: 211–216

Hoch-Ligeti C, Restrepo C, Stewart HL (1986) Comparative pathology of cardiac neoplasms in humans and in laboratory rodents: a review. JNCI 76: 127–142

Imhof W, Ivankovic S (1983) Karzinogene Wirkung von 1-Phenyl- und 1-(Pyridyl-3-)-3,3-dimethyltriazen sowie 1-Phenyl- und 1-(Pyridyl-3-)-3,3-diethyltriazen bei einmaliger prae- und postnataler Verabreichung an BD IX Ratten. Arch Geschwulstforsch 53: 557–569

Ivankovic S (1976) Tumours of the heart. In: Turusov VS (ed) Tumours of the rat. Part 2. IARC, Lyon, pp 313–319 (Pathology of tumours in laboratory animals, vol I)

Ketkar M, Reznik G, Haas H, Hilfrich J, Mohr U (1977) Tumors of the heart and stomach induced in European hamsters by intravenous administration of N-methyl-N-nitrosourea. JNCI 58: 1695–1699

Mennel HD (1971) Die Morphologie der mit neurotropen Karzinogenen erzeugten Herztumoren bei Ratten. Beitr Pathol 144: 221–230

Monroe B, Federman M, Balogh K (1984) Cardiac neurilemmoma. Report of a case with electron microscopic examination. Arch Pathol Lab Med 108: 300–304

Ragsdale BD (1973) Anitschkow nuclear structure in cardiac metastases. Am J Clin Pathol 59: 798–802

Robertson JL, Garman RH, Fowler EH (1982) Spontaneous cardiac tumors in eight rats. Vet Pathol 19: 30–37

Schreiber D, Batka H, Warzok R, Quentin E (1972) Induktion von Herztumoren bei Ratten durch Methylnitrosoharnstoff. Zentralbl Allg Pathol 115: 31–39

Simionescu N, Simionescu M (1977) The cardiovascular system. In: Weiss L (ed) Histology, 5th edn. Elsevier, New York, pp 430–431

Ursell PC, Albala A, Fenoglio JJ jr (1982) Malignant neurogenic tumor of the heart. Hum Pathol 13: 640–645

Van Zwieten MJ, Burek JD, Zurcher C, Hollander CF (1979) Aortic body tumours and hyperplasia in the rat. J Pathol 128: 99–112

Vesselinovitch SD, Mihailovich N (1968) The development of neurogenic neoplasms, embryonal kidney tumors, harderian gland adenomas, Anitschkow cell sarcomas of the heart, and other neoplasms in urethan-treated newborn rats. Cancer Res 28: 888–897

Wilens SL, Sproul EE (1938) Spontaneous cardiovascular disease in the rat. I. Lesions in the heart. Am J Pathol 14: 177–199

Parvovirus Infection, Rat

Robert O. Jacoby

Synonyms. Rat virus infection, Kilham rat virus infection, H-1 virus infection.

Gross Appearance

Rat parvovirus infection causes cerebellar hypoplasia and hemorrhagic encephalomyelopathy. The lesions occur separately or together in suckling rats, whereas adult rats are susceptible only to the hemorrhagic changes. Cerebellar hypoplasia is manifested by reduced size and foliar delineation that can be regional or pancerebellar. When lesions are diffuse, the cerebellum has an arcuate contour, and the corpora quadrigemina are exposed. Hemorrhagic encephalomyelopathy consists of small to large hemorrhages that can occur anywhere in the central nervous system, but especially in the cerebellum. Extensive hemorrhage is often accompanied by malacia.

Microscopic Features

Cerebellar hypoplasia is caused by viral destruction of the external germinal layer which results in depletion of the external granular layer of the developing cerebellum (granuloprival cerebellar hypoplasia) (Fig. 190) (Margolis et al. 1971). Rat parvoviruses cause lytic infection of other germinal cells in the central nervous system, especially in the ventricular zones, subependymal plate, caudate/putamen and olfactory bulbs, but histologic sequellae of these effects have not been described. Early stages of infection are characterized by necrosis of germinal cells preceded by development of basophilic intranuclear inclusions (Fig. 191) that contain viral antigen (Fig. 192) (Margolis et al. 1971; Jacoby et al. 1987a). Necrosis can be focal, segmental, panfoliar, or pancerebellar and is not accompanied by inflammation. There is resultant depletion or truncated development of the granular layer, but other cell layers are usually unaffected. However, heterotopic clusters of granule cells and disordered Purkinje's cells may be found.

Hemorrhagic encephalomyelopathy is characterized by multifocal hemorrhage in gray and white matter (Fig. 193) (El Dadah et al. 1967; Margolis and Kilham 1970). The hemorrhages vary in size from minute petechia to large extravasations accompanied by infarction and malacia (Fig. 194). Hemorrhage is usually acute, so blood breakdown products are not seen. Intranuclear viral inclusions can be detected in vascular endothelium (Fig. 195) and less commonly in vascular muscle tunics and meningocytes (Margolis and Kilham 1970; Cole et al. 1970). They are more easily visualized in early cases and in tissues fixed by perfusion rather than by immersion. Affected endothelium may be swollen or necrotic, and vascular lesions can include thrombosis.

Ultrastructure

Electron microscopy of the vascular lesions has revealed that virus-infected endothelial cells have marginated chromatin surrounding a lucent zone that corresponds to the inclusions seen by light microscopy (Baringer and Nathanson 1972).

Differential Diagnosis

The nervous system lesions of parvoviral infection are not found in other naturally occurring diseases of rats. Hemorrhage can occur from trauma, neoplasia, or chemical toxicity. Because such insults could conceivably unmask or accentuate underlying parvovirus infection (El Dadah et al. 1967), additional tests such as serology, immunohistochemistry, and virus isolation should be considered (Jacoby et al. 1987a). The same advice pertains to unexplained congenital malformations of the cerebellum.

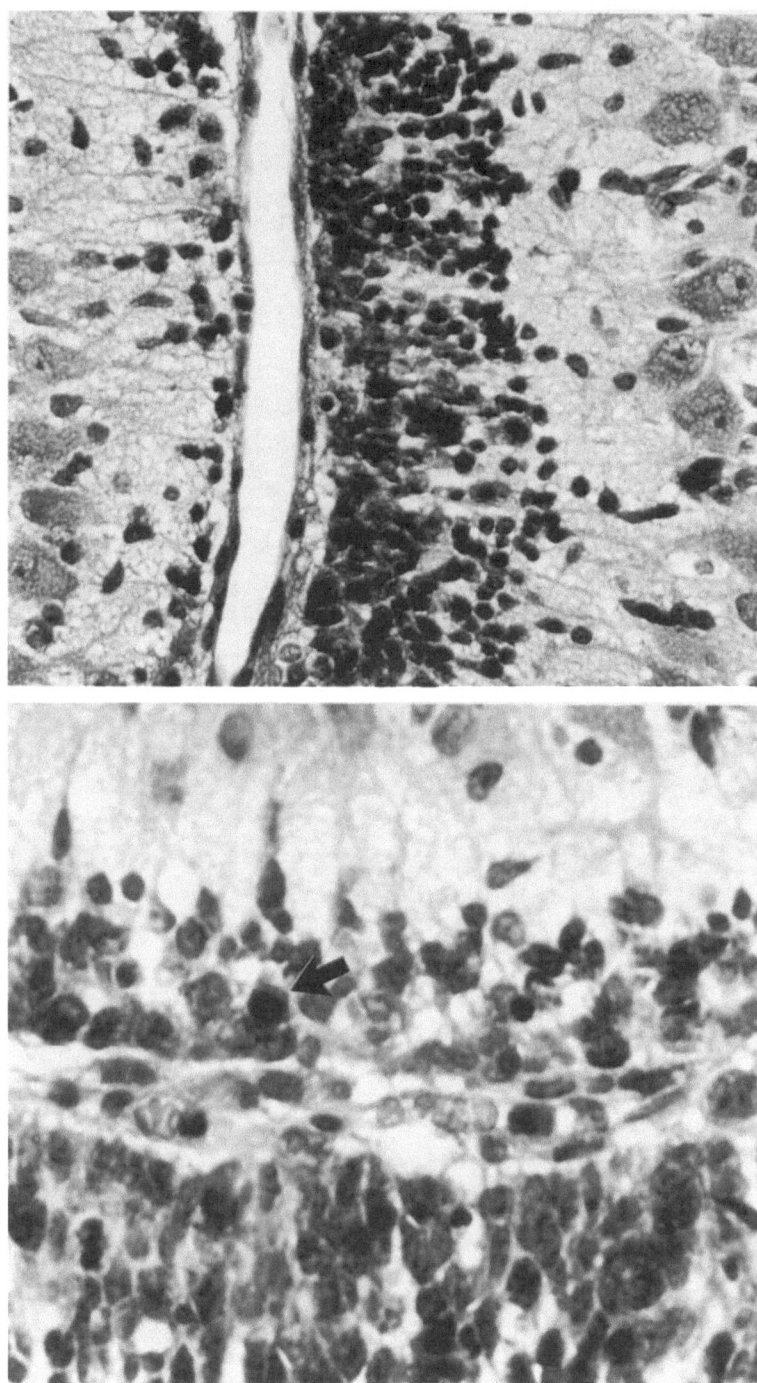

Fig. 190 *(above).* Cerebellum from a suckling rat with rat virus infection. Note multifocal necrosis in the external germinal layer that has resulted in especially severe depletion of germinal cells in the folium to the left. H and E, ×425

Fig. 191 *(below).* Intranuclear rat virus inclusion *(arrow)* in the external germinal layer of cerebellum. H and E, ×680

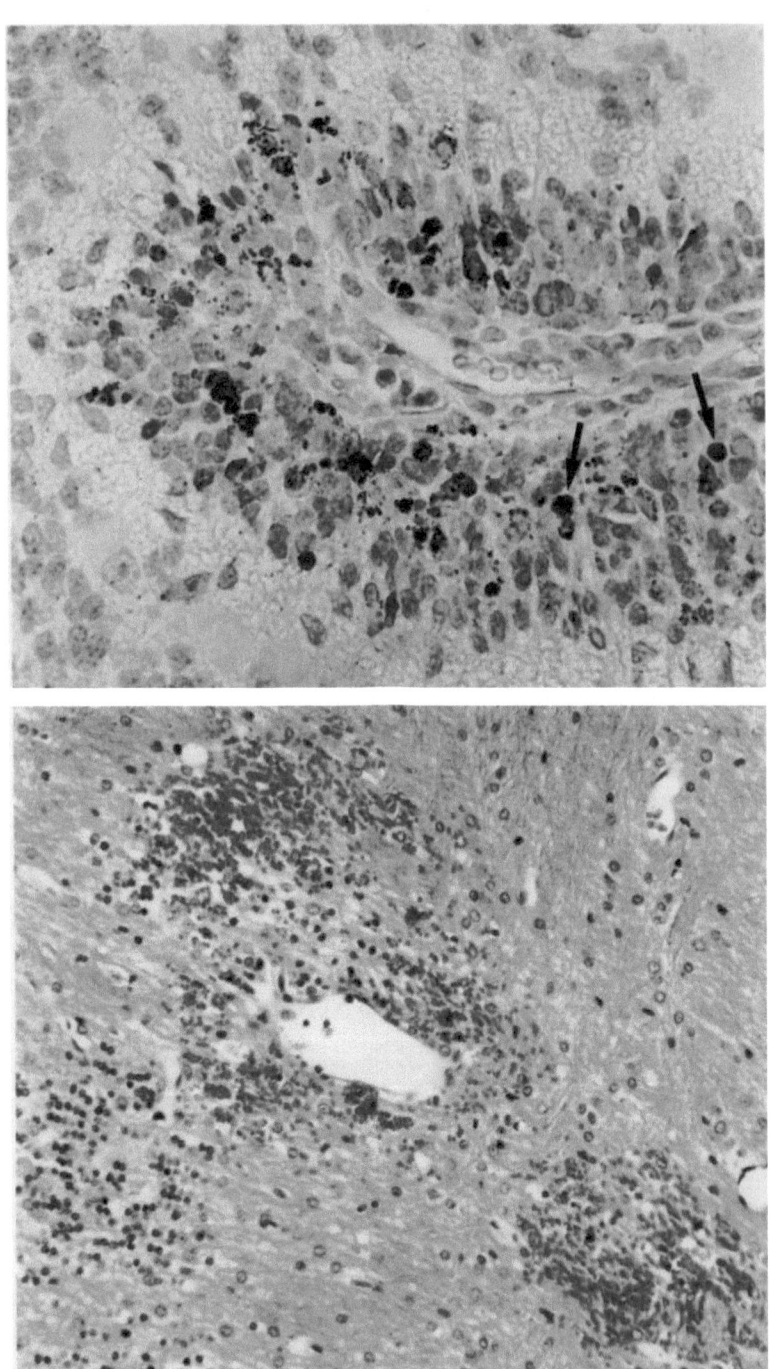

Fig. 192 *(above).* Rat virus antigen in the external germinal layer of cerebellum occurring as intranuclear staining *(arrows)* of morphologically intact cells and antigen-positive cell debris. Immunoperoxidase stain, × 425

Fig. 193 *(below).* Cerebellar hemorrhage in a suckling rat with rat virus infection. H and E, × 170

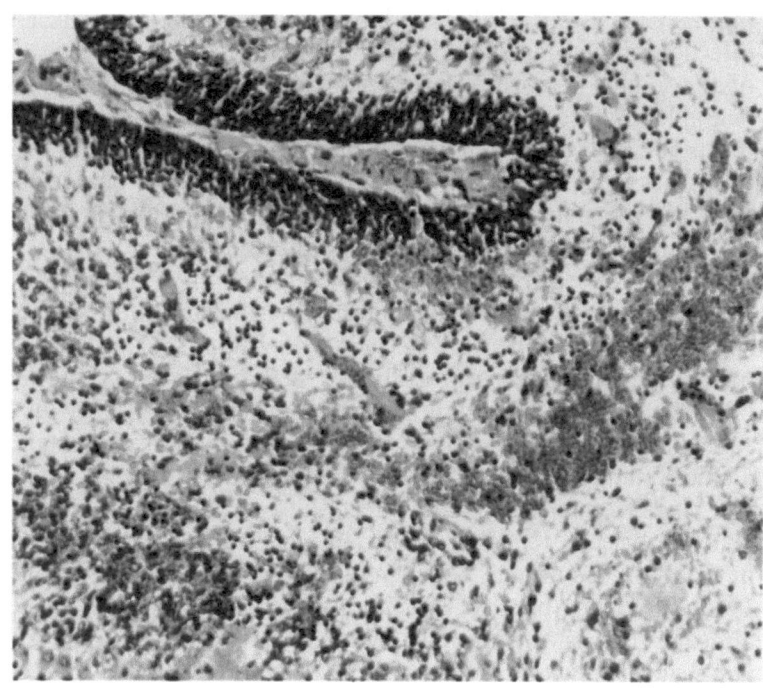

Fig. 194. Hemorrhage and malacia in the cerebellum of a suckling rat with rat virus infection. H and E, × 170

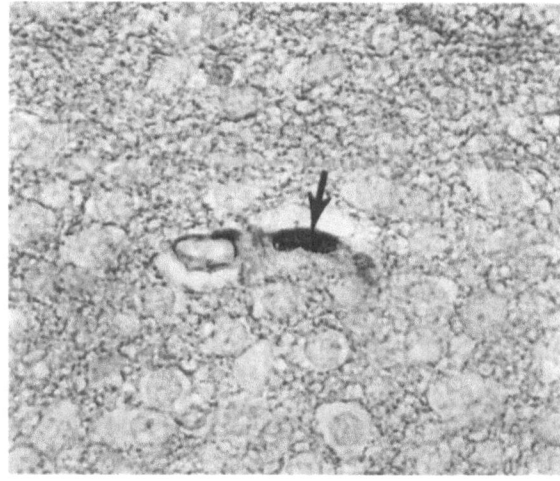

Fig. 195. Rat virus antigen in the nucleus *(arrow)* of a capillary endothelial cell in the brain of a suckling rat. Immunoperoxidase stain, × 425

Viral inclusions and viral antigen are widespread during early stages of infection, but tissue fixation methods influence the stability of the latter. Paraformaldehyde-lysine-periodate (PLP) fixative preserves murine parvoviral antigens better than neutral buffered formalin (Jacoby et al. 1987a). Although nervous system disease from parvoviruses is most prevalent in suckling rats, hemorrhagic lesions can occur in adults and cause sudden death (El Dadah et al. 1967; Coleman et al. 1983). Infections severe enough to cause nervous system lesions of either type in young rats will often induce necrosis in other tissues, notably liver (Kilham and Margolis 1966a; Margolis et al. 1968).

Biologic Features

Parvoviruses are extremely small (18–26 nm), single-stranded DNA viruses that require host cells in S-phase for replication (Tattersall and Cotmore 1986). Productive infection is lytic and accounts for the pathogenicity of these viruses for proliferating cells. Because such cells are plentiful in developing tissues, young animals are more susceptible than adults to severe or lethal infection. Parvoviruses of vertebrates consist of those that depend on adenovirus or herpesvirus coinfection for their own replication (dependovirus) and autonomous parvoviruses. All known rodent parvoviruses are autonomous, and viruses in two of the three serogroups, rat virus (RV) and H-1 virus, cause natural infection of laboratory-reared and wild rats (Kilham 1966). A third virus, minute virus of mice, is believed to cause natural infection only in mice. RV is the prototype virus of the family Parvoviridae and is highly prevalent in laboratory rats (Robey et al. 1968). H-1 virus is less prevalent, but shares many biologic properties with RV (Toolan 1960, 1968).

Rats are the only known natural hosts for rat parvoviruses, although infection has been experimentally induced in other species (Siegl 1984). Infection of fetal and neonatal hamsters has been studied extensively because it leads to developmental abnormalities, especially of teeth and bone (Toolan 1960). For this reason rat parvoviruses have been called "osteolytic" viruses.

Clinical manifestations of parvovirus infection in rats range from asymptomatic infection to severe or lethal disease, the latter occurring most often in fetal or infant rats (Kilham and Margolis 1966a). Suckling born to virus-immune mothers appear to be protected from lethal infection (Novotny and Hetrick 1970), but little else is known about the effects of host immunity on the course of infection. The incidence of clinical signs and lesions is low in naturally occurring infection of rats, but infection is highly contagious, so its attack rate of infection in rat colonies is normally high (Robinson et al. 1968). Transmission can occur in utero or by contact (Novotny and Hetrick 1970; Lipton et al. 1972; Jacoby et al. 1987b) and virus can persist in and be excreted by seropositive rats (Lipton et al. 1972; Jacoby et al. 1987a).

The pathogenesis of cerebellar hypoplasia is well understood. The external germinal layer develops a high level of mitotic activity in late prenatal and early postnatal life. During this replicative period germinal cells are highly susceptible to attack by rat parvoviruses. External germinal cells migrate inwards to form the internal granular layer. Destruction of all or part of the progenitor population leads to depletion of the granular layer.

The pathogenesis of hemorrhagic encephalomyelopathy is not completely known, but there has been speculation that it results from the combined effects of viral infection on endothelium leading to thrombosis and hemorrhage, a deficiency of clotting factors secondary to viral hepatitis and viral attack megakaryocytes (Margolis and Kilham 1970, 1972). Rat parvoviruses possess hemagglutinins, but the importance of hemagglutination to the vascular lesions is unknown.

Comparison with Other Species

Cerebellar hypoplasia occurs in kittens infected with feline panleukopenia virus (Kilham and Margolis 1966b), in calves infected with the virus of bovine virus diarrhea (Brown et al. 1973) and in pigs infected with hog cholera virus (Emerson and Delez 1965). Minute virus of mice has the potential to produce similar lesions, but they rarely, if ever, occur. Cerebellar hypoplasia from experimental inoculation of parvoviruses has been reported for hamsters and ferrets (reviewed by Siegl 1984). Cerebellar hypoplasia, apparently of hereditary origin, has been reported in various species of domestic animals (Jones and Hunt 1983). Parvoviral lesions of human cerebellum have not been reported nor has viral hemorrhagic encephalopathy been found in humans or in mammals other than the rat.

References

Baringer RJ, Nathanson N (1972) Parvovirus hemorrhagic encephalopathy of rats. Electron microscopic observations of the vascular lesions. Lab Invest 27: 514–522

Brown TT, De Lahunte A, Scott FW (1973) Virus induced congenital anomalies of the bovine fetus. II. Histopathology of cerebellar degeneration (hypoplasia) induced by the virus of bovine diarrhea-mucosal disease. Cornell Vet 63: 561–578

Cole GA, Nathanson N, Rivet H (1970) Viral hemorrhagic encephalopathy of rats. II. Pathogenesis of central nervous system lesions. Am J Epidemiol 91: 339–350

Coleman GL, Jacoby RO, Bhatt PN, Smith AL, Jonas AM (1983) Naturally occurring lethal parvovirus infection of juvenile and young rats. Vet Pathol 20: 49–56

El Dadah AH, Nathanson N, Smith KO, Squire RA, Santos GW, Melby EC (1967) Viral hemorrhagic encephalopathy of rats. Science 156: 392–394

Emerson JL, Delez AL (1965) Cerebellar hypoplasia, hypomyelinogenesis and congenital tremors of pigs, associated with prenatal hog cholera vaccination of sows. J Am Vet Med Assoc 147: 47–54

Jacoby RO, Bhatt PN, Gaertner DJ, Smith AL, Johnson EA (1987a) The pathogenesis of rat virus infection in infant and juvenile rats after oronasal inoculation. Arch Virol 95: 251–270

Jacoby RO, Gaertner DJ, Bhatt PN, Paturzo FX, Smith AL (1987b) Transmission of experimentally induced rat virus infection. Lab Anim Sci (in press)

Jones TC, Hunt RD (1983) Veterinary pathology, 5th edn, Lea and Febiger, Philadelphia, pp 420–424, 1656–1660

Kilham L (1966) Viruses of laboratory and wild rats. NCI Monogr 20: 117–135

Kilham L, Margolis G (1966a) Spontaneous hepatitis and cerebellar "hypoplasia" in suckling rats due to congenital infection with rat virus. Am J Pathol 49: 457–475

Kilham L, Margolis G (1966b) Viral etiology of spontaneous ataxia of cats. Am J Pathol 48: 991–1011

Lipton H, Nathanson N, Hodous J (1972) Enteric transmission of parvoviruses: pathogenesis of rat virus infection in adult rats. Am J Epidemiol 96: 443–446

Margolis G, Kilham L (1970) Parvovirus infections, vascular endothelium and hemorrhagic encephalopathy. Lab Invest 22: 478–488

Margolis G, Kilham L (1972) Rat virus infection of megakaryocytes: a factor in hemorrhagic encephalopathy. Exp Mol Pathol 16: 326–340

Margolis G, Kilham L, Ruffolo PR (1968) Rat virus disease an experimental model of neonatal hepatitis. Exp Mol Pathol 8: 1–20

Margolis G, Kilham L, Johnson RH (1971) The parvoviruses and replicating cells: insights into the pathogenesis of cerebellar hypoplasia. Prog Neuropathol 1: 168–201

Novotny JF, Hetrick FM (1970) Pathogenesis and transmission of Kilham rat virus infection in rats. Infect Immun 2: 298–303

Robey RE, Woodman DR, Hetrick FM (1968) Studies on the natural infection of rats with the Kilham rat virus. Am J Epidemiol 88: 139–143

Robinson GW, Nathanson N, Hodous J (1968) Sero-epidemiological study of rat virus infection in a closed laboratory colony. Am J Epidemiol 94: 91–100

Siegl G (1984) Biology and pathogenicity of autonomous parvovirus. In: Berns KI (ed) The parvoviruses. Plenum, New York, pp 297–362

Tattersall P, Cotmore SF (1986) The rodent parvoviruses. In: Bhatt PN, Jacoby RO, Morse HC, New AE (eds) Viral and mycoplasmal infections of laboratory rodents: effect on biomedical research. Academic, New York, pp 305–348

Toolan HW (1960) Experimental production of mongoloid hamsters. Science 131: 1446–1448

Toolan HW (1968) The picodna viruses: H, RV and AAV. Int Rev Exp Pathol 6: 135–180

Encephalomyelitis, Theiler's Virus, Mouse

Robert O. Jacoby

Synonyms. Mouse poliomyelitis, Theiler's disease.

Gross Appearance

Gross lesions are not seen.

Microscopic Features

Histologic lesions of naturally occurring mouse encephalomyelitis consist of neuronal necrosis, neuronophagia, nonsuppurative inflammation, and gliosis in the gray matter of the brain and spinal cord (Olitsky and Schlesinger 1941; Lipton 1975). These lesions are most prominent in posterior regions of the brain and in the spinal cord (Fig. 196). They are also more severe in lower centers than in the cerebrum, and the cerebellum is typically spared. Although neuronal necrosis can be widespread in the spinal cord, it most commonly occurs in ventral horn (motor) neurons of the spinal cord and is accompanied by perivascular infiltration of mononuclear cells (Figs. 197, 198). In severe cases mononuclear cells and polymorphonuclear leukocytes are found throughout the gray matter and the leptomeninges and they are accompanied by mic-

rogliosis. Cowdry type B intranuclear inclusions have been found in affected neurons at the onset of clinical signs (paralysis) (Olitsky and Schlesinger 1941), but they are not a consistent feature of infection. Inflammation may persist for up to several months after necrosis subsides and, in such cases, is accompanied by astrocytosis and focal mineralization.

The acute lesions of mouse encephalomyelitis can be induced experimentally by inoculation of mice with highly virulent strains of virus (Theiler and Gard 1940a). Less virulent strains can induce an early poliomyelitic phase followed by chronic demyelination (Daniels et al. 1952; Lipton 1975), but demyelinating lesions have not been observed in the naturally occurring disease. They are associated with persistent infection and a shift in viral replication from cells in gray matter to cells in white matter (Dal Canto and Lipton 1982). Several cell types are infected including oligodendrocytes and infiltrating mononuclear cells. Demyelination is most pronounced in the spinal cord but may also occur in brain stem and cerebellum (Fig. 199). Axonal remyelination and astrocytosis follow as inflammation subsides.

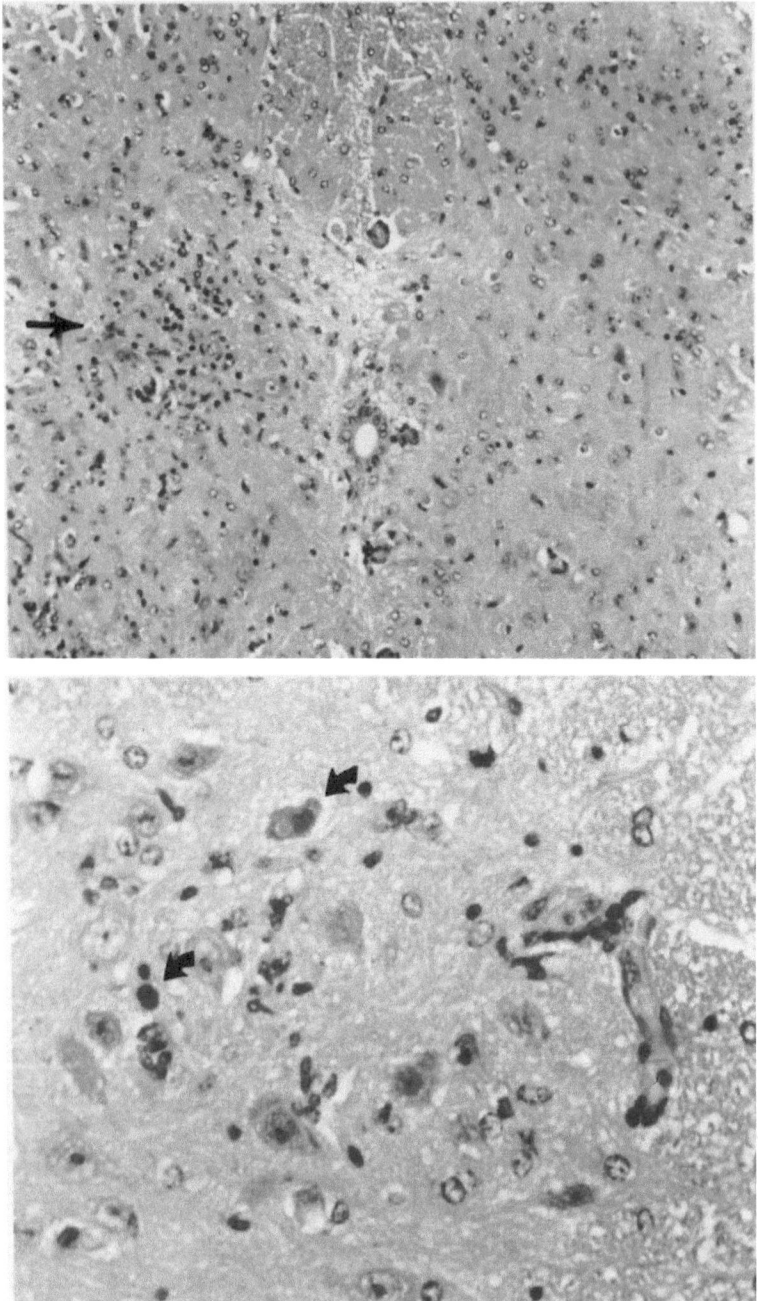

Fig. 196 *(above)*. Lumbar spinal cord, mouse. Lesions from a paralyzed mouse with naturally occurring mouse encephalomyelitis virus infection. Note inflammation and necrosis affecting the ventral horn. Lesions are more severe in one horn *(arrow)* than in the other. H and E, × 170

Fig. 197 *(below)*. Ventral horn of lumbar spinal cord with neuronal necrosis *(arrows)*, mild nonsuppurative infiltration and mild gliosis. H and E, × 425

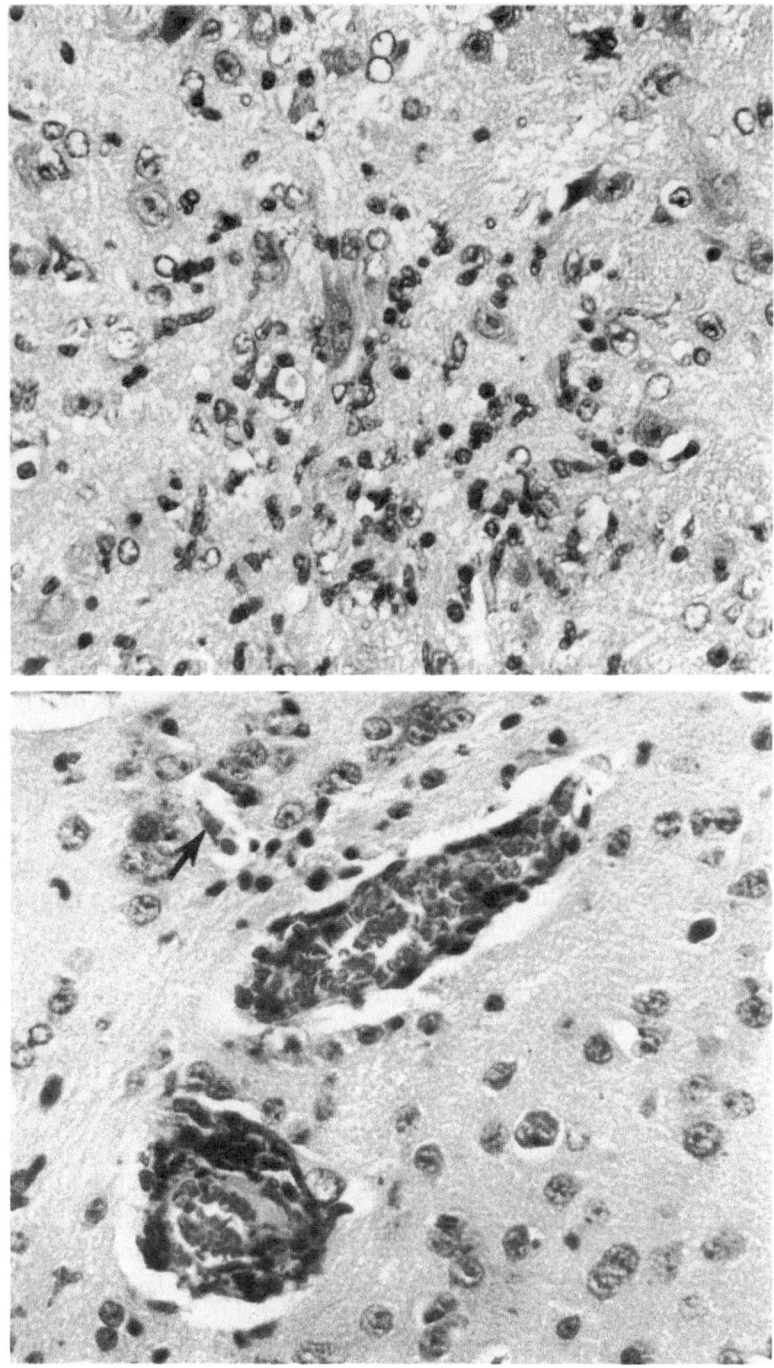

Fig. 198 *(above).* Ventral horn of lumbar spinal cord with prominent gliosis. H and E, × 425

Fig. 199 *(below).* Thalamus with neuronal necrosis *(arrow)* and nonsuppurative inflammation. H and E, × 425

Ultrastructure

Ultrastructural characterization of acute mouse encephalomyelitis is incomplete. Studies of spinal cord indicate that viral replication is primarily in large neurons, but smaller neurons in the intermediate and dorsal horns can be infected (Dal Canto and Lipton 1975, 1982). In early stages of acute disease, virus is found primarily in neuronal cell bodies, whereas later it is detected in axons and dendrites. It is, however, virtually impossible to identify virions by routine electron microscopy unless they are compartmentalized such as in crystalline arrays. Therefore special techniques, such as immunoelectron microscopy, are required to localize sites of infection (Dal Canto and Lipton 1982). In chronic demyelinating disease virus can be detected in macrophages in demyelinating lesions. Demyelination results from stripping of myelin lamellae by mononuclear cell processes, whereas virus-infected oligodendrocytes do not degenerate (Dal Canto and Lipton 1975).

Differential Diagnosis

Mouse encephalomyelitis must be differentiated from other encephalitides of mice, especially those due to viral infection. Mouse hepatitis virus encephalitis can induce necrosis and inflammation in brain and spinal cord, and some strains cause chronic demyelination. The acute lesions of mouse hepatitis, however, affect anterior and posterior areas of brain and, in spinal cord, are not confined to gray matter. Reovirus-3 can cause severe necrotizing encephalitis in neonatally inoculated mice, but lesions of the nervous system are not characteristic of naturally acquired infection and do not involve spinal cord. Lymphocytic choriomeningitis is characterized by lymphocytic inflammation of the meninges and choroid plexuses whereas necrosis is scant. In addition, it occurs after intracerebral inoculation of immunocompetent mice and rarely, if ever, occurs during natural infection. Neurologic impairment caused by bacterial infection (including rolling disease due to *Mycoplasma neurolyticum* exotoxins), trauma, intoxication, or genetic defects are unlikely to have characteristic ventral horn lesions.

Mouse encephalomyelitis infection can be confirmed in several ways. Apart from clinical signs and lesions, viral antigen can be detected in lesions by immunohistochemistry (Liu et al. 1967;

Dal Canto and Lipton 1982; Rodriguez et al. 1983), and virus can be isolated from the central nervous system or intestines of clinically affected mice (Lipton and Rozhon 1986). However, during asymptomatic infection virus will likely be found only in intestine. The disease can be detected serologically (Shaw 1956; Lipton 1978), but seroconversion alone may not reveal whether infection is active or historical.

Biologic Features

Theiler's mouse encephalomyelitis virus is a member of the Picornaviridae and is a natural pathogen of mice. Antibodies to the virus have been detected in rats, but clinical signs and lesions have not been found. It is highly prevalent in mouse colonies and usually produces asymptomatic enteric infection that is detected by seroconversion (Dean 1951; Descoteaux et al. 1977). Rarely, and by mechanisms that are not understood, high-titer viremia occurs, and virus infects the nervous system where it causes encephalomyelitis. The severity and character of lesions after experimental inoculation is influenced by virus strain, route of inoculation, and host age and genotype (reviewed by Downs 1982; Lipton and Rozhon 1986). Highly virulent strains (e.g., GDVII, FA) cause acute encephalomyelitis after inoculation intracerebrally or by routes mimicking natural infection (oral, intranasal). Less virulent strains (TO, DA) cause disease only after intracerebral inoculation and result in biphasic disease including chronic demyelination. Young mice are more susceptible to encephalitis than adult mice, and mouse strain-dependent susceptibility to chronic demyelinating disease has been demonstrated (Lipton and Dal Canto 1979).

The typical sign of naturally occurring infection is posterior flaccid paralysis in mice that are otherwise clinically normal. Affected mice can survive if they have easy access to food and water, otherwise they can die from dehydration or malnutrition. The encephalitic form of the disease may be expressed clinically by hyperexcitability and convulsion prior to death.

Acute disease is caused by lethal viral attack on neurons accompanied by an inflammatory response and, in surviving animals, by gliotic repair.

Chronic demyelinating disease appears to have immunopathologic components, despite the fact that oligodendrocytes are infected (Lipton and Dal Canto 1976).

Under natural conditions mice acquire infection by ingestion and virus is thought to replicate in the intestine from whence it is subsequently excreted (Theiler and Gard 1940b), so the disease usually spreads by ingestion of infected feces. Immune mice can harbor virus, and it has been recovered from the intestine for up to 53 days postinfection (Theiler and Gard 1940a, b). In addition, virus is relatively resistant to environmental inactivation. Therefore, although infection may spread slowly, it may do so persistently. There is no evidence for in utero transmission.

Comparison with Other Species

Mouse encephalomyelitis closely resembles human poliomyelitis (Theiler 1941; Olitsky 1945), and the demyelinating lesion has been proposed as a model for multiple sclerosis (reviewed by Lipton and Rozhon 1986). Pigs are susceptible to viral polioencephalomyelitis that morphologically resembles human poliomyelitis (Manuelidis et al. 1954).

References

Dal Canto MC, Lipton HL (1975) Primary demyelination in Theiler's virus infection. An ultrastructural study. Lab Invest 33: 626-637

Dal Canto MC, Lipton HL (1982) Ultrastructural immunohistochemical localization of virus in acute and chronic demyelinating Theiler's virus infection. Am J Pathol 106: 20-29

Daniels JB, Pappenheimer AM, Richardson S (1952) Observations on encephalomyelitis of mice (DA strain). J Exp Med 96: 517-530

Dean DJ (1951) Mouse encephalomyelitis: immunologic studies of a non-infected colony. J Immunol 66: 347-359

Descoteaux JP, Grignon-Archambault D, Lussier G (1977) Serologic study of the prevalence of murine viruses in five Canadian mouse colonies. Lab Anim Sci 27: 621-626

Downs WG (1982) Mouse encephalomyelitis virus. In: Foster HL, Small JD, Fox JG (eds) The mouse in biomedical research. II. Diseases. Academic, New York, pp 341-352

Lipton HL (1975) Theiler's virus infection in mice: an unusual biphasic disease process leading to demyelination. Infect Immun 11: 1147-1155

Lipton HL (1978) Characterization of the TO strains of Theiler's mouse encephalomyelitis viruses. Infect Immun 20: 869-872

Lipton HL, Dal Canto MC (1976) Theiler's virus-induced demyelination: prevention by immunosuppression. Science 192: 62-64

Lipton HL, Dal Canto MC (1979) Susceptibility of inbred mice to chronic central nervous system infection by Theiler's murine encephalomyelitis virus. Infect Immun 26: 369-374

Lipton HL, Rozhon EJ (1986) The Theiler's murine encephalomyelitis viruses. In: Bhatt PN, Jacoby RO, Morse HC, New AE (eds) Viral and mycoplasmal infections of laboratory rodents: effects on biomedical research. Academic, Orlando, pp 253-275

Liu C, Collins J, Sharp E (1967) The pathogenesis of Theiler's GD VII encephalomyelitis virus infection in mice as studied by immunofluorescent technique and infectivity titrations. J Immunol 98: 46-55

Manuelidis EE, Sprinz H, Horstmann DM (1954) Pathology of Teschen disease. Virus encephalomyelitis of swine. Am J Pathol 30: 567-597

Olitsky PK (1945) Certain properties of Theiler's virus, especially in relation to its use as a model for poliomyelitis. Proc Soc Exp Biol Med 58: 77-81

Olitsky PK, Schlesinger RW (1941) Histopathology of CNS of mice infected with virus of Theiler's disease (spontaneous encephalomyelitis). Proc Soc Exp Biol Med 47: 79-83

Rodriguez M, Leibowitz JL, Lampert DW (1983) Persistent infection of oligodendrocytes in Theiler's virus-induced encephalomyelitis. Ann Neurol 13: 426-433

Shaw M (1956) Serologic studies of Theiler's mouse encephalomyelitis virus. Proc Soc Exp Biol Med 92: 390-392

Theiler M (1941) Studies on poliomyelitis. Medicine (Baltimore) 20: 443-462

Theiler M, Gard S (1940a) Encephalomyelitis of mice. I. Characteristics and pathogenesis of the virus. J Exp Med 72: 49-67

Theiler M, Gard S (1940b) Encephalomyelitis of mice. III. Epidemiology. J Exp Med 72: 79-90

Mouse Hepatitis Virus Infection, Brain, Mouse

Stephen W. Barthold

Synonyms. Mouse hepatitis virus (MHV); hepato-encephalitis virus; murine hepatitis virus; mouse coronavirus infection.

Gross Appearance

Infection of most adult mice is usually subclinical, with no gross lesions. In susceptible mice, gross lesions can occur in multiple organs, including multiple focal areas of necrosis or hemorrhage in liver, intestinal ulceration or mucosal thickening, lymphoadenomegaly and splenomegaly. Gross brain lesions are not visible, but encephalitic signs can include tremor, incoordination, and convulsions (Piazza 1969). Some mice can manifest posterior paresis (Bailey et al. 1949; Sebesteny and Hill 1974), and athymic nude mice develop cachexia (wasting disease) due to chronic infections (Sebesteny and Hill 1974).

Microscopic Features

The features of microscopic lesions are dependent upon route of virus inoculation, virus strain, mouse genotype, mouse age, and stage of infection. Only natural routes of virus inoculation (oral/nasal) and neurotropic virus strains pertain to this review. Following intranasal inoculation of neurotropic virus, adult immunocompetent mice develop acute mild necrotizing rhinitis and neuritis of submucosal olfactory nerves. Inflammation extends into the lamina fibrosa, then to the inner layers of the olfactory bulbs of the brain. Marked necrosis with malacia of olfactory bulbs can occur (Fig. 200, 201). Necrotizing inflammation extends posteriorly along the ventral meninges, piriform cortex, olfactory tracts, septum pellucidum, anterior commissures, lateral ventricles, periependymal tissues and hippocampus. Initially, this is accompanied by infiltrates of polymorphonuclear leukocytes, followed by lymphocytes, with capillary endothelial swelling. Rarely, virus-induced giant cells (syncytia) are present in meningeal connective tissue, endothelium, or leukocytes. Necrosis of neurons, glia, and ependymal cells are seen in the early encephalitic stage of infection.

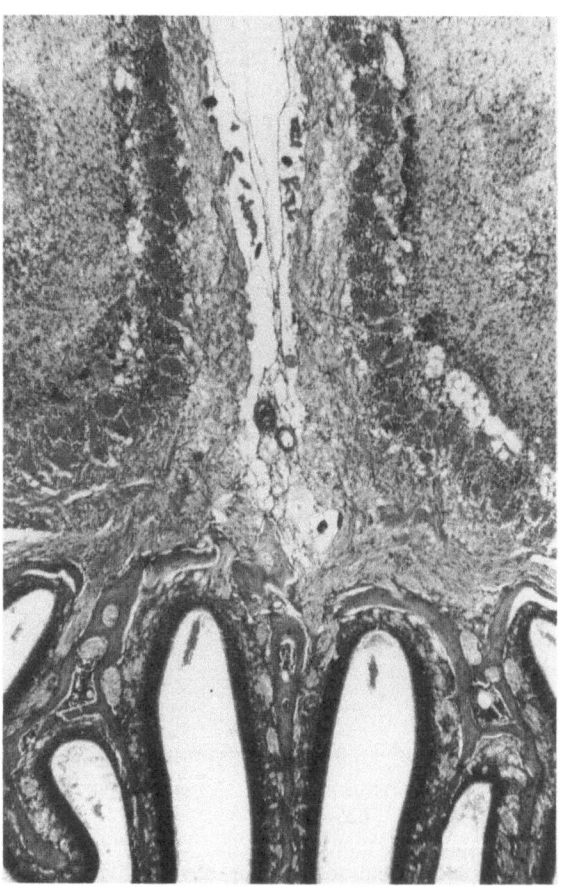

Fig. 200. Posterior nose and olfactory bulbs of an adult mouse 28 days after intranasal inoculation with MHV-A59. Note necrotizing inflammation and malacia of olfactory bulbs. H and E, × 43

As infection progresses, necrotizing lesions wane, followed by mild astrocytosis. Spongiosis and demyelination appear in the brain stem and spinal cord with varying degrees of perivascular lymphocyte infiltration (Figs. 202, 203). Ependymal necrosis can occur in the cervical and thoracic spinal cord. Focal meningitis, with extension of infection into adjacent fiber tracts occurs in an irregular distribution (Bailey et al. 1949; Barthold and Smith 1987; Goto et al. 1977). In mice inoculated intracerebrally, demyelination can occur in the pons, internal capsule, corpus callosum, hippocampal commissure, and subcortical white matter (Weiner 1973). In demyelinating areas, there is preservation of axons and nerve cells with glial proliferation and leukocytic

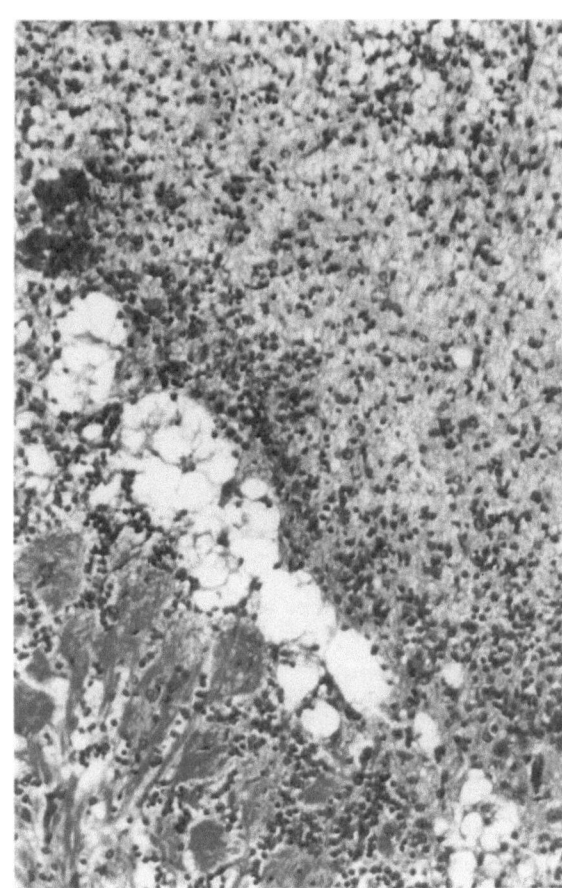

Fig. 201 *(upper left).* Olfactory bulb from mouse represented in Fig. 200. H and E, × 172

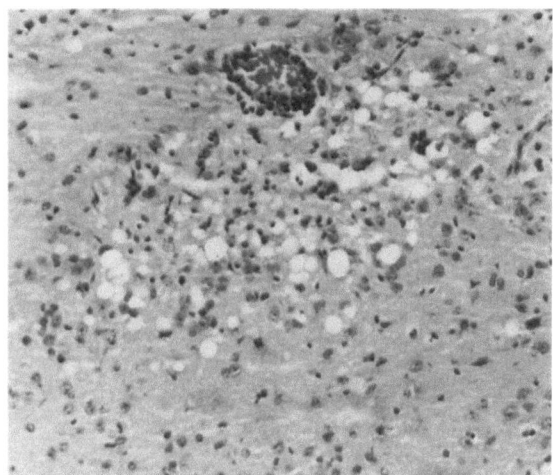

Fig. 202 *(upper right).* Brain stem, adult mouse, 28 weeks after intranasal inoculation with MHV-S. Note spongiosis, perivascular lymphocytes, and demyelination. (From Barthold and Smith 1983.) H and E, × 120

Fig. 203 *(below).* Section of mouse lumbar spinal cord, 60 days after intracerebral inoculation with MHV-A59. Note demyelination of white matter, characterized by pallor and spongiosis. (From Lavi et al. 1984.) × 80

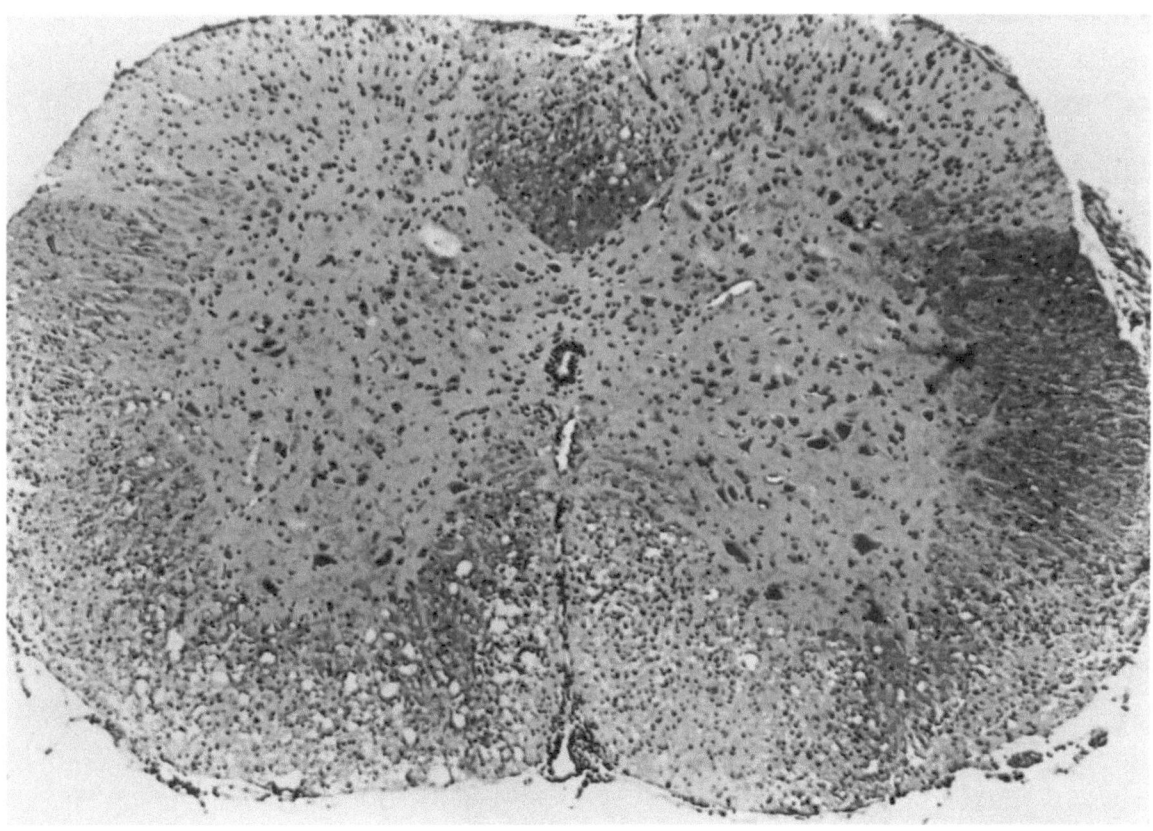

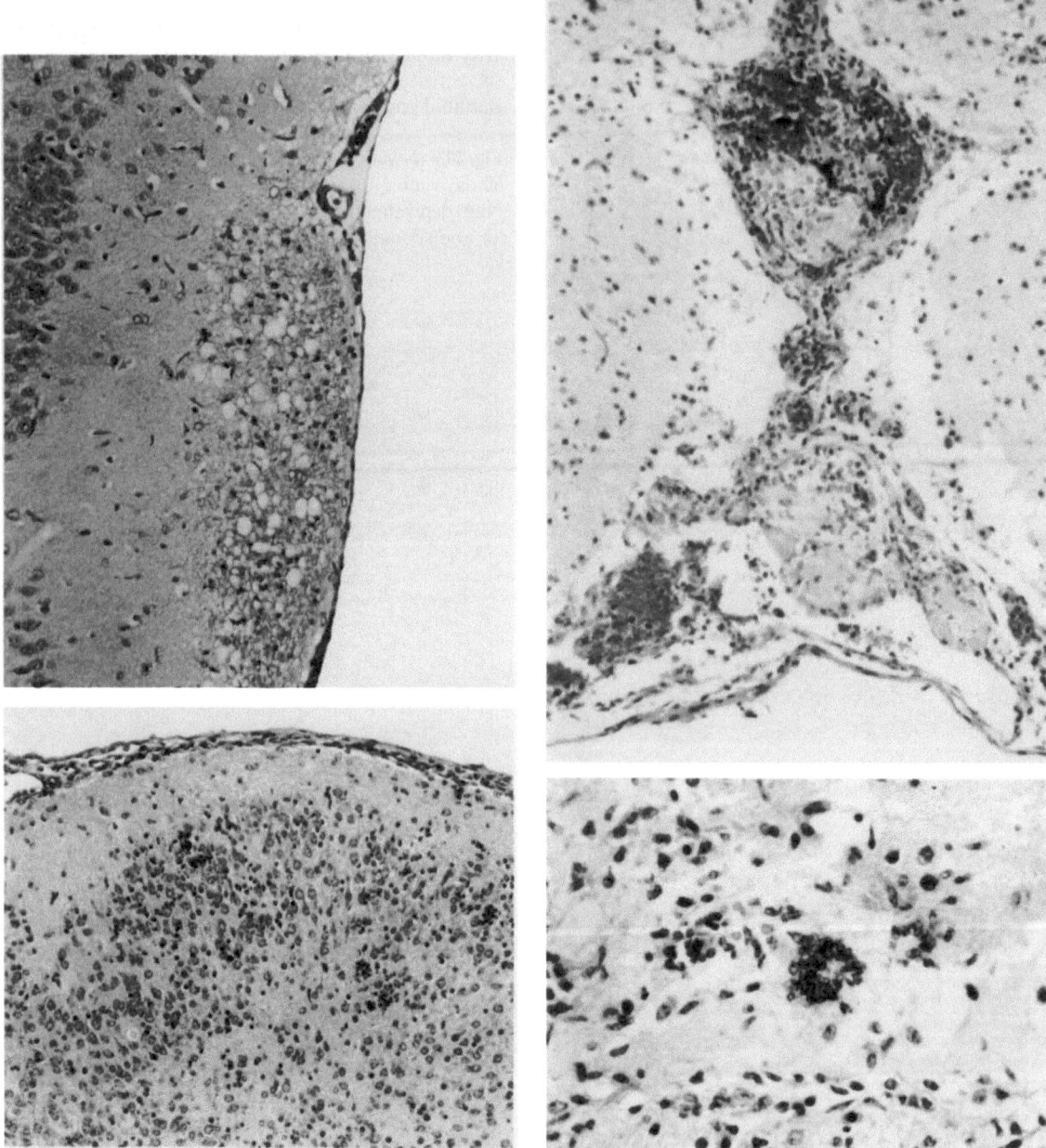

Fig. 204 *(upper left)*. Brain, mouse infected intranasally with MHV-3. Mild meningitis and demyelination, selectively involving the olfactory tract of the anteroventral cerebral cortex. (From Barthold et al. 1986.) H and E, × 135

Fig. 205 *(lower left)*. Cerebral cortex, neonatal mouse, 4 days after oronasal inoculation with MHV-S. Acute encephalitis. H and E, × 120

Fig. 206 *(upper right)*. Blood vessels at the base of the brain of a nude mouse naturally infected with MHV. Note endothelial syncytia and thrombosis. H and E, × 172

Fig. 207 *(lower right)*. Hippocampus of a nude mouse naturally infected with MHV. Note glial syncytium. H and E, × 286

infiltration (Lampert et al. 1973). In mice infected intranasally with some non-neurotropic MHV strains, mild demyelination and meningitis occur only in the anterior olfactory pathways (Barthold et al. 1986) (Fig. 204).

In contrast to adult mice, neonates develop panencephalitis involving all parts of the brain, due to diffuse hematogenous dissemination (Barthold and Smith 1984, 1987) (Fig. 205). Viral syncytia are more readily observed in neonates (Goto et al. 1979). Athymic nude mice frequently develop brain lesions when infected with mouse hepatitis virus, but published descriptions are not well detailed (Sebesteny and Hill 1974; Tamura et al. 1976). Vascular lesions predominate, with secondary extension into adjacent brain. Affected vessels have endothelial swelling, syncytium formation, and thrombosis (Fig. 206). Vessels in the meninges, base of the brain, and choroid plexus are most frequently affected. Neural lesions consist of necrosis, gliosis, and formation of syncytia from neurons, glia, and leukocytes (Fig. 207). Degenerating cells and syncytia possess prominent basophilic aggregates of karyorrhectic material. Brain stem spongiosis, demyelination, meningitis, and ependymitis, as seen in euthymic mice, can also be found.

Ultrastructure

Electron microscopy of spinal cord and brain of paralyzed mice has revealed virus particles in satellite cells adjacent to neurons in the gray matter and astrocytes, oligodendrocytes and phagocytic cells in white matter. Virus particles appear within membrane-bound vacuoles or budding into endoplasmic reticulum of infected cells. Typical virions average 80 nm in diameter, with a central electron-lucent core and multiple 20 nm projections (peplomers) on their surface. Infected cells possess excess microtubules, smooth and rough endoplasmic reticulum, mitochondria, and large aggregates of reticular electron-dense material near areas of virus formation. Oligodendroglia contain myelin figures and multiple anomalous connections to myelin sheaths. Infiltration of myelin sheaths, with stripping of lamellae by leukocytes and phagocytosis of myelin debris, particularly in later stages of infection, are associated with demyelination. As a result, bare axons are found in myelinated tracts (Fig. 208). Polymorphonuclear leukocytes, lymphocytes, macrophages, and multinucleate giant cells occur in affected areas. In late infection, proliferation of astrocytes containing excess glial filaments and remyelination are found (Herndon et al. 1975; Lampert et al. 1973; Powell and Lampert 1975).

Differential Diagnosis

Clinical manifestations of central nervous system disease can be caused by mouse encephalomyelitis virus, neurotropic retrovirus, labyrinthitis, or neoplasia. Microscopic features of mouse encephalomyelitis virus infection are described elsewhere in this volume (p. 175). Several ecotropic retroviruses cause progressive hindlimb paralysis in wild mice due to noninflammatory spongiform degeneration with proliferation of astroglia (Gardner 1978). Reovirus 3 can cause encephalitis in neonatal mice (Kundin et al. 1966). Athymic nude mice can develop paralytic disease when infected with polyoma virus, which infects oligodendrocytes causing demyelination. Polyoma virus can also induce vertebral bone tumors that compress the spinal cord (McCance et al. 1983). Cachexia, or wasting disease, in nude mice is most frequently due to mouse hepatitis virus, but can also be caused by chronic infections with Sendai virus (Ward et al. 1976), pneumonia virus of mice (Richter et al. 1986), polyoma virus (McCance et al. 1983), and *Pneumocystis carinii* (Weir et al. 1986), among others. Definitive diagnosis of mouse hepatitis virus infection can be achieved by virus isolation, confirmation of viral antigens in tissues by immunohistochemistry, as well as seroconversion of recovered mice or gnotobiotic mice inoculated with suspect material (mouse antibody production test).

Biologic Features

Natural History. Mouse hepatitis virus seems to be highly contagious and is spread by respiratory and orofecal routes. It can also be a contaminant of biologic material such as transplantable tumors. Vertical transmission of virus from dam to fetus can occur under certain circumstances. Because of its highly mutable nature, there are numerous strains of virus which vary widely in virulence and organotropism. Most virus strains are only mildly pathogenic and tend to produce subclinical infections in adult, immunocompetent mice. More severe disease can occur in immunologically incompetent mice, such as neonates, athymic mice, and immunosuppressed mice. A variety of other stressors can also exacerbate disease.

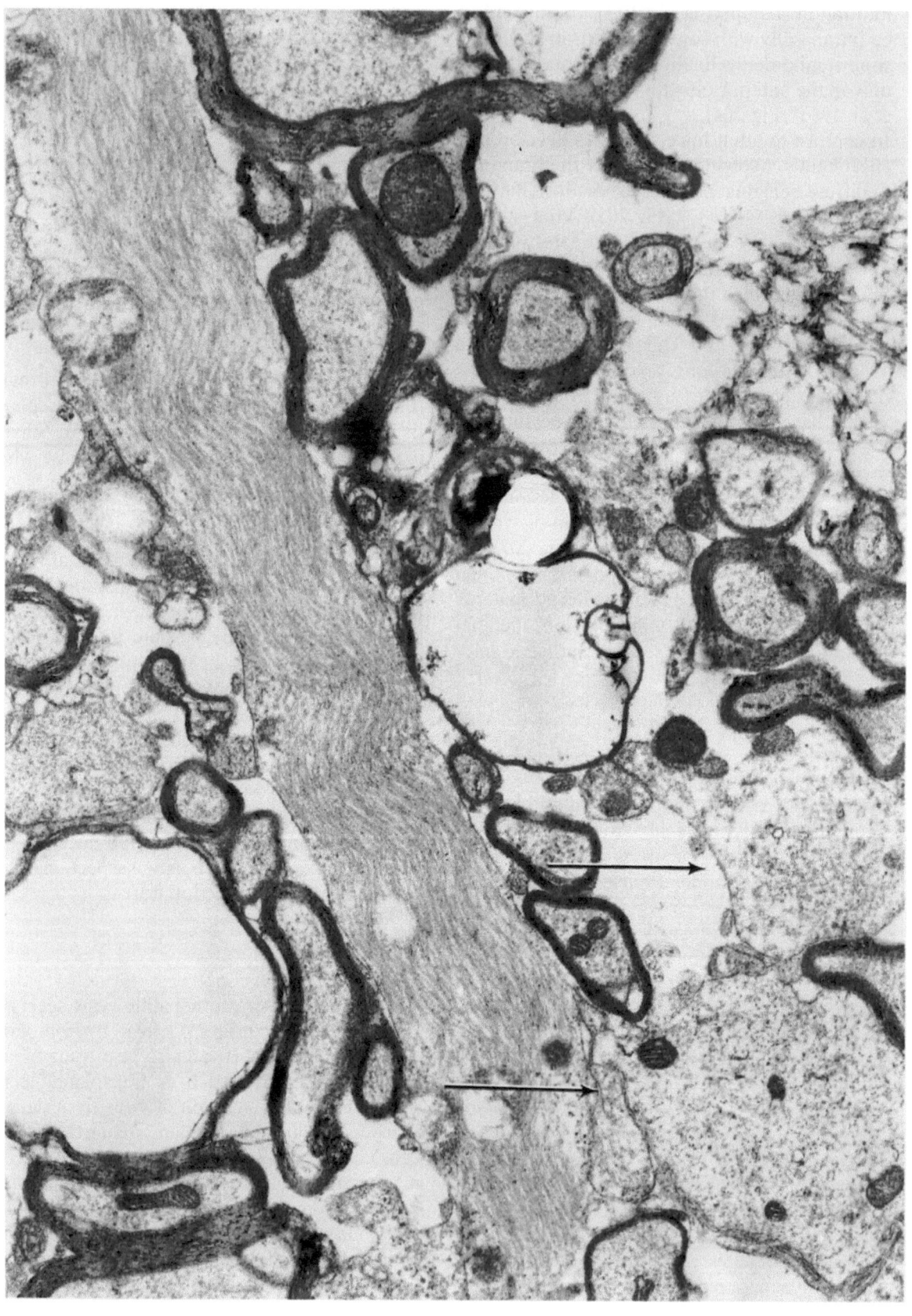

Fig. 208. White matter of spinal cord from a mouse, 60 days after intracerebral inoculation with MHV-A59. Note several bare axons *(arrows),* as well as normal myelinated axons. (From Lavi et al. 1984.) TEM, × 7000

Infections are usually short term, with no carrier state, but persistent infections, particularly of the central nervous system, can occur in experimentally infected mice. Athymic nude mice develop chronic, progressive infections when infected with low virulence strains that do not kill them acutely (Barthold 1986). Recovered immunocompetent mice are immune to reinfection with the homologous strain of virus, but are susceptible to infection with an antigenically heterologous virus strain. Because of the antigenic diversity and large number of virus strains, there is a high likelihood of multiple infections of a single mouse, analogous to the common cold in man (Barthold and Beck 1987).

Pathogenesis. The primary target for mouse hepatitis virus is either nasal or intestinal epithelium, depending on virus strain. Enterotropic virus strains are largely restricted to the intestine, with limited dissemination to other organs, even in susceptible neonates or nude mice. The brain is unlikely to be infected in most enterotropic mouse hepatitis virus infections. In susceptible mice, nonenterotropic virus strains readily disseminate by viremia from the primary nasal mucosal target to multiple organs, including lymphoid organs and liver. Dissemination of virus is dependent on the virulence of the infecting virus as well as on host genotype, age, and immune status. Despite viremic dissemination to other organs, there appears to be an effective blood-brain barrier in immunocompetent adult mice. However, hematogenous infection of brain occurs in neonatal mice and athymic nude mice (Barthold 1986; Barthold and Smith 1984, 1987; Barthold et al. 1986).

The major means of brain infection in adult, immunocompetent mice is naso-olfactory spread of virus. Infection of the brain directly along olfactory pathways is dependent on virus strain and can occur in the apparent absence of dissemination to other organs. Conversely, oral inoculation of virus results in disseminated infection without brain involvement. Mouse hepatitis virus initially replicates in nasal respiratory and olfactory mucosa, then spreads along olfactory nerve fibers and perineurium, through the ethmoid cribriform plate into the olfactory bulbs within 2 days of intranasal inoculation. Once in the brain, virus spreads along the anteroventral meninges, olfactory tracts, and lateral ventricles. Thus, the cerebral cortices and cerebellum are usually not affected. Virus titers peak in the brain around 4–5 days after intranasal inoculation, when en-

cephalitis and mortality are most severe. Encephalitis resolves in surviving mice but spongiform demyelinating lesions persist for 30–60 days. Virus is usually cleared from the brain during these intervals (Barthold 1987; Barthold and Smith 1987; Goto et al. 1977). Persistent brain infections have been reported in mice inoculated intracerebrally or intraperitoneally with selected strains of virus (Herndon et al. 1975; Knobler et al. 1982; Lavi et al. 1984; Virelizier et al. 1975). In mice, demyelination is primary due to virus damage to oligodendroglia.

Etiology. Mouse hepatitis virus is a coronavirus that has numerous constantly changing strains that vary in virulence, organotropism, and genetic/antigenic relatedness. All strains cross-react antigenically, but have strain-specific antigenic moeities as well. Effective host immunity is directed at strain-specific antigens. Antigenic relatedness does not predict biologic behavior of virus strains (Barthold 1986).

Frequency. Mouse hepatitis virus occurs among mice in a majority of biomedical research institutions throughout the world. When present within a population, the rate of infection is very high, as judged by seroconversion. Clinical disease is uncommon or mild in most adult mice, and lesions are usually subtle. Significant disease is most likely to be encountered in neonatal, stressed, immunosuppressed, or athymic mice, or when the virus is first introduced to a breeding colony. Under these circumstances, acute brain and cord lesions are likely to be seen. Demyelinating disease in adult, immunocompetent mice frequently occurs following intracerebral inoculation with selected virus strains, but is otherwise rare.

Comparison with Other Species

Mouse hepatitis virus, like coronaviruses of other species, produces enteric, respiratory, and generalized disease in susceptible hosts (Barthold 1986). Rats are susceptible to experimental infection with mouse hepatitis virus and develop demyelinating disease, but its pathogenesis differs from disease in mice. In rats, demyelination is immune mediated, as in experimental allergic encephalomyelitis (Watanabe et al. 1983; p. 6 this volume). Mouse hepatitis virus is genetically and antigenically closely related to several other coronaviruses, including bovine coronavirus, hemagglutinating encephalomyelitis virus of swine, human coronavirus of the OC43 subgroup and rat coronaviruses. The significance of this close relationship is unknown. Nonhuman primates inoculated intracerebrally with mouse hepatitis virus develop brain lesions (Kersting and Pette 1956), and humans have been found to develop antibodies to mouse hepatitis virus (Barthold 1986).

References

Bailey OT, Pappenheimer AM, Cheever FS, Daniels JB (1949) A murine virus (JHM) causing disseminated encephalomyelitis with extensive destruction of myelin. II. Pathology. J Exp Med 90: 195-212

Barthold SW (1986) Mouse hepatitis virus biology and epizootiology. In: Bhatt PN, Jacoby RO, Morse HC, New AE (eds) Viral and mycoplasmal infections of laboratory rodents. Effects on biomedical research. Academic, Orlando, pp 572-601

Barthold SW (1987) Olfactory neural pathway in mouse hepatitis virus nasoencephalitis. (in preparation)

Barthold SW, Beck DS (1987) Intranasal challenge immunity of mice to antigenically homologous and heterologous strains of mouse hepatitis virus. Proceedings of third international symposium on corona virus. Plenum, New York

Barthold SW, Smith AL (1983) Mouse hepatitis virus in weanling Swiss mice following intranasal inoculation. Lab An Sci 33: 355-360

Barthold SW, Smith AL (1984) Mouse hepatitis virus strain-related patterns of tissue tropism in suckling mice. Arch Virol 81: 103-112

Barthold SW, Smith AL (1987) Response of genetically susceptible and resistant mice to intranasal inoculation with mouse hepatitis virus JHM. Virus Res 7: 225-239

Barthold SW, Beck DS, Smith AL (1986) Mouse hepatitis virus nasoencephalopathy is dependent upon virus strain and host genotype. Arch Virol 91: 247-256

Gardner MB (1978) Type-C viruses of wild mice: characterization and natural history of amphotropic, ecotropic and xenotropic murine leukemia viruses (MuLV). Curr Top Microbiol Immunol 79: 215-259

Goto N, Hirano N, Aiuchi M, Hayashi T, Fujiwara K (1977) Nasoencephalopathy of mice infected intranasally with a mouse hepatitis virus, JHM strain. Jpn J Exp Med 47: 59-70

Goto N, Takahashi K, Huang K-J, Katami K, Fujiwara K (1979) Giant cell formation in the brain of suckling mice infected with mouse hepatitis virus, JHM strain. Jpn J Exp Med 49: 169-177

Herndon RM, Griffin DE, McCormick U, Weiner L (1975) Mouse hepatitis virus-induced recurrent demyelination. A preliminary report. Arch Neurol 32: 32-35

Kersting G, Pette E (1956) Zur Pathohistologie und Pathogenese der experimentellen JHM-Virus Encephalomyelitis des Affen. Dtsch Z Nervenheilkd 174: 283-304

Knobler RL, Tunison LA, Lampert PW, Oldstone MBA (1982) Selected mutants of mouse hepatitis virus type 4 (JHM strain) induce different CNS diseases. Pathobiology of disease induced by wild type and mutants ts8 and ts15 in BALB/c and SJL/J mice. Am J Pathol 109: 157-168

Kundin WD, Liu C, Gigstad J (1966) Reovirus infection in suckling mice: immunofluorescent and infectivity studies. J Immunol 97: 393-401

Lampert PW, Sims JK, Kniazeff AJ (1973) Mechanism of demyelination in JHM virus encephalomyelitis. Electron microscopic studies. Acta Neuropathol (Berl) 24: 76-85

Lavi E, Gilden DH, Highkin MK, Weiss SR (1984a) Persistence of mouse hepatitis virus A59 RNA in a slow virus demyelinating infection in mice as detected by in situ hybridization. J Virol 51: 563-566

Lavi E, Gilden DH, Wroblewska Z, Rorke LB, Weiss SR (1984b) Experimental demyelination produced by the A59 strain of mouse hepatitis virus. Neurology 34: 597-603

McCance DJ, Sebesteny A, Griffin BE, Balkwill F, Tilly R, Gregson NA (1983) A paralytic disease in nude mice associated with polyoma virus infection. J Gen Virol 64: 57-67

Piazza M (1969) Experimental viral hepatitis. Thomas, Springfield

Powell HC, Lampert PW (1975) Oligodendrocytes and their myelinplasma membrane connections in JHM mouse hepatitis virus encephalomyelitis. Lab Invest 33: 440-445

Richter CB, Thigpen JE, Small JD (1986) Fatal wasting disease caused by PVM in naturally infected nu/nu mice (abstr). Lab Anim Sci 36: 575

Sebesteny A, Hill AC (1974) Hepatitis and brain lesions due to mouse hepatitis virus accompanied by wasting in nude mice. Lab Anim 8: 317-326

Tamura T, Ueda K, Hirano N, Fujiwara K (1976) Response of nude mice to a mouse hepatitis virus isolated from a wasting nude mouse. Jpn J Exp Med 46: 19-30

Virelizier JL, Dayan AD, Allison AC (1975) Neuropathological effects of persistent infection of mice by mouse hepatitis virus. Infect Immun 12: 1127-1140

Ward JM, Houchens DP, Collins MJ, Young DM, Reagan RL (1976) Naturally-occurring Sendai virus infection of athymic nude mice. Vet Pathol 13: 36-46

Watanabe R, Wege H, ter Meulen V (1983) Adoptive transfer of EAE-like lesions from rats with coronavirus-induced demyelinating encephalomyelitis. Nature 305: 150-153

Weiner LP (1973) Pathogenesis of demyelination induced by a mouse hepatitis virus (JHM virus). Arch Neurol 28: 298-303

Weir EC, Brownstein DG, Barthold SW (1986) Spontaneous wasting disease in nude mice associated with *Pneumocystis carinii* infection. Lab Anim Sci 36: 140-144

Lymphocytic Choriomeningitis, Mouse

Kathryn E. Wright and Michael J. Buchmeier

Gross Appearance

Tissue from the central nervous system of affected mice undergoes no alteration which is recognizable macroscopically.

Microscopic Features

The classical lesion of lymphocytic choriomeningitis occurs in adult mice only and is characterized by extensive infiltration of mononuclear cells into the meninges and choroid plexus (Rivers and Scott 1936; Lillie and Armstrong 1945). Infiltration is focal, and reports differ as to whether the third and fourth (Lillie and Armstrong 1945) or the lateral ventricles (Walker et al. 1975) are more affected. The ventricular spaces can contain both polymorphonuclear and mononuclear cells (Tosolini and Mims 1971; Walker et al. 1975). Inflammatory cells are rarely observed in the parenchyma except for some perivascular cuffing of blood vessels in mice that survive the major lesion (Rivers and Scott 1936; Walker et al. 1975). Necrosis of the neurons is equally rare (Walker et al. 1975). The spinal cord is generally free from disease, but occasionally some mononuclear infiltration of the meninges can be noted (Rivers and Scott 1936; Lillie and Armstrong 1945).

A second lesion in the central nervous system can occur in young mice if infected at 4 days of age (Cole et al. 1971; Cole and Nathanson 1974). In addition to acute choriomeningitis, cerebellar granule cell necrosis with some hemorrhage is observed. There is inflammation of neural membranes and small vessels (Cole et al. 1971; Cole and Nathanson 1974). Similar lesions can also be seen in the cerebral cortex, hippocampus, and olfactory bulb (Cole and Nathanson 1974).

Mice infected with the causative agent lymphocytic choriomeningitis virus congenitally or neonatally can be persistently infected without overt gross or microscopic lesions. Indeed this observation, first made by Traub (1936a, b), was the first description of a persistent virus infection. This virus has been the subject of a large number of experimental studies which have illuminated basic concepts in biology (Buchmeier et al. 1980).

Ultrastructure

The major ultrastructural feature of the acute lesion is the presence of electron-dense intracytoplasmic inclusions of polyribosomes in the epithelial cells of the choroid plexus and other affected areas. Infected epithelial cells appear normal in all other respects. Enveloped virions containing multiple electron-dense granules characteristic of the virus can be observed budding into the cerebrospinal fluid from the microvillus surfaces of the choroid plexus (Walker et al. 1975). Infiltrating mononuclear cells accumulate at the endothelial basement lamina and beneath the basal margin of choroid epithelial cells and in general, are present in areas where virus is budding (Walker et al. 1975). The architectures of the meninges and choroid plexus are normal and without ultrastructurally evident lesions (Walker et al. 1975). Reports conflict regarding the presence (Doherty and Zinkernagel 1974) or absence (Walker et al. 1975) of edema.

Differential Diagnosis

Acute lymphocytic choriomeningitis is unlikely to be confused with other diseases. The characteristic lesion develops only after intracranial infection of adult immunocompetent mice with the specific virus. Outward symptoms appear at day 4 or 5 after infection, depending on the viral dose, and include ruffling of the fur, a hunched posture, and facial edema. These symptoms worsen, the animal loses weight and becomes sluggish and sensitive to loud noises. Death occurs at day 7-9 of tonic convulsions with extended rear limbs, flexed forelimbs, and thoracic spine. Characteristic tonic convulsions can be induced in symptomatic mice by spinning them by the tail. Infection with some strains of murine hepatitis virus and anaphylactic shock can lead to similar signs (Hotchin 1962); however, no other condition results in the mononuclear infiltrate observed after intracranial infection with the virus. Inoculation of blood or tissue homogenates from infected animals intracranially to adult mice will result in the disease whereas the same material will cause asymptomatic persistent infection in neonates. Diagnosis of infection can be

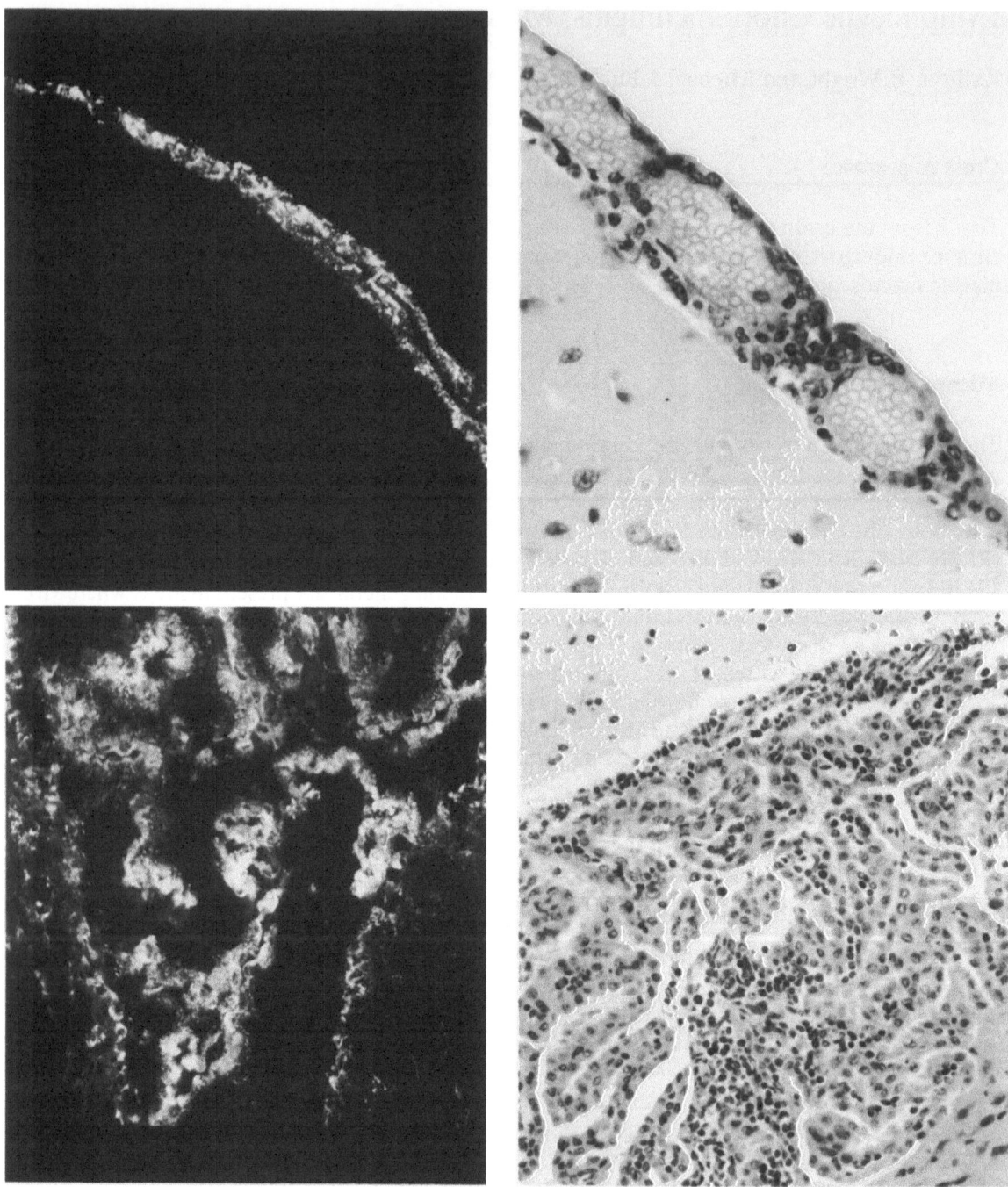

Fig. 209 *(upper left)*. Viral antigens in the brains of acutely infected mice using FITC-conjugated guinea pig antiserum to lymphocytic choriomeningitis viruses. Early expression of lymphocytic choriomeningitis viral antigen in the meninges of a mouse infected 5 days earlier. × 250

Fig. 210 *(lower left)*. Viral antigens in the brains of acutely infected mice using FITC-conjugated guinea pig antiserum to lymphocytic choriomeningitis viruses. Antigen in ependymal cells of the choroid plexus of a mouse infected 7 days earlier with the lymphocytic choriomeningitis viruses. × 250

Fig. 211 *(upper right)*. Acute lymphocytic choriomeningitis. Congestion and mild perivascular meningeal infiltrate early in disease. H and E, × 400

Fig. 212 *(lower right)*. Acute lymphocytic choriomeningitis. Moderate inflammatory focus in the choroid plexus of the third ventricle of a mouse infected 6 days earlier with lymphocytic choriomeningitis viruses. H and E, × 100

confirmed most readily by detection of cytoplasmic viral nucleocapsid protein antigen in the brain and other tissues by immunofluorescence with virus-specific antiserum. Demonstration of characteristic intracytoplasmic inclusions in neurons and budding virions from ependymal cells are helpful, but require electron-microscopic examination.

Biologic Features

Natural History and Pathogenesis. Lymphocytic choriomeningitis develops within 6 days after intracranial infection of adult, immunocompetent mice with the virus. Viral antigen is first detected in the meninges and choroid plexus around day 2 post infection (Fig. 209); by day 4 or 5 nearly all epithelial cells in both tissues are infected (Walker et al. 1975) (Fig. 210). The first signs of cellular infiltrate occur in the meninges at day 3 or 4 (Fig. 211) and extend to the choroid plexus by day 6 (Fig. 212). The ventricles may also contain inflammatory cells at this point (Lillie and Armstrong 1945; Walker et al. 1975). Death occurs at day 7-9. In surviving animals, inflammatory cells may progress into the parenchyma, but this phenomenon is never extensive (Rivers and Scott 1936; Walker et al. 1975).

Development of the lesion requires competent cellular immunity. Suppression of the cellular immune response in adult mice by irradiation (Rowe 1956), neonatal thymectomy (Rowe et al. 1963), or treatment with antithymocyte sera (Hirsch et al. 1968) or cyclophosphamide (Gilden et al. 1972) abrogated the disease and the mononuclear infiltrate associated with it. Transfer of immune T splenocytes but not immune serum to these infected mice resulted in disease and death (Cole et al. 1971, 1972; Cole and Nathanson 1974). T cells expressing cytotoxic function have been implicated in causing the disease as lymphocytes expressing the T cell antigen, Thy 1.2, and having lymphocytic choriomeningitis virus-specific cytotoxic activity in vitro have been isolated from the central nervous system of mice with lymphocytic choriomeningitis (Zinkernagel and Doherty 1973). Cells expressing Thy 1.2 can be observed in infiltrates in the ventricular spaces (Fig. 213).

Etiology and Frequency. Classic lymphocytic choriomeningitis can only be induced experimentally by inoculation of immunocompetent mice with the arenavirus, lymphocytic choriomeningi-

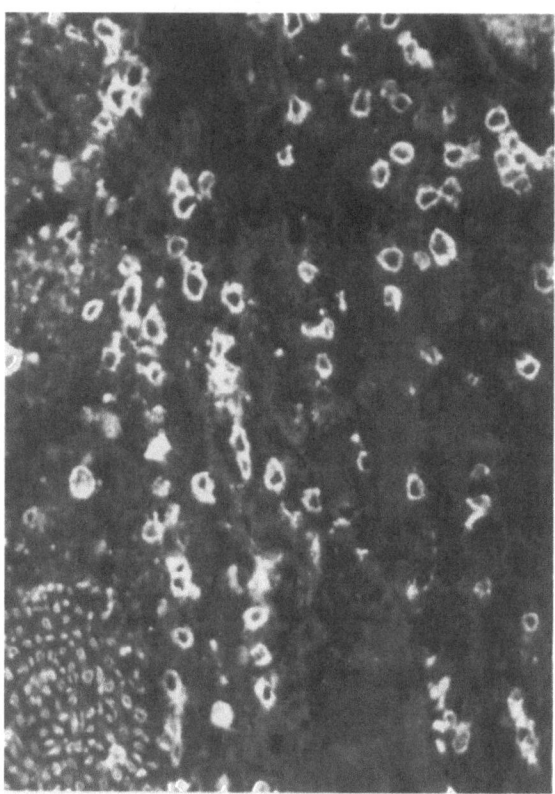

Fig. 213. Thy 1.2 positive lymphocytes in an inflammatory lesion in the ventricle of a mouse infected 7 days earlier with lymphocytic choriomeningitis virus. Rat anti-thy 1.2 staining visualized with FITC-conjugated mouse anti-rat IgG. × 400

tis virus by the intracranial route. Inoculation of adult mice by a peripheral route usually results in an asymptomatic infection that is rapidly cleared. However, certain strains of the virus cause extensive lesions in the viscera and death after intraperitoneal infection (Lehmann-Grube 1971), and certain strains of mice are particularly susceptible to neonatal infection and appear to die due to hormonal imbalances (Oldstone et al. 1982). Although virus is reported to reach the central nervous system in adult animals infected peripherally (Rivers and Scott 1936), only occasionally is slight meningitis or choroiditis observed (Lillie and Armstrong 1945).

Inoculation of neonatal mice by all routes results in a life-long persistent infection that mirrors the persistent infection observed in mice in the wild (Hotchin 1962; Casals 1984). Infectious virus and viral antigen can be detected in most tissues of the body, including the brain, until death. The distribution of viral antigen in the brains of carrier mice is distinct from that observed in acutely

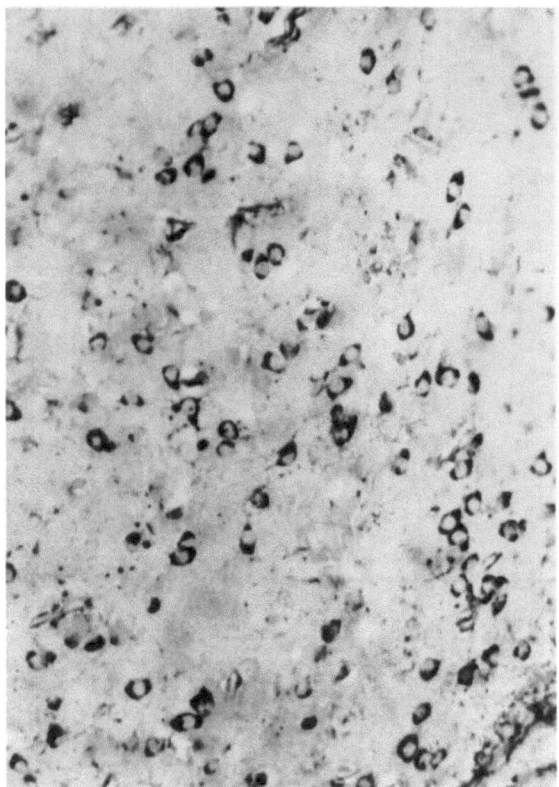

Fig. 214. Persistent lymphocytic choriomeningitis virus infection in cortical neurons of a mouse infected neonatally 4 months earlier. Abundant viral antigen is evident in neuronal cell bodies throughout the cortex by this time. Monoclonal antibody to viral nucleocapsid protein detected with guinea pig peroxidase antiperoxidase (PAP). (Courtesy Dr. M. Rodriguez.) × 250

infected adult mice. There is extensive infection of neuronal cells in the parenchyma, and, as animals age, more neurons and Purkinje's cells become infected (Mims 1966; Rodriguez et al. 1983) (Fig. 214). At later stages, immune complexes can be demonstrated in the brain (Oldstone 1984). One study claims that persistently infected carrier mice display behavioral abnormalities (Hotchin and Seegal 1977), but most strains of mice show no discernable signs until late in life when they develop a wasting syndrome due to immune complex disease (Hotchin 1962). Histologically, at all ages, the brains of carrier mice are normal, with only occasional slight meningitis shortly after infection (Traub 1936a) or mild perivascular round cell infiltrate (Oldstone and Dixon 1970).

In the wild, infection is passed vertically from mother to offspring in utero or, less likely, by naso-oral infection after contact with nasal secretions and/or excreta from infected mice (Traub 1936b, 1939). The distribution of viral antigen and lack of microscopic lesions in animals infected in utero are indistinguishable from animals experimentally infected neonatally (Wilsnack and Rowe 1964).

Comparison with Other Species

The natural reservoir for the virus is feral mice, but occasionally laboratory mice become infected through experimental or accidental introduction of the virus or virus-infected tumor cells (Parker 1986; van der Zeijst et al. 1983). Once the infection is established in a colony, it is perpetuated by congenital and/or vertical transmission to offspring. Persistent infections also occur in hamsters with both vertical and horizontal transmission (Parker et al. 1976). When young hamsters are inoculated, infection persists with prolonged viruria; older animals tend to clear infection (Smadel and Wall 1942; Lewis et al. 1965). There are no reports of pathologic lesions within the central nervous system in infected hamsters.

Humans can also become infected although they rarely transmit the disease (Parker 1986). The means of human infection is through contact with infected rodents, pet hamsters being a particular source in recent years (Buchmeier et al. 1980). Generally the virus infection is asymptomatic or produces a nonmeningeal influenza-like illness in man. Less frequent severe cases may occur as aseptic meningitis and meningoencephalitis (Scott and Rivers 1936; Buchmeier et al. 1980; Casals 1984).

Neural lesions can be induced in rats if infected at an early age (Cole et al. 1971). Rats inoculated intracranially with the virus prior to 14 days of age developed marked cerebellar hypoplasia with minimal inflammation. Treatment of suckling rats with antithymocyte serum prevented cerebellar lesions, hence the lesion appeared to be immune mediated. Guinea pigs, monkeys, and dogs have been infected experimentally, but little has been done to examine the lesions in the central nervous system after infection (Parker 1986).

References

Buchmeier MJ, Welsh RM, Dutko FJ, Oldstone MBA (1980) The virology and immunobiology of lymphocytic choriomeningitis virus infection. Adv Immunol 30: 275-331

Casals J (1984) Arenaviruses. In: Evans AS (ed) Viral infections of humans: epidemiology and control. Plenum Medical, New York

Cole GA, Nathanson N (1974) Lymphocytic choriomeningitis. Prog Med Virol 18: 94-110

Cole GA, Gilden DH, Monjan AA, Nathanson N (1971) Lymphocytic choriomeningitis virus: pathogenesis of acute central nervous system disease. Fed Proc 30: 1831-1841

Cole GA, Nathanson N, Prendergast RA (1972) Requirement for theta-bearing cells in lymphocytic choriomeningitis virus-induced central nervous system disease. Nature 238: 335-337

Doherty PC, Zinkernagel RM (1974) T-cell-mediated immunopathology in viral infections. Transplant Rev 19: 89-120

Gilden DH, Cole GA, Monjan AA, Nathanson N (1972) Immunopathogenesis of acute central nervous system disease produced by lymphocytic choriomeningitis virus. I. Cyclophosphamide-mediated induction of the virus-carrier state in adult mice. J Exp Med 135: 860-873

Hirsch MS, Murphy FA, Hicklin MD (1968) Immunopathology of lymphocytic choriomeningitis virus infection of newborn mice. J Exp Med 127: 757-766

Hotchin J (1962) The biology of lymphocytic choriomeningitis infection: virus-induced immune disease. Cold Spring Harbor Symp Quant Biol 27: 479-499

Hotchin J. Seegal R (1977) Virus-induced behavioral alteration of mice. Science 196: 671-674

Lewis AM Jr, Rowe WP, Turner HC, Huebner RJ (1965) Lymphocytic choriomeningitis virus in hamster tumor: spread to hamsters and humans. Science 150: 363-364

Lehmann-Grube F (1971) Lymphocytic choriomeningitis virus. Springer, Berlin Heidelberg New York, pp 3-173 (Virology monographs, vol 10)

Lillie RD, Armstrong C (1945) Pathology of lymphocytic choriomeningitis in mice. Arch Pathol 40: 141-152

Mims CA (1966) Immunofluorescence study of the carrier state and mechanism of vertical transmission in lymphocytic choriomeningitis virus infection in mice. J Pathol Bacteriol 91: 395-402

Oldstone MBA (1984) Virus-induced immune complex formation and disease: definition, regulation, importance. In: Notkins AL, Oldstone MBA (eds) Concepts in viral pathogenesis. Springer, Berlin Heidelberg New York, pp 201-209

Oldstone MBA, Dixon FJ (1970) Pathogenesis of chronic disease associated with persistent lymphocytic choriomeningitis viral infection. II. Relationship to tissue injury in chronic lymphocytic choriomeningitis disease. J Exp Med 131: 1-19

Oldstone MBA, Sinha YN, Blount P, Tishon A, Rodriguez M, von Wedel R, Lampert PW (1982) Virus-induced alterations in homeostasis: alterations in differentiated functions of infected cells in vivo. Science 218: 1125-1127

Parker JC (1986) Lymphocytic choriomeningitis virus. In: Allen AM, Norjouri T (eds) Manual of microbiologic monitoring of laboratory animals. US Dept of Health and Human Services, Public Health Service, NIH, pp IC-1-IC-5

Parker JC, Igel HJ, Reynolds RK, Lewis AM, Rowe WP (1976) Lymphocytic choriomeningitis virus infection in fetal, newborn and young adult Syrian hamsters (Mesocricetus auratus). Infect Immun 13: 967-981

Rivers TM, Scott TFM (1936) Meningitis in man caused by a filterable virus. II. Identification of the etiological agent. J Exp Med 63: 415-432

Rodriguez M, Buchmeier MJ, Oldstone MBA, Lampert PW (1983) Ultrastructural localization of viral antigens in the CNS of mice persistently infected with lymphocytic choriomeningitis virus (LCMV). Am J Pathol 110: 95-100

Rowe WP (1956) Protective effect of pre-irradiation on lymphocytic choriomeningitis infection in mice. Proc Soc Exp Biol Med 92: 194-198

Rowe WP, Black PH, Levey RH (1963) Protective effect of neonatal thymectomy on mouse LCM infection. Proc Soc Exp Biol Med 114: 248-251

Scott TFM, Rivers TM (1936) Meningitis in man caused by a filterable virus. I. Two cases and the method of obtaining a virus from their spinal fluids. J Exp Med 63: 397-414

Smadel JE, Wall MJ (1942) Lymphocytic choriomeningitis in the Syrian hamster. J Exp Med 75: 581-591

Tosolini FA, Mims CA (1971) Effect of murine strain and viral strain on the pathogenesis of lymphocytic choriomeningitis infection and a study of footpad responses. J Infect Dis 123: 134-144

Traub E (1936a) An epidemic in a mouse colony due to the virus of acute lymphocytic choriomeningitis. J Exp Med 63: 533-546

Traub E (1936b) The epidemiology of lymphocytic choriomeningitis in white mice. J Exp Med 64: 183-200

Traub E (1939) Epidemiology of lymphocytic choriomeningitis in a mouse stock observed for four years. J Exp Med 69: 801-817

van der Zeijst BAM, Noyes BE, Mirault M-E, Parker B, Osterhaus AD, Swyryd EA, Bleumink N, Horzinek MC, Stark GR (1983) Persistent infection of some standard cell lines by lymphocytic choriomeningitis virus: transmission of infection by an intracellular agent. J Virol 48: 249-261

Walker DH, Murphy FA, Whitfield SG, Bauer SP (1975) Lymphocytic choriomeningitis: ultrastructural pathology. Exp Mol Pathol 23: 245-265

Wilsnack RE, Rowe WP (1964) Immunofluorescent studies of the histopathogenesis of lymphocytic choriomeningitis virus infection. J Exp Med 120: 829-840

Zinkernagel RM, Doherty PC (1973) Cytotoxic thymus-derived lymphocytes in cerebrospinal fluid of mice with lymphocytic choriomeningitis. J Exp Med 138: 1266-1269

Encephalitozoonosis, Central Nervous System, Rat, Mouse

Karen S. Regan and John A. Shadduck

Synonyms. Nosematosis *(Nosema cuniculi)*

Gross Appearance

Gross lesions are not evident in the central nervous system in encephalitozoonosis.

Microscopic Features

The number, size, and histologic appearance of lesions in the central nervous system of mice vary with the strain of mouse. In euthymic mice the lesions consist of multiple small granulomata and/or multiple glial aggregates throughout the brain and spinal cord. The granulomata contain lymphocytes and mononuclear cells and may have a central area of necrosis (Fig. 215). Astrocytic hypertrophy is evident at the periphery of the lesions. Collections of small macrophages and lymphocytes occur in Virchow-Robin spaces of vessels in areas adjacent to the glial nodules, and foci of inflammatory cells frequently accumulate in the meninges near cortical lesions. The inflammatory foci are seen with equal frequency in the gray and white matter and are most often adjacent to blood vessels. Organisms can be found free or within glial cells in and around the inflammatory foci; they are also present in parasitophorous vacuoles in the neuropil without an accompanying inflammatory reaction (Fig. 216). It is the latter which can be easily missed without diligent search and the use of appropriate diagnostic techniques.

The spores of *Encephalitozoon cuniculi* measure 1.5×2.5 μm and are gram-positive, slightly curved rods with rounded ends. They are difficult to detect with routine hematoxylin and eosin stains, as is illustrated in Fig. 217. The organisms are best revealed with Gram's stain or its Brown-Brenn modification, but also stain satisfactorily with Giemsa's stain or carbolfuchsin (Attwood and Sutton 1965). Some immature forms of the parasite within the vacuoles will stain gram-negatively. Periodic acid Schiff reaction or silver impregnation do not reveal a cyst wall.

The organism does not appear to have a specific site of predilection in the brain, although some authors report an increased frequency of menin-

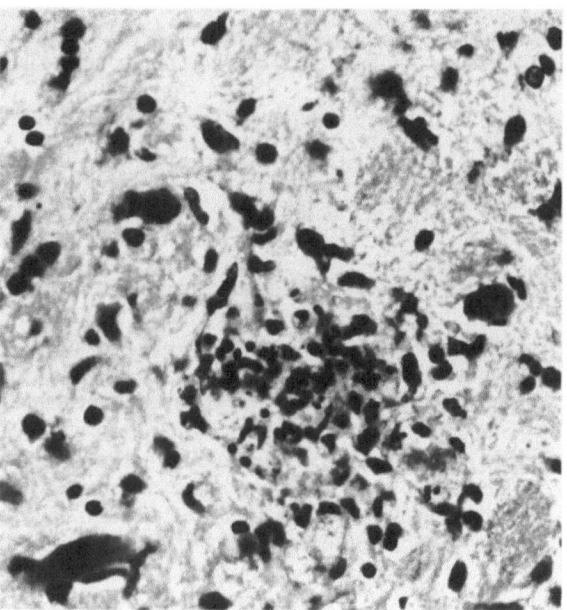

Fig. 215. Brain, mouse infected 33 days earlier with *E. cuniculi.* Subcortical glial nodule with central necrosis. Parasites are not seen in this section. H and E, × 450

geal lesions near the base of the brain and in the interhemispheric and hippocampal fissures of the cerebrum (Jortner and Percy 1978).

The disease in athymic mice follows a different course than in their euthymic counterparts and this is reflected in the histologic appearance of the lesions. Groups of parasites are situated throughout the brain and spinal cord and are usually not accompanied by an inflammatory response (Fig. 216). However, small foci of suppuration in the neuropil and meninges sometimes accompany the parasite foci (Fig. 218). Occasional glial nodules may have necrotic centers; parasites can frequently be identified at the periphery of these lesions.

Lesions of encephalitozoonosis in the rat are similar to those in euthymic mice, but, as reported by Attwood and Sutton (1965) and Majeed and Zubaidy (1982), are typically granulomatous and can contain epithelioid macrophages. Giant cells have been reported in some lesions.

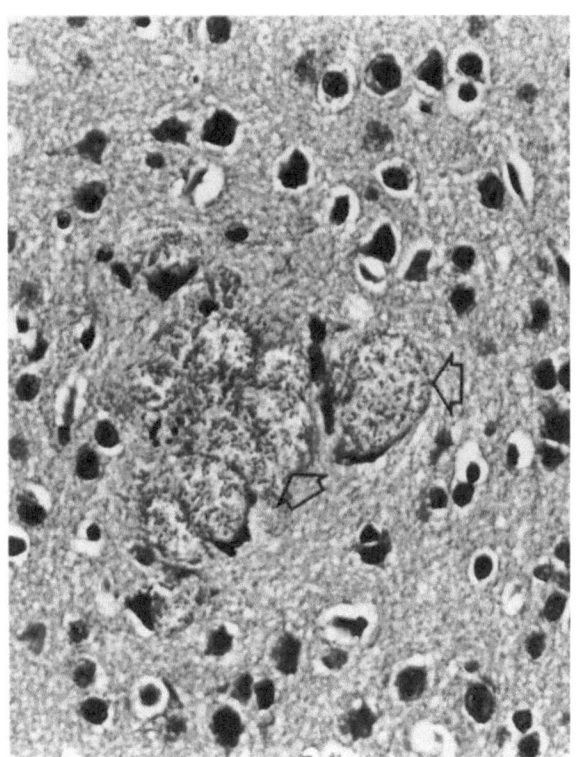

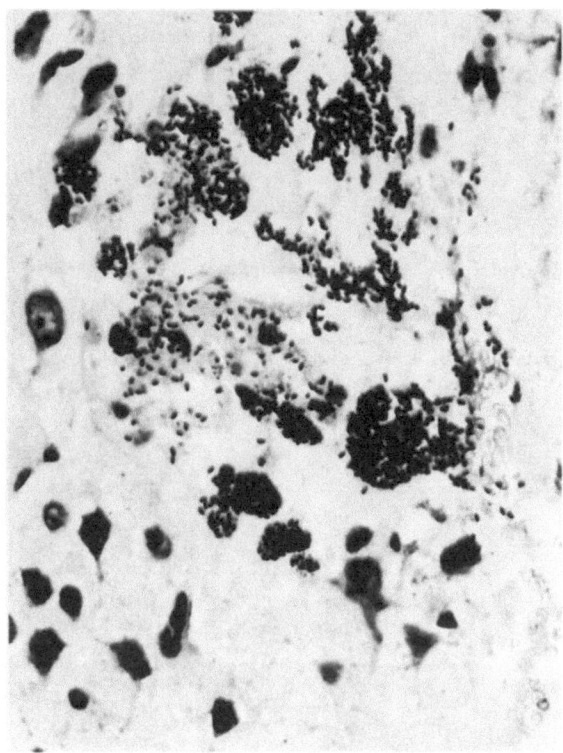

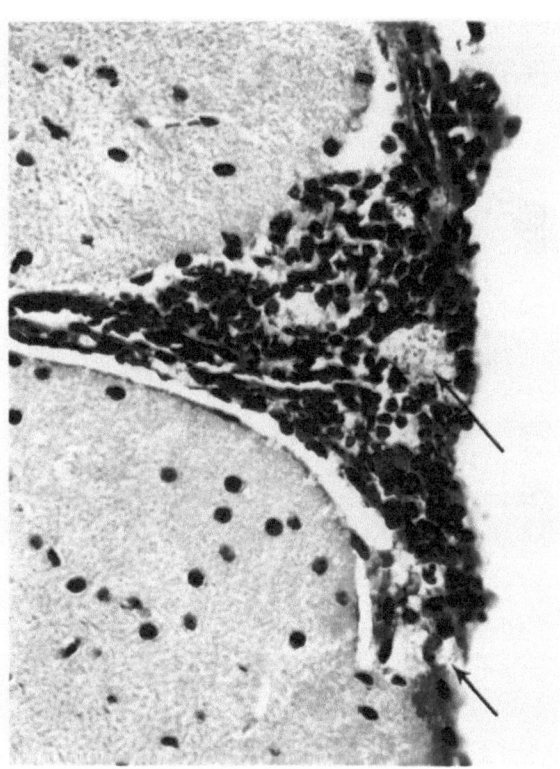

Fig. 216 *(upper left).* Brain, nude mouse infected 35 days earlier with *E. cuniculi.* Multiple parasitophorous "vacuoles" *(arrows)* within the cortical gray matter. The parasitophorous "vacuoles" are sharply delimited, but do not have a distinct wall, and the organisms, although numerous, do not stain well with hematoxylin and eosin and are difficult to visualize. Note absence of inflammation. H and E, × 400

Fig. 217 *(upper right).* Brain, nude mouse. Cortical gray matter with numerous *E. cuniculi* organisms. The parasites stain strongly gram positive. Compare with Fig. 216. Brown and Brenn, × 400

Fig. 218 *(lower right).* Brain, athymic, nude, mouse on postinfection day 23. Suppurative cerebellar meningitis with *E. cuniculi* in parasitophorous "vacuoles" *(arrows).* H and E, × 400

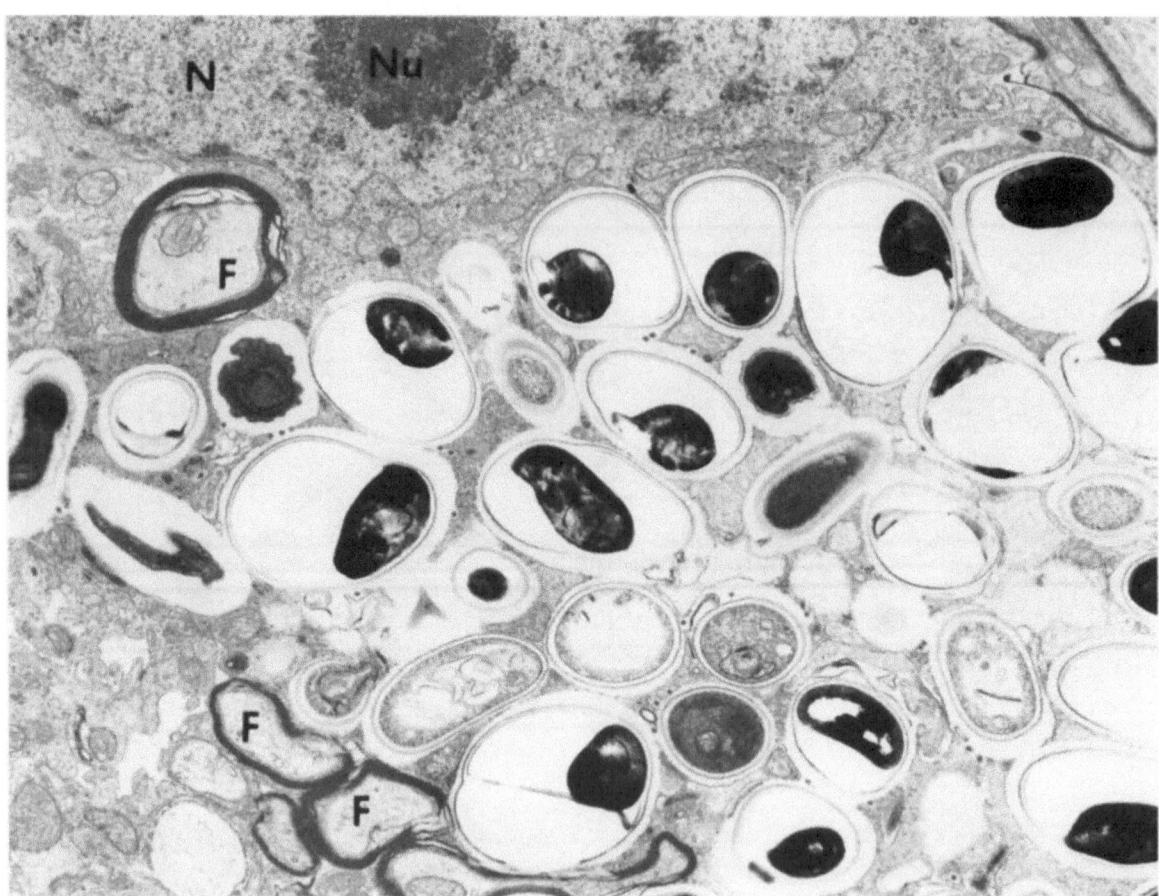

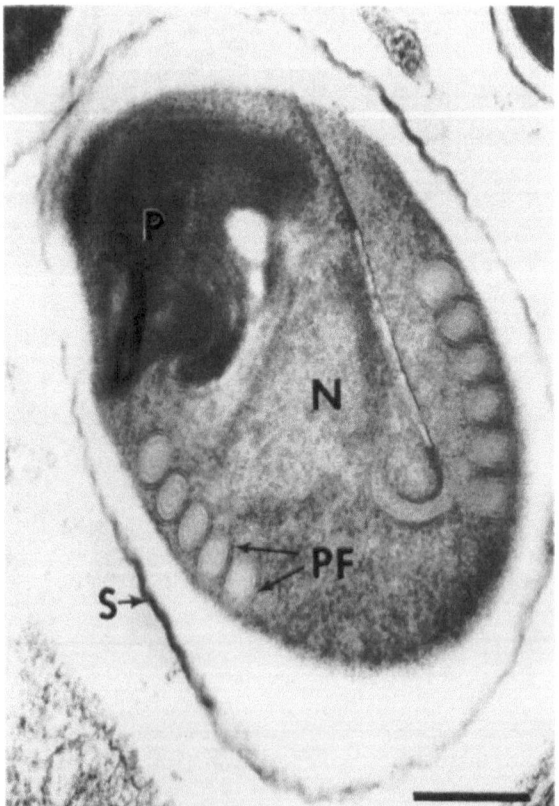

Fig. 219 *(above)*. *E. cuniculi* in the cerebral white matter of an athymic mouse. Multiple organisms in various stages of maturation are present. The large space around and within many of the spores is shrinkage artifact. The limits of the vacuole are not distinct. *N*, host cell nucleus; *Nu*, host cell nucleolus; *F*, host myelinated nerve fibers. TEM, ×15750

Fig. 220 *(below)*. Mature *E. cuniculi* spore with five to six coils of the polar filament *(PF)*. *P*, polar plast; *N*, nucleus; *S*, spore wall. *Bar* = .25 mm. TEM, ×65500

Ultrastructure

The ultrastructure of the developmental and spore stages of *E. cuniculi* has been described (Pakes et al. 1975) and has been well summarized by Canning et al. (1986). The ultrastructural characteristics of *E. cuniculi* are useful in separating this parasite from other protozoan parasites which may occur in the vertebrate central nervous system. Characteristics common to the Microsporidia include the presence of a coiled polar filament and the lack of mitochondria. Specific features of spores of *E. cuniculi* which can be used to differentiate them from other Microsporidia include: the presence of a thick endospore, a corrugated exospore, a single nucleus, a posterior vacuole, and a polar filament containing 4.5 to 5 coils (Figs. 219 and 220).

Biologic Features

Natural History. *E. cuniculi* is an obligate intracellular protozoan parasite. Spontaneous cases of encephalitozoonosis have been reported in many species of wild and domestic rodents, carnivores, nonhuman primates, and man. In laboratory animals, it is most frequently a chronic, latent disease, and lesions are only discovered incidentally (Perrin 1943). Natural transmission of the parasite is thought to occur both horizontally and vertically. In most species, the parasite invades the renal tubular epithelial cells and subsequently escapes into the tubular lumena when the host cell degenerates. The spores can then be passed in the urine, where they can be detected by direct examination of the urine sediment (Goodman and Garner 1972). Urine contamination of the environment provides a source of spores which can be ingested by another host. Carnivorous species can also acquire the infection by eating animals infected with *E. cuniculi*. Cannibalism is also thought to be a source of infection. Transplacental transmission has been postulated and evidence for it has been presented in blue foxes (Mohn et al. 1982), rabbits (Hunt et al. 1972), and mice (Innes et al. 1962). Because of the subclinical nature of the disease in rodents and the multiplicity of routes of transmission, infection in a colony can persist.

Pathogenesis. Many of the details of the life cycle of *E. cuniculi* have been extensively reviewed by Canning et al. (1986). Spores of the the parasite are ingested by the host, but the route by which they are disseminated within the host is unclear. The parasite may penetrate a host epithelial cell and begin replication prior to dissemination (Lainson et al. 1964). Alternatively, the parasite may first enter or be taken up by host macrophages and be transported throughout the host tissues via the lymph and eventually the blood (Cox et al. 1979). Spores may also directly penetrate the host intestinal wall and directly enter the vascular system (Gannon 1980). The presence of many lesions in highly vascular organs (liver, lungs, kidney) and the frequency of lesions found perivascularly suggest that a parasitemia does occur at some time during the course of infection.

The spores may enter the host cell by an active process or may be phagocytized and taken up into a membrane-bound vesicle. The spore is capable of actively penetrating a cell by forceful extrusion of the polar filament through the membrane of the host cell. This process does not disrupt the integrity of the membrane (Canning et al. 1986). The infective sporoplasm is then transferred into the cell via the polar filament (Kramer 1960) and begins replicating inside a parasitophorous vacuole. The vacuole is bound by a limiting membrane of presumed host origin (Weidner 1975). Within this vacuole the parasite first develops into meronts which replicate by binary fission. Meronts develop into sporonts and then into sporoblasts. As the sporoblasts go through the final stages of development into a spore, they accumulate in the center of the ever-expanding vacuole. The host cell eventually degenerates and ruptures, releasing the spores and allowing them to spread to adjacent cells.

Etiology. "Encephalitozoon cuniculi" is the name originally given to the organism by Levaditi, Nicolau, and Schoen in 1923. They described the organism as being a Microsporidia present in the kidneys and brains of rabbits, and reproduced the disease in mice and other species. Subsequently, the organism was reported by other authors in numerous other animals, including man. In many of these reports the parasite was not precisely identified, and different species names and occasionally genus names were assigned to the same parasite. Thus *E. rabei* (Manouelian and Viala 1924), *E. negrii* (Manouelian and Viala 1927), *E. muris* (Garnham and Roe 1954), *Glugea rabei* (Levaditi et al. 1926), and *G. lyssae* (Levaditi et al. 1924) are all considered by Canning et al. (1986) to be *E. cuniculi*.

In 1964, the genus name of the parasite was changed to *Nosema* (Lainson et al. 1964) based on morphologic criteria. This gave rise to the name "nosematosis" for the disease entity in mammals which we today know as "encephalitozoonosis." Differences between the genera *Nosema* and *Encephalitozoon* were subsequently determined (Cali 1971), and the organism was reassigned to the genus *Encephalitozoon*.

Frequency. Because encephalitozoonosis is a subclinical and latent disease in many of the animal species in which it occurs, recognition of the presence of the disease in a colony has been difficult. Reports of the frequency of the disease were based on the histologic lesions and demonstration of the parasite in tissue sections. Since these studies are infrequent, so also are accurate reports on the incidence of the disease. Existing literature reports disease prevalence ranging from 20% to 50% in mice and rats (Attwood and Sutton 1965; Innes et al. 1962; Lainson 1954).

Recently, there has been an increasing awareness on the part of laboratory workers, researchers, and veterinarians of diseases which can affect the quality or confuse the results of in vivo or in vitro experiments. With the development of reliable serologic tests for the detection of antibody to *E. cuniculi*, infected animals can be detected prior to the start of a research project. These screening tests allow a more accurate assessment of the frequency of encephalitozoonosis in laboratory colonies. Several recent serologic surveys of mouse colonies disclosed them all to be free of antibodies to *E. cuniculi*, suggesting that well-managed colonies can be maintained free of this parasite.

Comparison with Other Species

Infection with *E. cuniculi* is similar in rodents and lagomorphs, with the exception that rabbits occasionally develop clinical signs of the disease, whereas mice and rats rarely do. Lesions in rabbits are most similar to those in rats, since they typically have more granulomata in the central nervous system than mice. Encephalitozoonosis in carnivores, however, is a clinical disease of the neonate in which the host demonstrates severe nervous signs (Shadduck et al. 1978; van Dellen et al. 1978; Nordstoga and Westbye 1976). Histologically, the lesions in the central nervous system of carnivores consist of multifocal microgranulomas and a granulomatous vasculitis which can resemble polyarteritis nodosa.

Attempts have been made in several reports to link *E. cuniculi* to cases of human encephalitis. In most cases in these reports the causative organism has been subsequently determined not to be *E. cuniculi*, but in two such cases (Matsubayashi et al. 1959; Bergquist et al. 1984) the presence of *E. cuniculi* was confirmed. In both of these, the patients were children who exhibited neurologic disturbances and subsequently recovered. Antibodies to *E. cuniculi* have been demonstrated in select groups of people (Bergquist et al. 1985; Singh et al. 1982), but whether these results are indicative of exposure to and/or infection with *E. cuniculi* or represent cross reactions with other microsporidian parasites is unclear.

References

Attwood HD, Sutton RD (1965) Encephalitozoon granulomata in rats. J Pathol Bacteriol 89: 735–738

Bergquist NR, Stintzing G, Smedman L, Waller T, Andersson T (1984) Diagnosis of encephalitozoonosis in man by serological tests. Br Med J [Clin Res] 288: 902

Bergquist R, Morfeldt-Manson L, Pehrson PO, Petrini B, Wasserman J (1984) Antibody against *Encephalitozoon cuniculi* in Swedish homosexual men. Scand J Infect Dis 16: 389–391

Cali A (1971) Morphogenesis in the genus *Nosema*. Proc IVth Int Coll Insect Pathol, Maryland 1970, pp 431–438

Canning EU, Lom J, Dykova I (1986) The Microsporidia of birds and mammals. In: Canning EU, Lom J (eds) The Microsporidia of vertebrates. Academic, Orlando, pp 189–238

Cox JC, Pye D (1975) Serodiagnosis of nosematosis by immunofluorescence using cell culture grown organisms. Lab Anim 9: 297–304

Cox JC, Hamilton RC, Attwood HD (1979) An investigation of the route and progression of *Encephalitozoon cuniculi* infection in adult rabbits. J Protozool 26: 260–265

Gannon J (1980) The course of infection of *Encephalitozoon cuniculi* in immunodeficient and immunocompetent mice. Lab Anim 14: 189–192

Goodman DG, Garner FM (1972) A comparison of methods for detecting *Nosema cuniculi* in rabbit urine. Lab Anim Sci 22: 568–572

Hunt RD, King NW, Foster HL (1972) Encephalitozoonosis: evidence for vertical transmission. J Infect Dis 126: 212–214

Innes JRM, Zeman W, Frenkel JK, Borner G (1962) Occult, endemic encephalitozoonosis of the central nervous system of mice (Swiss Bagg-O'Grady strain). J Neuropathol Exp Neurol 21: 519–533

Jortner BS, Percy DH (1978) The nervous system. In: Benirschke K, Garner FM, Jones TC (eds) Pathology of laboratory animals. Springer, Berlin Heidelberg New York, pp 319–442

Kramer JP (1960) Observations on the emergence of the microsporidian sporoplasm. J Insect Pathol 2: 433–439

Lainson R (1954) Natural infection of *Encephalitozoon* in the brain of laboratory rats. Trans R Soc Trop Med Hyg 48: 51

Lainson R, Garnham PCC, Killick-Kendrick R, Bird RG (1964) Nosematosis, a microsporidial infection of rodents and other animals, including man. Br Med J 2: 470–472

Levaditi C, Nicolau S, Schoen R (1923) L'étiologie de l'encephalite épizootique du lapin dans ses rapports avec l'étude experimentale de encephalite léthargique du *Encephalitozoon cuniculi* (nov.spec.). C R Soc Biol (Paris) 177: 985

Majeed SK, Zubaidy AJ (1982) Histopathological lesions associated with *Encephalitozoon cuniculi* (nosematosis) infection in a colony of Wistar rats. Lab Anim 16: 244–247

Matsubayashi H, Koike T, Mikata T, Hagiwara S (1959) A case of *Encephalitozoon*-like body infection in man. AMA Arch Pathol 67: 181–187

Mohn SF, Nordstoga K, Moller OM (1982) Experimental encephalitozoonosis in the blue fox. Transplacental transmission of the parasite. Acta Vet Scand 23: 211–220

Nordstoga K, Westbye K (1976) Polyarteritis nodosa associated with nosematosis in blue foxes. Acta Pathol Microbiol Scand [A] 84: 291–296

Pakes SP, Shadduck JA, Cali A (1975) Fine structure of *Encephalitozoon cuniculi* from rabbits, mice and hamsters. J Protozool 22: 481–488

Perrin TL (1943) Spontaneous and experimental *Encephalitozoon* infection in laboratory animals. Arch Pathol 36: 559–567

Shadduck JA, Benedele R, Robinson GT (1978) Isolation of the causative organism of canine encephalitozoonosis. Vet Pathol 15: 449–460

Singh M, Kane GJ, Mackinlay L, Quaki I, Yap EH, Ho BC, Ho LC, Lim KC (1982) Detection of antibodies to *Nosema cuniculi* (Protozoa: Microsporidia) in human and animal sera by the indirect fluorescent antibody technique. Southeast Asian J Trop Med Public Health 13: 110–113

van Dellen AF, Botha WS, Boomker J, Warnes WEJ (1978) Light and electron microscopical studies on canine encephalitozoonosis: cerebral vasculitis. Onderstepoort J Vet Res 45: 165–186

Weidner E (1975) Interaction between *Encephalitozoon cuniculi* and macrophages. Parasitophorous vacuole growth and the absence of lysosomal fusion. Z Parasitenkd 47: 1–9

Toxoplasmosis, Nervous System, Mouse and Hamster

Karen S. Regan and John A. Shadduck

Gross Appearance

The gross appearance of the brain and spinal cord in acute or chronic toxoplasmosis is frequently normal. Occasionally, small foci of hemorrhage and/or malacia may be present in any area (Koestner and Cole 1960; Innes and Saunders 1962).

Microscopic Features

The histologic appearance of paraffin-embedded sections of brain and spinal cord from infected mice and hamsters varies with the stage and route of the infection, the parasite strain and dose, and the immunologic state of the host (Dubey and Frenkel 1973; Fernando 1982). In acute infection, merozoites (tachyzoites) may rarely be found within neurons, astrocytes, or glial cells or free in the neuropil. These parasitic forms are arcuate and measure $5-8 \times 1-2$ μm; they can be visualized best in Giemsa-stained sections. Frequently, organisms are absent or sparse, necessitating serial sectioning for visualization. Mild, scattered neuronal degeneration may be present and accompanied by a generalized increase in glial cells and the formation of glial nodules (Frenkel 1956; Ito and Tsunoda 1968). Mild focal lymphoplasmacytic perivascular encephalitis and meningitis may also be found (Kittas et al. 1984).

Lesions of chronic toxoplasmosis are by far the most common and develop as sequelae to acute infection. Multiple glial nodules, some with necrotic centers containing cyst remnants, are scattered throughout the brain and spinal cord (Fig. 221). Astrocytes at the periphery of the nodules are frequently hypertrophied (Frenkel 1956). Lymphocytic or lymphoplasmacytic infiltrates distend the subarachnoid space and the Virchow-Robin spaces of adjacent vessels. Fibrinoid necrosis of vessel walls may be seen in association with microthrombi in the centers of small necrot-

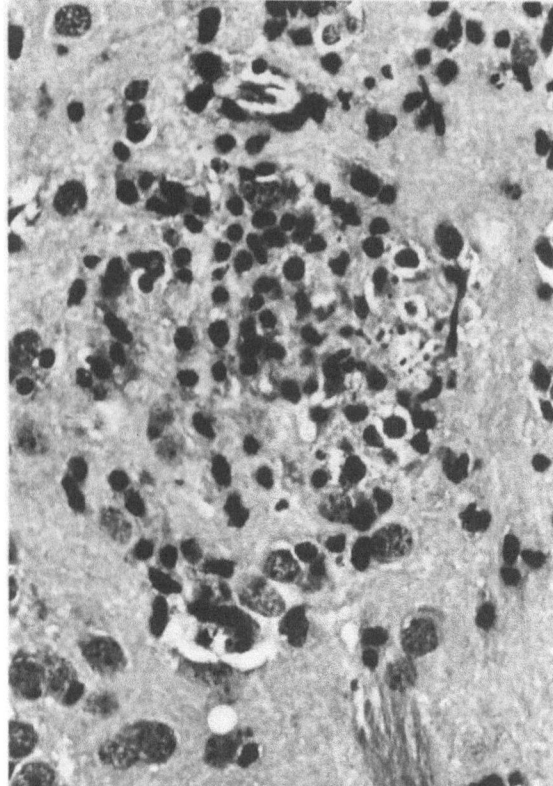

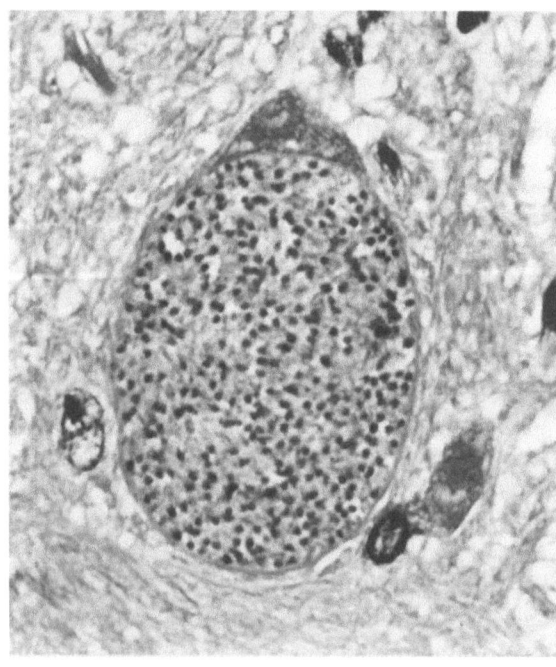

Fig. 221 *(above).* Glial nodule in the cerebral subcortical white matter from a hamster infected 30 days previously with *Toxoplasma gondii*. H and E, × 450

Fig. 222 *(below).* Intact *T. gondii* cyst in the subcortical white matter of a chronically infected mouse. The cyst has a prominent wall and is filled with bradyzoites. Note lack of inflammatory response in adjacent neuropil. H and E, × 950

ic foci (Frenkel 1956; Hay et al. 1985). Intact cysts of *Toxoplasma* merozoites (bradyzoites) can be found in the cytoplasm of cells at the periphery of the glial nodules and necrotic foci or in areas unassociated with an inflammatory response, as seen in Fig. 222 (Frenkel 1956; Uga et al. 1980). Lesions in athymic mice may completely lack inflammatory infiltrates and consist solely of small necrotic foci and scattered *Toxoplasma* cysts (Buxton 1980). The cysts have an argyrophilic, periodic acid Schiff-positive wall that is less than 1 μm thick (Fig. 223). Cysts vary in number and size with the host and the age of the lesion. Cysts in mice become larger with time (Uga et al. 1980), whereas cysts from similarly aged lesions will be larger in hamsters than in mice (Frenkel 1973). Merozoites within the cysts contain PAS-positive granules.

In murine hosts, many authors have described a predilection of the parasite for the gray matter and, more specifically, for the neocortex (Verma and Bowles 1967; Uga et al. 1980), the deep gray matter, and the brain stem (Sasaki et al. 1981; Hay et al. 1984). White matter and cerebellum are also involved, but contain fewer lesions and associated parasitic cysts.

Mice with congenital toxoplasmosis have similar histologic lesions to those with chronic acquired infection. In addition, lymphoplasmacytic infiltrates are frequently present in the stroma of the choroid plexus, and occasionally foci of dystrophic calcification are seen (Graham et al. 1984; Hay et al. 1985).

Ultrastructure

The ultrastructure of the merozoites and tissue cysts of *Toxoplasma* is useful to distinguish it from other protozoal organisms which can be found in the nervous system. *Toxoplasma* is a member of the phylum Apicomplexa; this includes organisms which at some stage possess an apical complex consisting of polar rings, rhoptries, micronemes, a conoid, and subpellicular microtubules (Levine 1982). Other cytoplasmic organelles include a nucleus, mitochondria, Golgi complex, endoplasmic reticulum, and ribosomes (Tichy and Peychl 1968) (Fig. 224). The parasite is enclosed in a pellicle which consists of three unit membranes. The cyst is limited by a single unit membrane which is highly folded and is directly adjacent to the host cell structures (Chobotar and Scholtyseck 1982) (Fig. 223). The cyst is not divided into compartments (Mehlhorn and Frenkel 1980).

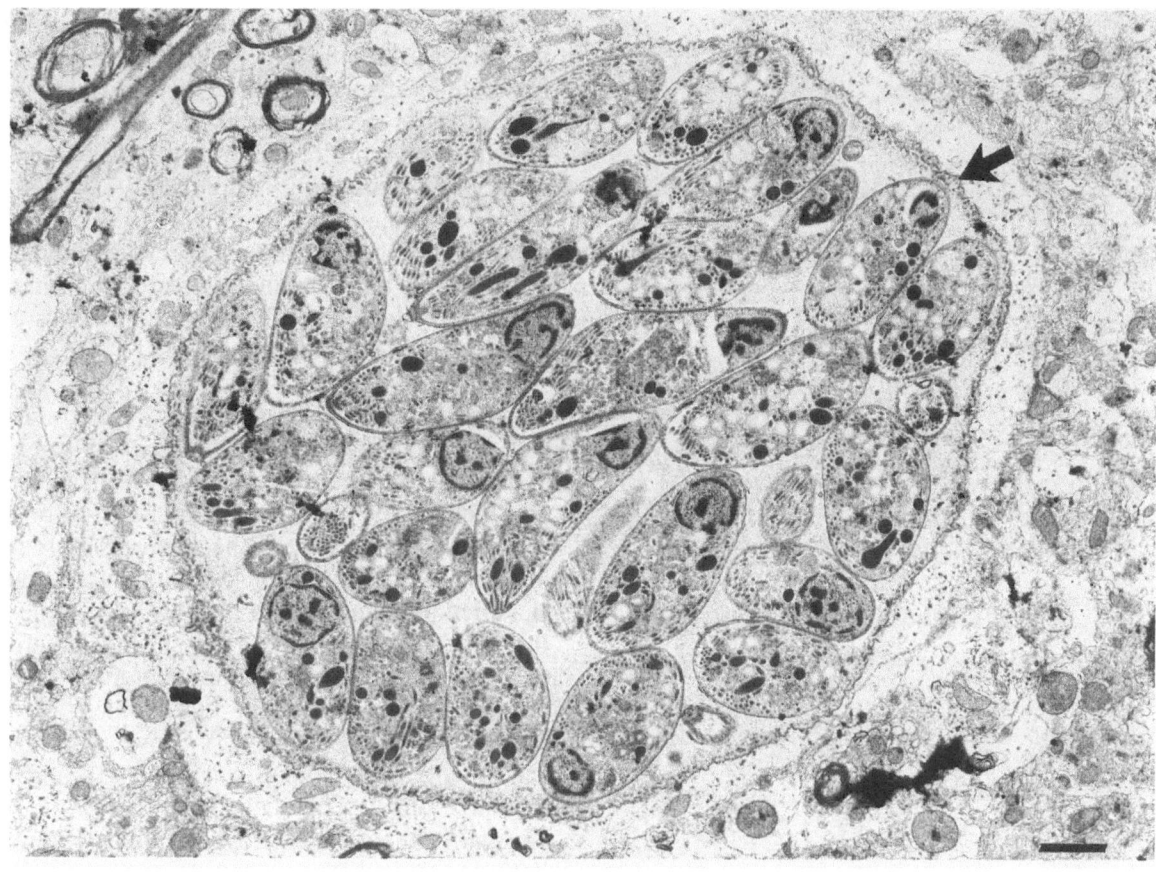

Fig. 223. Cyst containing multiple merozoites of *T. gondii* in the cerebrum of a chronically infected mouse. The cyst wall is prominent *(arrow)*. *Bar* = 1 mm. TEM, × 8830

Differential Diagnosis

Cysts of *Toxoplasma* must be differentiated from cysts and pseudocysts of other protozoa. *Frenkelia sp.* forms large multilobulated cysts in the brain and spinal cord of mice; these cysts contain two stages of the parasite, metrocytes and merozoites (Frenkel 1971, 1977). *Encephalitozoon cuniculi* can often be differentiated on tinctorial and morphological criteria. Spores of *Encephalitozoon* are slightly smaller (1.5–2.5 × 1–2 μm), have rounded ends, are gram positive, stain purple with carbolfuchsin, and lack an argyrophilic cyst wall. Ultrastructurally, *Encephalitozoon* lacks the apical complex found in *Toxoplasma* (Moller 1968). Amastigote stages of *Trypanosoma sp.* and *Leishmania sp.* are much smaller (1.5–4 μm diameter), have a kinetoplast, and stain with methylene blue. By electron microscopy, a kinetosome can be seen (Levine 1985).

Biologic Features

Natural history. *Toxoplasma gondii* was first discovered in a North African rodent by Nicolle and Manceaux in 1908. It has since been found to infect birds and most mammals including man, all common domestic species, many zoo and wild species, and most laboratory rodents. The modes of transmission and the life cycle of the parasite have been well characterized and have been presented in detail by Frenkel (1985). Members of the cat family are the only known definitive hosts, but nearly any species, including cats, can serve as intermediate hosts. In the definitive host the parasite undergoes an enteroepithelial life cycle which culminates in the formation of oocysts. The oocysts are passed unsporulated in the feces, sporulate in 1–21 days in the environment and are then infective for both definitive and intermediate hosts. Horizontal transmission occurs via ingestion of the oocysts in the environment or, in carnivores, by ingestion of tis-

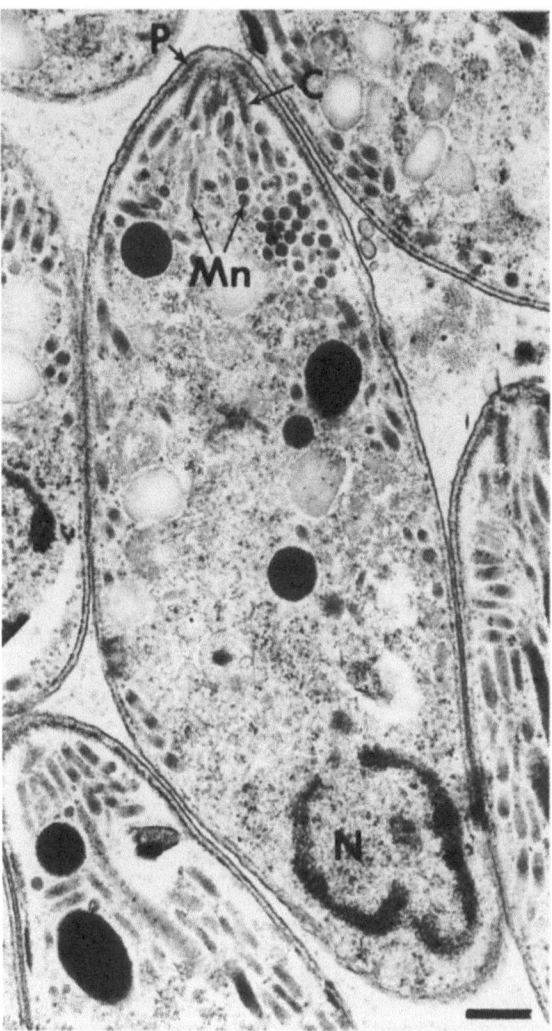

Fig. 224. Higher magnification of a *T. gondii* merozoite from Fig. 223, with nucleus *(N)* and some structures of the apical complex which can be used to distinguish this parasite from others not in the phylum Apicomplexa. *C,* conoid; *P,* polar ring; *Mn,* micronemes. *Bar* = .25 mm. TEM, × 36 000

sues of an infected host. Vertical transmission (in utero – mother to offspring) has been demonstrated in many species, including rodents, dogs, sheep, cattle, and man (Beverly 1959, 1973; Fernando 1982).

Pathogenesis. In the extraintestinal stages of the infection, the sporozoites released from the ingested oocysts or the bradyzoites released from the ingested cysts enter the lamina propria and mesenteric lymph nodes of the host and produce tachyzoites (Frenkel 1973). These forms multiply rapidly by endodyogeny within a host cell vacuole until the host cell disintegrates and the ta-

chyzoites are released. The organisms spread via the blood and lymph to multiple sites and can replicate in many types of host cells. The formation of cysts occurs within one to two weeks postinfection and coincides with the development of host immunity (Frenkel 1973). Within the intracellular cysts, the bradyzoites slowly multiply by endodyogeny. The cysts frequently do not evoke an inflammatory response from the host unless the cyst wall ruptures. The cysts can persist for the life of the host.

Etiology. Historically, *T. gondii* has been confused with *Leishmania* and *Encephalitozoon*. It was recognized as a human pathogen by Wolf, Cowen, and Paige in 1939 and was later shown to be serologically identical with the *Toxoplasma* found in animals (Frenkel 1973). The organism is now classified in the protozoan phylum Apicomplexa. It is classified with those organisms requiring two hosts, one for the development of the sexual stages and another for the development of the asexual stages (Levine 1985). However, as has been mentioned, Felidae can serve as both the definitive and intermediate host. *Toxoplasma* is unusual in that it lacks host specificity (Frenkel 1970; Henry and Beverley 1973).

Many naturally occurring strains of *Toxoplasma* have been isolated and most of these are of low virulence, as is indicated by the high prevalence of serum antibody titers in animals and man, but the low incidence of clinical disease (Koestner and Cole al. 1960; Jones 1973; Krick and Remington 1978; Turner 1978). Although most cases of toxoplasmosis are subclinical, primary infection or reactivation of a latent infection in an immunologically compromised host can be fatal. Reactivation of latent toxoplasmosis in hamsters by administration of cortisone and radiation has been demonstrated (Frenkel 1957). Likewise, the incidence of clinical toxoplasmosis in human patients with acquired immune deficiency syndrome is increasing (Sun et al. 1986).

Frequency. It has been estimated that approximately 50% of the human population of the United States are infected with the chronic asymptomatic form of toxoplasmosis (Krick and Remington 1978). Similarly, regional studies in animals report that 24%–50% of normal rabbits, 62% of cats, and 42% of dogs have antibodies to *Toxoplasma* (Shadduck und Pakes 1971). However, recent reports of spontaneous toxoplasmosis resulting in clinical illness and/or death in laboratory animals are sparse. The infection can persist undetected in animal colonies because of the subclinical nature of the disease and because of the potential for horizontal transmission via cannibalism and vertical transmission via the placenta. However, a number of serologic tests have been developed to detect subclinical carriers and lead to *Toxoplasma*-free colonies. In natural outbreaks of clinical disease in a laboratory facility, all sources of food, water, and bedding should be inspected for possible fecal contamination by cats. The oocysts withstand drying and remain infectious in food and bedding.

Comparison with Other Species

In most species including man, toxoplasmosis is a similar disease and can vary from a chronic inapparent infection to an acutely fatal one. Asymptomatic infections are the most common (Levine 1985). Aside from strain variations, other factors which may account for the prevalence of asymptomatic infections include the immune status of the host and host innate or genetic resistance to infection. Young animals with immature immune systems more frequently develop overt clinical disease than their adult counterparts (Frenkel 1970). Immunocompromised animals, such as those infected with known immunosuppressive agents or those receiving immunosuppressive therapy are also more likely to develop clinical disease.

In humans, congenital toxoplasmosis is a common form of the disease. The symptoms include encephalitis, intracranial calcification, hydrocephalus (Remington and Desmonts 1976), and retinochoroiditis, among others. A search for an animal model of congenital toxoplasmosis which displays all of the features of the human infection has so far been unsuccessful. In particular, one of the characteristic features of human congenital toxoplasmosis is periventricular and periaqueductal inflammation with subsequent obstruction of the aqueduct. The mouse models examined have subacute to chronic meningoencephalitis, but do not have the characteristic features of the human disease (Graham et al. 1984). The mouse model for human congenital ocular toxoplasmosis likewise displays similar but not identical histopathologic changes (Hay et al. 1984, 1985). Further development of this model may reveal more dissimilarities in pathogenesis than are currently thought to exist between species.

Acknowledgement. We gratefully acknowledge the generosity of J.K. Frenkel, who provided the mouse and hamster brains from which the light and electron micrographs were prepared.

References

Beverley JKA (1959) Congenital transmission of toxoplasmosis through successive generations of mice. Nature 183: 1348–1349
Beverley JKA (1973) Proceedings: vertical transmission of *Toxoplasma gondii.* J Med Microbiol 6: Pxxii
Buxton D (1980) Experimental infection of athymic mice with *Toxoplasma gondii.* J Med Microbiol 13: 307–311
Chobotar B, Scholtyseck E (1982) Ultrastructure. In: Long PL (ed) The biology of the coccidia. University Park Press, Baltimore, pp 101–165
Dubey JP, Frenkel JK (1973) Experimental *Toxoplasma* infection in mice with strains producing oocysts. J Parasitol 59 (3): 505–512
Fernando MA (1982) Pathology and pathogenicity. In: Long PL (ed) The biology of the coccidia. University Park Press, Baltimore, pp 287–327
Frenkel JK (1956) Pathogenesis of toxoplasmosis and of infections with organisms resembling *Toxoplasma.* Ann NY Acad Sci 64: 215–251
Frenkel JK (1957) Effects of cortisone, total body irradiation, and nitrogen mustard on chronic, latent toxoplasmosis. Am J Pathol 33: 618–619
Frenkel JK (1970) Pursuing *Toxoplasma.* J Infect Dis 122: 553–559
Frenkel JK (1971) Protozoal diseases of laboratory animals. In: Marcial-Rojas RA (ed) Pathology of protozoal and helminthic diseases with clinical correlations. Williams and Wilkins, Baltimore, pp 318–369
Frenkel JK (1973) Toxoplasmosis: parasite life cycle, pathology, and immunology. In: Hammond DM, Long PL (eds) The coccidia. *Eimeria, Isospora, Toxoplasma,* and related genera. University Park Press, Baltimore, pp 344–410
Frenkel JK (1977) *Besnoitia wallacei* of cats and rodents: with a reclassification of other cyst-forming isosporoid coccidia. J Parasitol 63: 611–628
Frenkel JK (1985) Toxoplasmosis, lung, mouse and hamster. In: Jones TC, Mohr U, Hunt RD (eds) Respiratory system. Springer, Berlin Heidelberg New York Tokyo, pp 227–230 (Monographs on pathology of laboratory animals)
Graham DI, Hay J, Hutchinson WM, Siim J Chr (1984) Encephalitis in mice with congenital ocular toxoplasmosis. J Pathol 142: 265–277
Hay J, Hair DM, Graham DI (1984) Localization of brain damage in mice following *Toxoplasma* infection. Ann Trop Med Parasitol 78 (6): 657–659
Hay J, Graham DI, Hutchison WM, Siim JC (1985) Meningoencephalitis accompanying retinochoroiditis in a murine model of congenital toxoplasmosis. Ann Trop Med Parasitol 79 (1): 21–29
Henry L, Beverley JK (1973) Proceedings: comparative pathology of toxoplasma infections. J Med Microbiol 6: XXI–XXII

Innes JRM, Saunders LZ (1962) Protozoan infections: toxoplasmosis. In: Innes JRM, Saunders LZ (eds) Comparative neuropathology. Academic, New York, pp 489–492

Ito S, Tsunoda K (1968) Distribution of *Toxoplasma gondii*, Beverley strain, in infected mice as determined by the fluorescent antibody technique and the histopathology of toxoplasmosis. Natl Inst Anim Health Q 8: 81–91

Jones SR (1973) Toxoplasmosis: a review. J Am Vet Med Assoc 163: 1038–1042

Kittas S, Kittas C, Paizi-Biza P, Henry L (1984) A histological and immunohistochemical study of the changes induced in the brains of white mice by infection with *Toxoplasma gondii*. Br J Exp Pathol 65: 67–74

Koestner A, Cole CR (1960) Neuropathology of canine toxoplasmosis. Am J Vet Res 21: 831–844

Krick JA, Remington JS (1978) Toxoplasmosis in the adult - an overview. N Engl J Med 298 (10): 550–553

Levine ND (1982) Taxonomy and life cycles of coccidia. In: Long PL (ed) The biology of the coccidia. University Park Press, Baltimore, pp 1–33

Levine ND (1985) Flagellates. The hemoflagellates. In: Veterinary protozoology. Iowa State University Press, Ames, pp 19–58

Mehlhorn H, Frenkel JK (1980) Ultrastructural comparison of cysts and zoites of *Toxoplasma gondii, Sarcocystis muris,* and *Hammondia hammondi* in skeletal muscle of mice. J Parasitol 66: 59–67

Moller T (1968) A survey on toxoplasmosis and encephalitozoonosis in laboratory animals. Z Versuchstierkd 10: 27–38

Nicolle C, Manceaux L (1908) Sur une infection à corps de Leishman (ou organismes voisins) du gondi. C R Acad Sci (D) (Paris) 147: 763–766

Remington JS, Desmonts G (1976) *Toxoplasmosis.* In: Remington JS, Klein JO (eds) Infectious diseases of the fetus and newborn infant. Saunders, Philadelphia, pp 191–332

Sasaki S, Miyagami T, Suzuki N (1981) Study on experimental toxoplasmic meningoencephalomyelitis. Its infectious route and lesions in CNS. Zentralbl Bakteriol Mikrobiol Hyg [A] 250: 167–172

Shadduck JA, Pakes SP (1971) Encephalitozoonosis (nosematosis) and toxoplasmosis. Am J Pathol 64: 657–674

Sun T, Greenspan J, Tenenbaum M, Farmer P, Jones T, Kaplan M, Peacock J (1986) Diagnosis of cerebral toxoplasmosis using fluorescein-labeled antitoxoplasma monoclonal antibodies. Am J Surg Pathol 10 (5): 312–316

Tichy J, Peychl L (1968) Electronmicroscopic findings in the spleen of mice in acute toxoplasmosis. Pathol Microbiol 31: 307–318

Turner GVS (1978) Some aspects of the pathogenesis and comparative pathology of toxoplasmosis. J S Afr Vet Assoc 49: 3–8

Uga S, Okada S, Matsumura T (1980) Proliferation of *Toxoplasma gondii* and its cyst-formation in mouse brains. Kobe J Med Sci 26: 253–267

Verma MP, Bowles L (1967) Concentration of *Toxoplasma gondii* in the brain tissue of animals: a histological study confirmed by biological isolations. J Parasitol 53: 254–257

Wolf A, Cowen D, Paige BH (1939) Toxoplasmic encephalitis. III. A new class of granulomatous encephalomyelitis due to a protozoon. Am J Pathol 15: 657–694

Spontaneous Radiculoneuropathy, Aged Rats

Georg J. Krinke

Synonyms. Spinal nerve root degeneration; spinal radiculoneuropathy; radicular myelinopathy; proximal demyelination; spontaneously occurring posterior paralysis.

Gross Appearance

In the advanced stage of this age-related disease, atrophy of the skeletal muscles is apparent in the lumbar region and the hindlimbs (Burek 1978). The vital fat stain Sudan III, administered orally 12 h before the autopsy, will demonstrate the focal accumulation of lipid within the spinal nerve roots as macroscopically discernible red patches (Krinke 1983).

Microscopic Features

In hematoxylin and eosin-stained paraffin sections the spinal nerve roots of aging rats are vacuolated; the lumbosacral roots are usually more affected than those in the thoracic or cervical re-

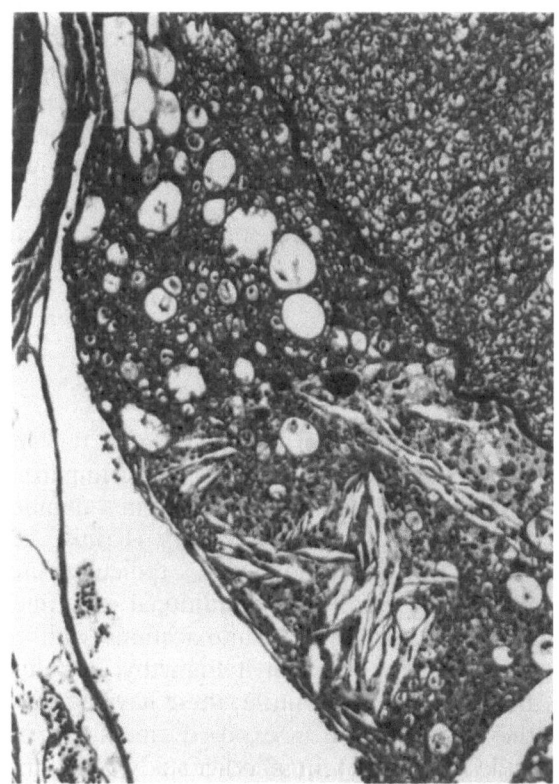

Fig. 225. Ventral spinal root, male rat, 26 months. Numerous round clear spaces and a focus of cholesterol clefts. H and E, × 150

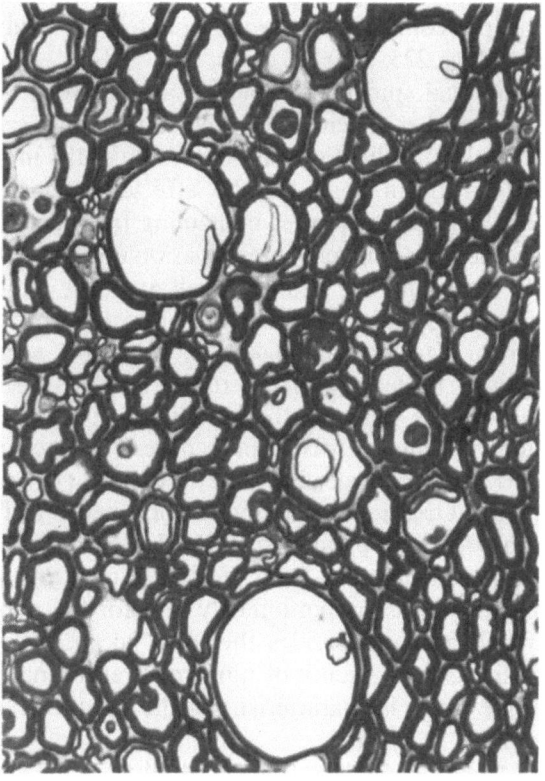

Fig. 226. Dorsal lumbar root, male rat, 16 months old. Several widely distended myelin sheaths encircle axons that are proportionately small for the sheath diameter. Epoxy resin, toluidine blue, × 600

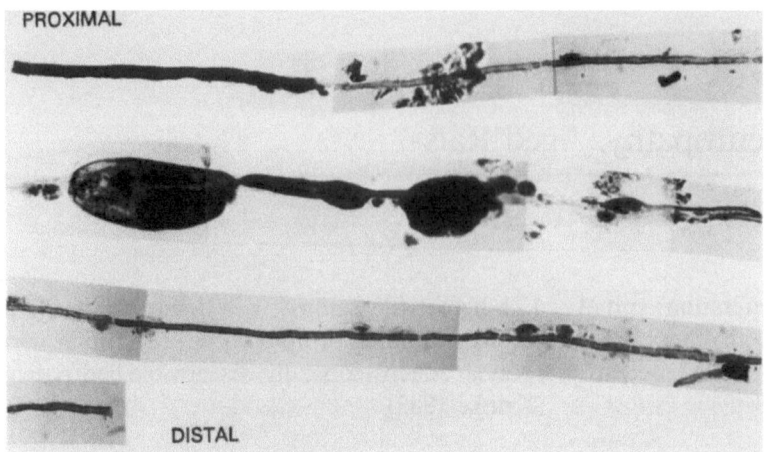

Fig. 227. Ventral lumbar root, male rat, 22 months old. Isolated, teased nerve fiber has a short proximal portion of normal myelin sheath. Distally, in the demyelinated fiber there are large fragments of distended sheath. Sudan black, glycerine, × 106

gions and the ventral more than the dorsal roots. On closer inspection, especially when using epoxy resin-embedded material sectioned at 1 µm, the vacuoles appear as distended myelin sheaths containing disproportionately small axons (Figs. 225, 226).

Individual spinal root fibers, examined with the "teased-fiber" technique, have undergone segmental demyelination with distention of the myelin sheath in some of the affected segments (Fig. 227). Macrophages containing fragments of disintegrating myelin are occasionally seen on the demyelinating axons as well as in the endoneurial space. Lipid material, released in the course of extensive breakdown of myelin, accumulates within the nerve roots; it forms focal thickenings visible in the bundles of spinal root fibers during the teasing procedure. The thickenings are birefringent in polarized light (Krinké 1983). Occasional rhomboid cholesterol clefts can be seen in paraffin sections (Fig. 225).

Each demyelinated axon receives a new myelin sheath that is proportionately thin for the axon diameter. Thus, besides the focal accumulation of lipid, the presence of numerous remyelinated nerve fibers is characteristic of the advanced lesion.

The presence of axonal degeneration in the spinal roots of aging rats has been reported (van Steenis and Kroes 1971; Gilmore 1972), but it is not the predominant change. Quantitative results demonstrate that no loss of spinal root axons occurs until a very advanced age (Krinke 1983).

Ultrastructure

The breakdown of myelin begins inside the distended portion of the sheath, where the myelin lamellae become separated from each other and turn into foamy material (Fig. 228). Macrophages remove the myelin debris while the axon persists within its endoneurial tube (Fig. 229). Schwann's cells cover the demyelinated axon and provide a new myelin wrapping (Fig. 230); the demyelination, however, is not preceded by structural changes in the Schwann's cells forming the affected sheaths.

Differential Diagnosis

The naturally occurring changes in the spinal nerve roots of aging rats are indistinguishable from the demyelination observed in a number of metabolic and toxic disorders (Krinke et al. 1981). Moreover, spontaneous radiculoneuropathy can be modified by additional experimental manipulations such as intoxications with compounds like acetylethyltetramethyl tetralin or B,B'-iminodipropionitrile; these have aggravated the demyelination in exposed animals (Spencer and Ochoa 1981). In an other study, X-ray irradiation of aging rats resulted in the excessive proliferation of Schwann's cells with the formation of concentric arrangements of supernumerary cells called "onion bulbs" (van der Kogel 1977).

Therefore, in experimental studies carried out on aging rats, such changes of spinal roots should be interpreted with great caution.

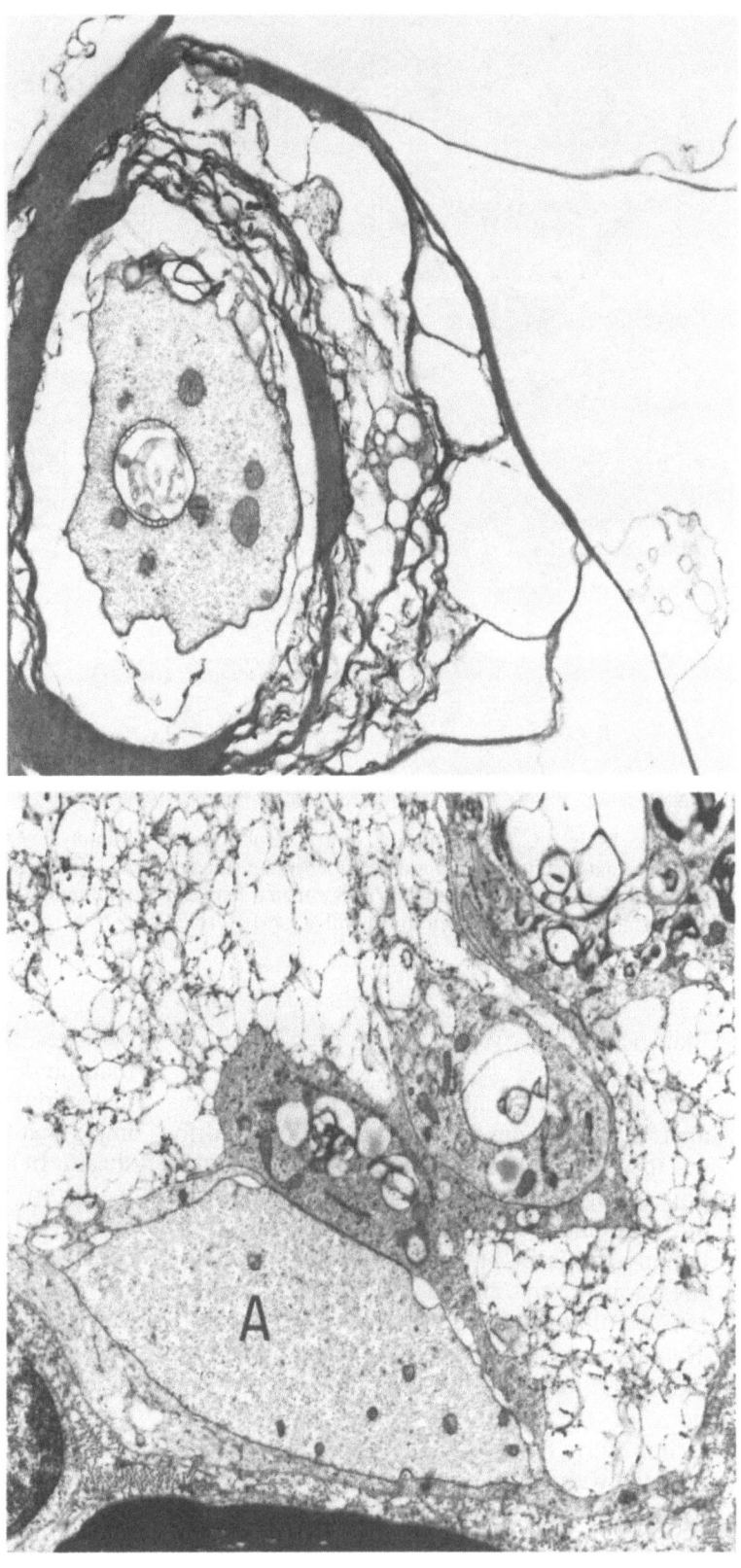

Fig. 228 *(above).* Dorsal lumbar root, male rat, 16 months old. Splitting and fine-vesicular degeneration of myelin sheath. Uranyl acetate and lead citrate, TEM, × 13 950

Fig. 229 *(below).* Dorsal lumbar root, male rat, 16 months old. Demyelinated axon *(A)* surrounded by macrophage processes engulfing the foamy debris. Uranyl acetate and lead citrate, TEM, × 10 230

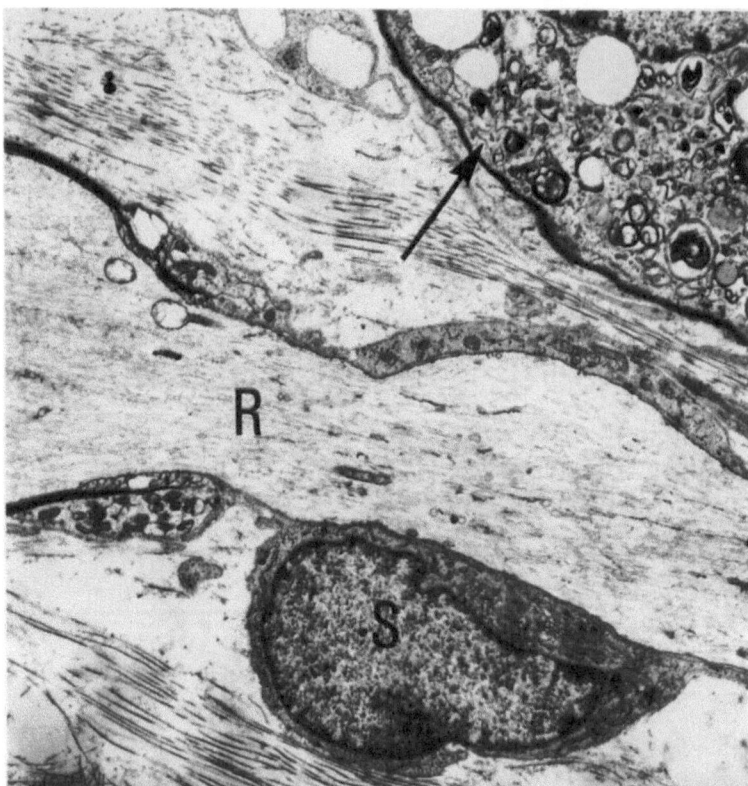

Fig. 230. Male rat, 27 months old, ventral lumbar root. Longitudinal section through a nerve fiber in the stage of remyelination. A node of Ranvier *(R)* is situated between two segments, one of them equipped with a newly formed thin myelin sheath, the other invested by a Schwann's cell *(S)*. The *arrow* points to an intramyelinic macrophage in another nerve fiber. Uranyl acetate and lead citrate, TEM, ×6600

Biologic Features

Natural History. Spontaneous changes in various areas of the nervous system of aging rats contribute to a complex neurologic syndrome. Distention of myelin sheaths with demyelination is most prominent in the ventral spinal roots at the lumbosacral level, but it is not restricted to these sites; spinal tracts and peripheral nerves are also affected although less severely.

The radioculoneuropathy is preceded by degeneration and loss of nerve fibers in the distal portions of the peripheral nerves (Spencer and Ochoa 1981; Krinke 1983). Nerve lesions are associated with changes in skeletal muscles, which are believed by some authors to represent neurogenic muscular atrophy (van Steenis and Kroes 1971; Burek 1978); other authors consider this myopathy to be independent of the neuropathy (Berg et al. 1962).

Pathogenesis. A characteristic feature of this lesion is the inverse relationship between the axon diameter and the myelin sheath distention, so that the thinnest axons appear inside the biggest distentions; this observation, however, does not imply that the axon is compressed by the swollen sheath. In healthy nerve fibers, the normal size of the axon is maintained by an intact myelin sheath; when the sheath is damaged the axon collapses, so that demyelinated (and remyelinated) nerve fibers are smaller than their original size (Raine 1982).

Distention of the myelin sheath of a kind similar to that observed in the spinal roots of aging rats occurs in experiments causing peripheral nerve lesions through crushing, transection, or compression. In such situations, some myelin segments proximal to the trauma accumulate fluid in the extracellular space formed by splitting of the sheath. This change, designated "myelin bubbling," is then followed by segmental demyelination (Spencer and Ochoa 1981). Since demyelination can occur with the formation of myelin bubbles as readily as without it, the bubbling may reflect a nonspecific disturbance in the selective permeability of the myelin-forming membrane.

Etiology. It is uncertain whether the demyelination of spinal roots in aged rats represents a primary myelin damage or whether it is a lesion secondary to other changes.

Axonal atrophy, resulting in an excessive disproportion between the size of the shrunken axon and its original myelin sheath, could account for the demyelination. There is quantitative evidence of axonal atrophy in the spinal roots of aging rats (Krinke 1983). Demyelination secondary to axonal has been reproduced in animal experiments employing nerve constriction or limb amputation, but myelin bubble formation was not noticed (Baba et al. 1982).

Despite the paucity of data on primary changes in the chemical structure or metabolism of myelin sheaths in aging rats, the possibility of such alterations should be considered. For instance, Uchida et al. (1986) have detected age-related changes in the composition of myelin proteins in the rat peripheral nerve. Such alterations could modify the physicochemical properties of myelin and facilitate demyelination.

Frequency. Solitary myelin bubbles occur in the rat spinal roots early in the 2nd year of life (Krinke 1983). A more severe lesion, called "radiculoneuropathy," is encountered from the end of the 2nd year onward.

The figures in Table 12 demonstrate the high susceptibility of several rat strains. In old animals the lesion becomes very frequent, to the extent that the number of affected individuals approaches 100%. A strain-related difference, at least in clinical signs, has been reported by Burek (1978). He observed a rather low susceptibility in the strains BN/Bi and WAG/Rij in comparison to the F1 rats (WAG × BN); clinical symptoms were more frequent in the male rats of the latter strain than in the females, despite the presence of radiculoneuropathy in both sexes.

According to Gilmore (1972), the lesions occur with equal frequency in both males and females. Similarly, Berg et al. (1962) have considered the frequency to be about equal in both sexes, although their figures indicate a slightly higher frequency in males (Table 12). Neuropathy was found to be more severe in males than in females by van Steenis and Kroes (1971). Taken in concert, the findings suggest that males may be more susceptible.

Table 12. Frequency of spontaneous radiculoneuropathy in different strains of aging rats

Strain	Age	Frequency[a] (%)	Reference
Sprague-Dawley			Berg et al. (1962)
Males	500– 699 days	28	
	700– 899 days	85	
	900–1100 days	100	
Females	600– 699 days	0	
	700– 899 days	82	
	900–1099 days	97	
	1100–1300 days	86	
Wistar	34 months	100	van Steenis and Kroes (1971)
Charles River	18 months	0	Gilmore (1972)
	18–20 months	67	
	>20 months	96	
(WAG × BN)F$_1$	6 months	0	Burek (1978)
	12 months	0	
	18 months	0	
	22 months	100	

[a] For the sake of simplicity the data originally available as absolute figures or fractions of percent are given as rounded percentage figures.

Behavioral Observations. Posterior paralysis (or severe paraparesis), loss of control of the tail, urinary incontinence, and atrophy of the skeletal muscles in the lumbar region and hindlimbs are present in some but not all of the rats afflicted by severe radiculoneuropathy. In this syndrome, the spinal root lesion may be only a contributory factor together with other changes in the spinal cord, peripheral nerves, and musculoskeletal system (Burek 1978).

Comparison with Other Species

The spinal nerve roots of old individuals have not been examined systematically in different species. Age-related segmental demyelination occurs in the dog (Griffiths and Duncan 1975) and the hamster (Spencer and Ochoa 1981). "Myelin bubbling" and demyelination are present in the ventral lumbosacral roots of old mice, but are less severe than in the rat (Krinke, unpublished observation). Focal demyelination of the spinal roots in humans suffering from chronic intervertebral disk degeneration (spondylosis) has been attributed to mechanical compression of the nerve fibers and restriction of the arterial blood supply rather than to old age (Bradley 1975).

References

Baba M, Fowler CJ, Jacobs JM, Gilliatt RW (1982) Changes in peripheral nerve fibers distal to a constriction. J Neurol Sci 54: 197–208

Berg BN, Wolf A, Simms HS (1962) Degenerative lesions of spinal roots and peripheral nerves in aging rats. Gerontology 6: 72–80

Bradley WG (1975) Diseases of the spinal roots. In: Dyck PJ, Thomas PK, Lambert EH (eds) Peripheral neuropathy, vol I. Saunders, Philadelphia, pp 645–658

Burek JD (1978) Pathology of aging rats. CRC, West Palm Beach, pp 153–160, 191–197

Gilmore SA (1972) Spinal nerve root degeneration in aging laboratory rats: a light microscopic study. Anat Rec 174: 251–257

Griffiths IR, Duncan ID (1975) Age changes in the dorsal and ventral lumbar nerve roots of dogs. Acta Neuropathol (Berl) 32: 75–85

Krinke G (1983) Spinal radiculoneuropathy in aging rats: demyelination secondary to neuronal dwindling? Acta Neuropathol (Berl) 59: 63–69

Krinke G, Suter J, Hess R (1981) Radicular myelinopathy in aging rats. Vet Pathol 18: 335–341

Raine CS (1982) Differences between the nodes of Ranvier of large and small diameter fibers in the PNS. J Neurocytol 11: 935–947

Spencer PS, Ochoa J (1981) The mammalian peripheral nervous system in old age. In: Johnson JE (ed) Aging and cell structure, vol I. Plenum, New York, pp 35–103

Uchida Y, Tomonaga M, Nomura K (1986) Age-related changes of myelin proteins in the rat peripheral nervous system. J Neurochem 46: 1376–1381

van der Kogel AJ (1977) Radiation-induced nerve root degeneration and hypertrophic neuropathy in the lumbosacral spinal cord of rats: the relation with changes in aging rats. Acta Neuropathol (Berl) 39: 139–145

van Steenis G, Kroes R (1971) Changes in the nervous system and musculature of old rats. Vet Pathol 8: 320–332

Peripheral Neuropathy in the Mutant Syrian Hamster

Asao Hirano and Masayuki Shintaku

Synonyms. Mutant Syrian hamster with hindleg paralysis; mutant Syrian hamster with sex-linked, hindleg paralysis.

Gross Appearance

Grossly visible lesions are not seen in the peripheral nerves although atrophy of the muscles of the hindlegs may be noted.

Microscopic Features

The lesions are virtually confined to the peripheral nervous system and are most prominent in the spinal anterior roots of the lumbar region and proximal portion of the sciatic nerve (proximal neuropathy or radiculoneuropathy). The skeletal muscles in the hindleg are generally well preserved, although neurogenic atrophy is noted in animals with advanced paralysis. Changes in the central nervous system are very mild, and the cell bodies of the anterior horn cells of the spinal cord are well preserved. Mild axonal and myelin abnormalities noted in the central nervous system are best explained by a secondary ascending degeneration (Hirano 1977).

Pathologic alterations in the peripheral nervous system include changes of diameter of the nerve fibers, axonal swelling or shrinkage, demyelination and remyelination, appearance of eosinophilic rod-like inclusion bodies in large myelinated fibers, proliferation of Schwann's cells and increase of endoneurial connective tissue (Maya et al. 1981). These changes are virtually confined to the heavily myelinated nerve fibers and undergo a progression in severity and extent of the changes with age. However, great variation exists among individual animals of the same age and between different anatomic sites, even in the same animal.

The most prominent finding is the appearance of highly refractile, eosinophilic rod-like inclusion bodies (Hirano bodies) in large myelinated fibers (Fig. 231) (Hirano and Dembitzer 1976). These inclusion bodies are found in both the anterior and posterior nerve roots. They are also found in normal control hamsters, though much less frequently.

A morphometric study of the peripheral nervous system revealed a decrease in the number of large myelinated fibers associated with an in-

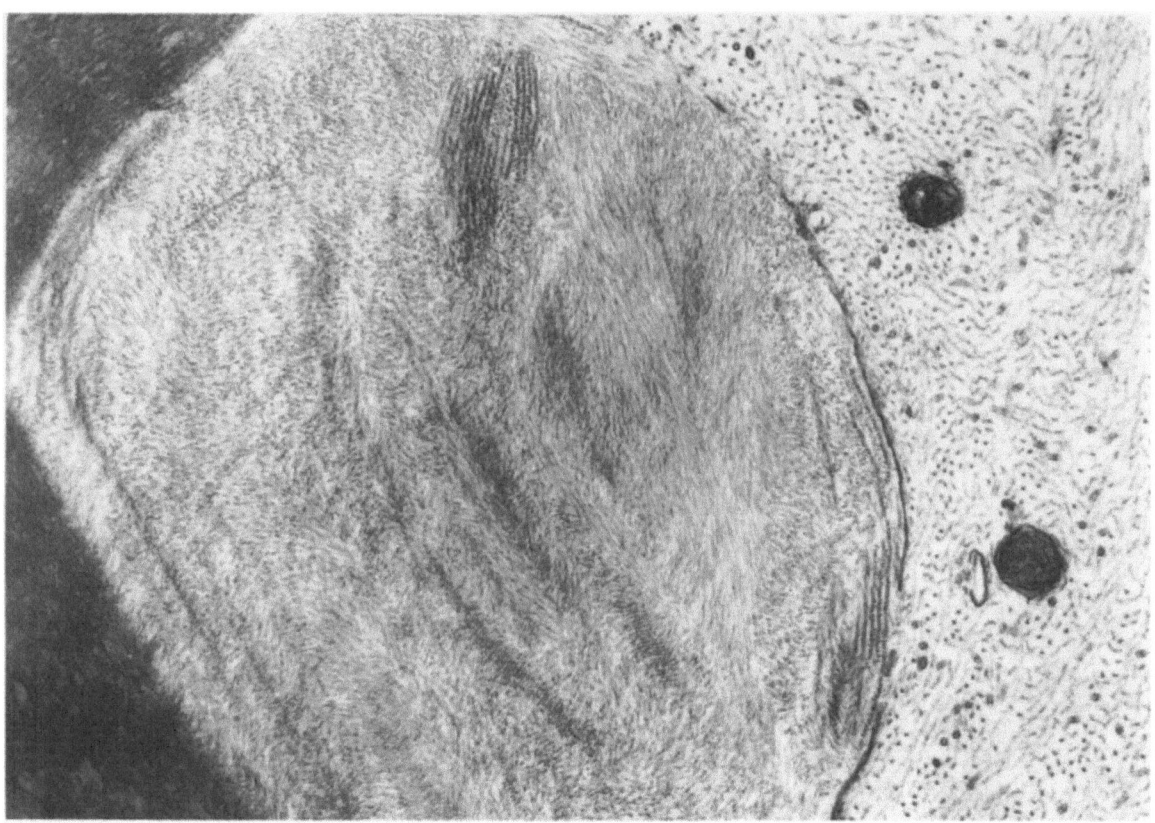

▲ **Fig. 232.** A remarkably distended inner loop of a myelin sheath in a mutant hamster is filled with 6-nm filaments which occasionally have a regular, "lattice-like" arrangement. (From Hirano 1978 a.) TEM, × 26 000

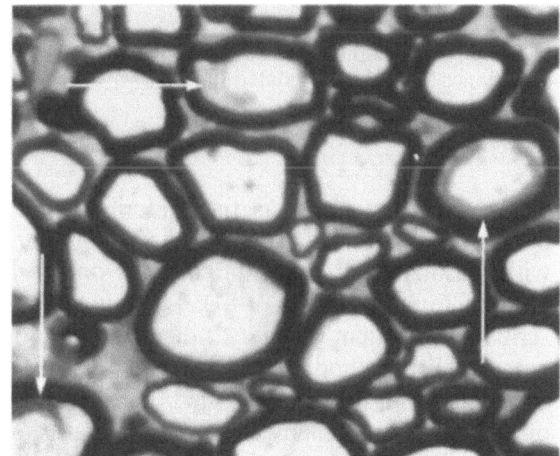

Fig. 231. Anterior root of a mutant hamster. Rod-like in- ▶ clusion bodies are seen *(arrows)*. (From Hirano and Dembitzer 1976.) Toluidine blue, Epon-embedded, × 2500

crease in the number of small myelinated fibers in the spinal roots (Maya et al. 1981).

Ultrastructure

Changes in the Inner Loop of the Schwann's Cell. The inner loop of the Schwann's cell is often markedly distended and contains focal accumulation of fine filaments approximately 6 nm in diameter (Fig. 232) (Hirano 1977). Similar fila-

mentous accumulation is also occasionally noted in the deeper portions of the Schmidt-Lanterman's clefts or cytoplasmic areas of the paranode (Hirano 1978 a). The arrangement of the individual filaments varies from random to elaborate crystalloid structures, occasionally with lattice-like features (Fig. 233) (Hirano and Dembitzer 1976). The latter correspond to the eosinophilic rod-like inclusion body observed in the light microscope. It is essentially similar to the Hirano body at both the light- and electron-microscopic

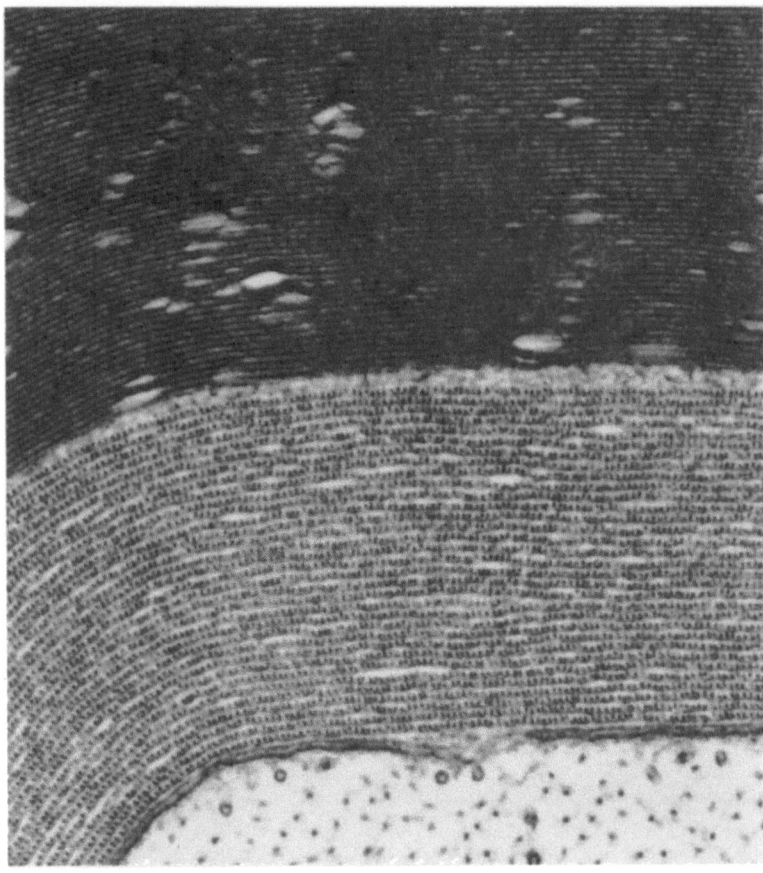

Fig. 233. Crystalloid inclusions, consisting of paired 6-nm filaments as well as regularly spaced densities between them, in an inner loop of a myelinated fiber. TEM, × 70 000

levels. This structure was first described in the pyramidal neurons of Ammon's horn in patients with parkinsonism-dementia complex on the island of Guam (Hirano 1981). Later it was described in a patient with Pick's disease and designated "Hirano body" (Schochet et al. 1968). Subsequent studies have revealed the appearance of this inclusion in many cell types in a variety of pathologic conditions in the human as well as in experimental animals (Hirano 1981; Peterson et al. 1985). Actin as a component of the Hirano body has been demonstrated by an immunocytochemical study (Goldman 1983).

Filamentous accumulations without lattice-like elements probably represent a stage in the formation of the lattice-like inclusions. Similar accumulations of filaments restricted to the adaxonal Schwann-cell cytoplasm of myelinated fibers has been described in the peripheral nerves of apparently normal rats (Jacobs and Cavanagh 1972) as well as in another experimental condition (Spencer and Thomas 1974).

Changes in the Myelin Lamellae. Most of the myelin lamellae appear normal in younger mutants. Following the accumulation of 6-nm filaments in the inner loop of the Schwann's cell, the myelin lamellae start to undergo disintegration (Hirano 1978 a). The sheath becomes distorted and irregular, filament-filled cytoplasmic areas are associated with degenerating myelin lamellae. Disintegrated myelin debris is ingested by phagocytes.

Fig. 234 *(above).* A demyelinated axon *(upper left)* invested by Schwann-cell cytoplasm in a mutant hamster. Fragments of disintegrated myelin are seen in the macrophages surrounding the Schwann's cell. (From Hirano 1978 a.) TEM, × 19 000

Fig. 235 *(below).* Two remyelinating axons in a mutant hamster. The relative thinness of the sheath is a reflection of the newly formed myelin. Each is also surrounded by a peripheral cuff of Schwann-cell cytoplasm or basal lamina. The sheath has an unusually large inner loop possibly indicating an ongoing pathologic process. (From Hirano 1978 a.) TEM, × 12 000

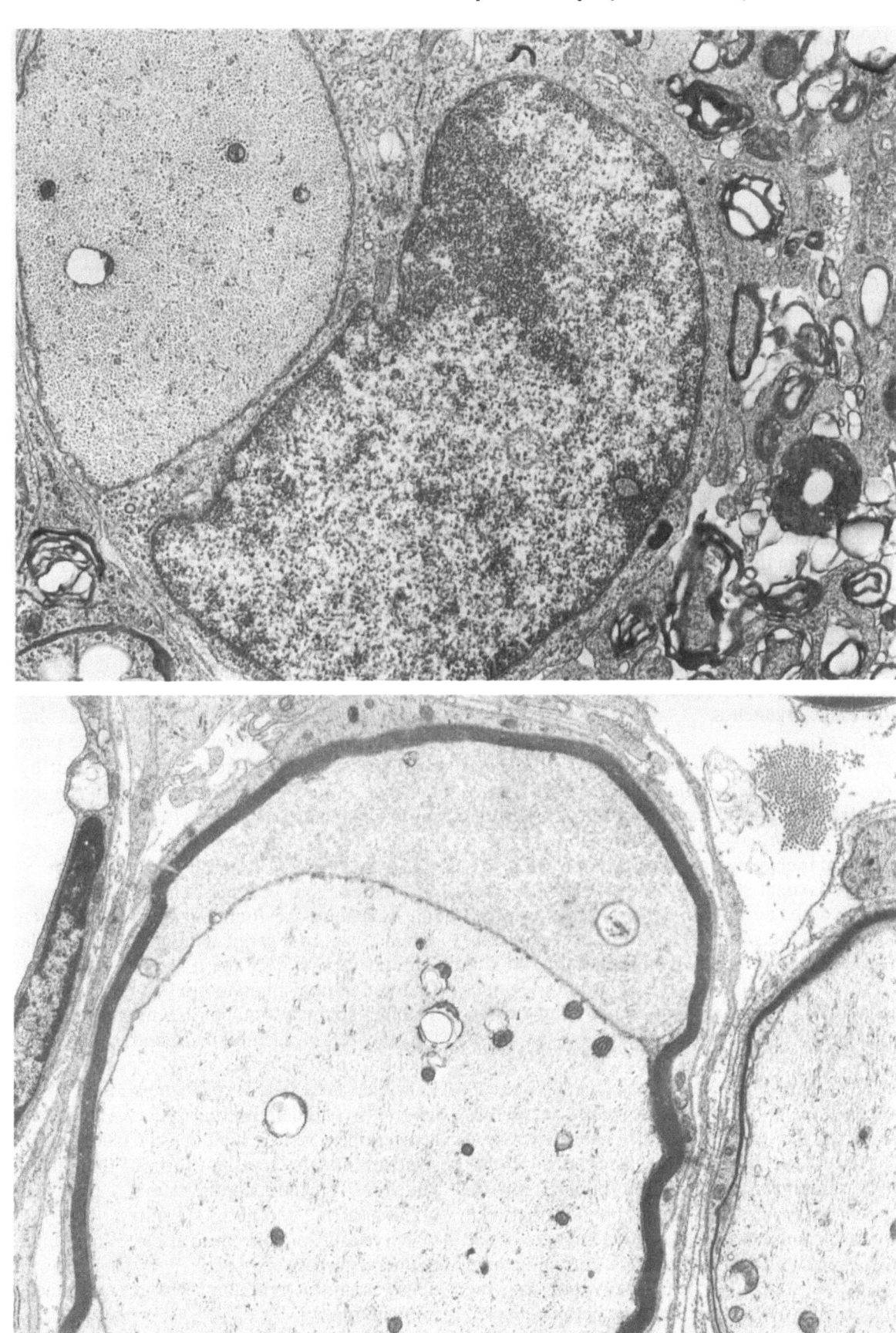

Finally, large caliber axons are completely de-nuded of myelin and are surrounded by cyto-plasm of a Schwann's cell (Fig. 234).

This demyelinating process is accompanied by the frequent appearance of remyelinating axons. These are characterized by the disproportionate thinness of the newly formed myelin sheath as compared to the larger caliber of the axons (Fig. 235). Evidence of recurrent demyelination and remyelination is observed in the form of on-ion bulb formations and abundant collagen fi-bers in the endoneurium (Hirano 1980).

Changes of the Axon. In addition to many normal-sized axons, both abnormally small and large (Fig. 236), myelinated axons are seen in the af-fected animals. The axoplasm displays a number of alterations (Hirano 1980). In some axons, the microtubules are arranged in small clusters. A fine filamentous or granular material is some-times present between the individual microtu-bules. Within the abnormally large axons, the pe-ripheral portion of the axoplasm frequently has an abnormally high accumulation of cytoplasmic organelles with a circumferential arrangement. On the other hand, the central region of the axon retains the normal longitudinal orientation of cy-toplasmic organelles.

Reaction of the Periaxonal Space to the Pathologic Process. The mutant Syrian hamster with hindleg paralysis has played a special role in the elucida-tion of the normal structure and pathologic alter-ations of the periaxonal space (Hirano 1983).

The periaxonal space in the peripheral nervous system of the normal animal is a narrow extracel-lular space between the axon and myelin-form-ing cell. It is less than 10 nm in width and sur-rounded completely by the Schwann-cell inner collar. While this space is separated from the par-enchymatous extracellular space by the trans-verse bands at the paranode of the myelin sheath, there are two theoretical pathways be-tween these two extracellular spaces: (a) the in-traperiod line; and (b) narrow channels between the transverse bands at the paranodes (Hirano 1983). Although there is no morphologically ap-parent specialized junctional apparatus between the axolemma and the plasma membrane of the Schwann's cell in the internode, the periaxonal space tends to retain its normal width, showing remarkable resistance to various pathologic pro-cesses.

Myelinated axons in the mutant hamster occa-sionally develop an enormous swelling. Even in

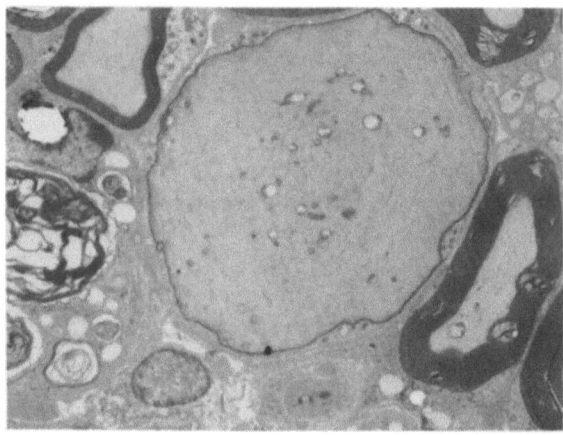

Fig. 236. A peripheral nerve in a mutant hamster. An ab-normally enlarged axon filled with neurofilaments and other organelles is surrounded by a thin myelin sheath. TEM, × 4000

this circumstance, the periaxonal space is not ap-preciably narrower than that of the normal nerve fiber (Hirano and Dembitzer 1981). Substantial enlargement of the inner loop is also not accom-panied by a narrowing of this space.

In other fibers, in which the axon is unusually small, the periaxonal space is sometimes, indeed, greatly enlarged. Under these conditions, how-ever, the axon is found at the edge of the periax-onal space separated from the inner collar by a distance corresponding to the width of the origi-nal periaxonal space (Fig. 237).

Changes in Neurons of the Peripheral Nervous Sys-tem. Three types of alterations of the endoplas-mic reticulum are found in the neurons of the spinal dorsal root ganglia and gasserian ganglion (Hirano 1978b). All these alterations are also found in normal animals, but to a lesser extent.

The first configuration consists of stacked, paral-lel lamellae of membrane-bound cisternae, re-sembling the "lamellar body" seen in human Purkinje's cells. The second one consists of con-centric or parallel cisternal spaces separated by spaces filled with a high-density material. This structure may be a variant form of the annulate lamellae. The third configuration is the "mem-brane-particle complex" (Pannese 1969), in which parallel or concentric arrays of membrane-bound cisternae are separated by single rows of dense granules (probably glycogen) unattached to membranes.

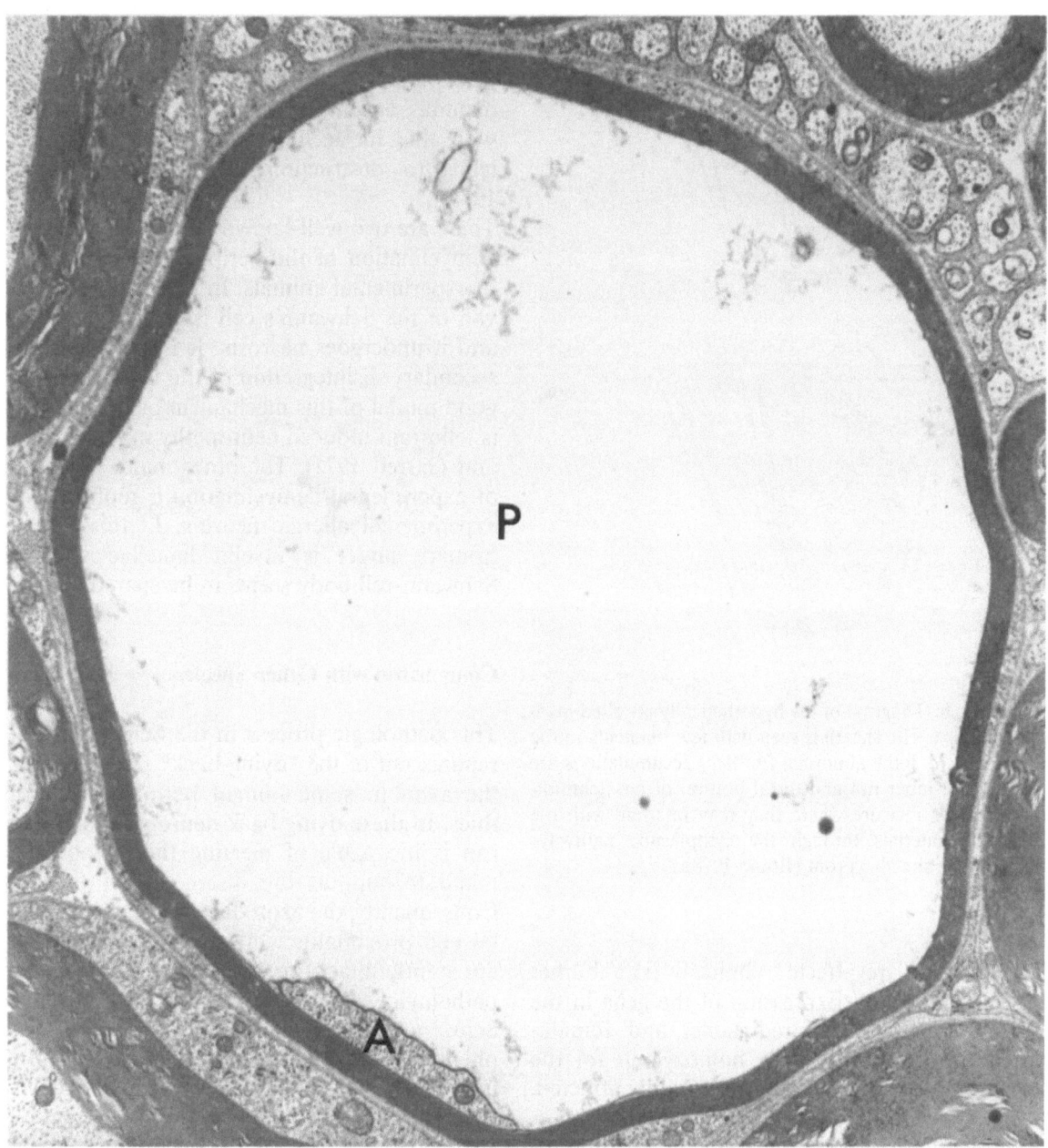

Fig. 237. An enlarged, fluid-filled periaxonal space *(P)* in an altered myelinatined fiber. The myelin sheath appears to be distended and is thinner than the adjacent sheaths. The axon *(A)* is attached to one part of the inner perimenter of the sheath. (From Hirano and Dembitzer 1981.) TEM, × 11500

Biologic Features

Behavioral Observations. A mutant Syrian hamster with sex-linked, hindleg paralysis was discovered and established by Nixon and Connelly (1968). This mutant hamster shows progressive paralysis of the hindleg beginning at 6–10 months after birth. The paralyzed hindlegs are rigidly extended straight back from the body. The progression of the disease finally tapers off and the severely paralyzed animals manage to survive for a relatively long time. Severity varies considerably in individual animals.

Etiology. This disorder was demonstrated to be transmitted as a recessive trait by a single gene (proposed symbol *pa*) which is located on the X-chromosome; therefore, all male animals carry-

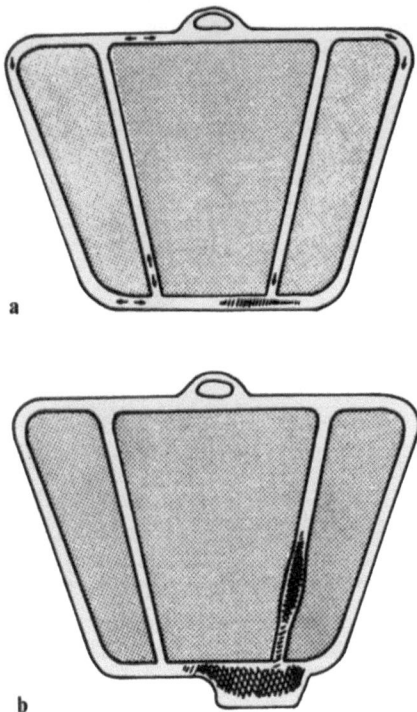

Fig. 238 a, b. Diagram of the hypothetically unrolled myelin sheath. **a** The sheath is seen with few filaments in the inner rim. In **b** the abnormal fibrillary accumulations are seen in the inner rim and distal portion of the Schmidt-Lanterman's incisure where they may interfere with the flow of materials through the cytoplasmic pathways through the sheath. (From Hirano 1978a)

ing the gene are affected clinically (Homburger and Bajusz 1970). Expression of the gene in the female animal is unpredictable, and females known to be genotypically homozygous for the gene may remain normal or only mildly affected.

Pathogenesis. The focal accumulation of 6-nm filaments in the inner loop appears to be the initial sign of the pathologic process in this mutant. Abnormal accumulations of fine filaments have also been observed in a variety of other pathologic conditions. They are, however, usually diffusely scattered and most obvious in the Schwann-cell perikaryon. In contrast, the filamentous accumulation in the mutant hamster is localized in the inner loop and distal portions of the Schmidt-Lanterman's clefts (Fig. 238). It is of interest to note that the thicker myelin sheaths are the ones affected, perhaps because it is in these sheaths that the inner loops are most remote from the Schwann-cell body. The continuous cytoplasmic pathway through the outer, lateral, and inner loops as well as Schmidt-Lanterman's clefts pre-

sumably plays an important role for the circulation of metabolites and certain small organelles. It is therefore reasonable to assume that the filamentous accumulation in these areas interferes with this intracellular circulation and thereby leads to destruction of the myelin (Hirano 1978a).

There are two well-known, major mechanisms of demyelination of the peripheral nervous system in experimental animals. In the first, the perikaryon of the Schwann's cell is damaged primarily and it undergoes necrosis. It is followed by the secondary disintegration of the myelin sheath. A good model of this mechanism of demyelination is tellurium-induced neuropathy in rats (Lampert and Garrett 1971). The other major mechanism of experimental demyelination is represented by experimental allergic neuritis. In this case, the primary target is myelin lamellae while the Schwann-cell body seems to be spared.

Comparison with Other Species

This pathologic process in the Schwann's cell is reminiscent of the "dying-back" phenomenon of the axon in some human peripheral neuropathies. In these dying-back neuropathies, the neuron is incapable of meeting the metabolic demand to support the distal end of the axon. Consequently, the axon degenerates from the distal end proximally, while the cell body remains apparently intact for a long time. The analogous pathologic process seems to occur in the Schwann's cell of the mutant hamster. A similar phenomenon is described in the oligodendrocyte in the cuprizone-induced demyelinating disease of mice (Ludwin and Johnson 1981), and the term "dying-back gliopathy" is proposed for that process by the authors.

The relevance of the changes seen in the mutant hamster with hindleg paralysis to those seen in the hereditary peripheral neuropathy of the human is still obscure. As far as we are aware, there is no publication describing a similar situation in the human being.

This mutant hamster was initially considered a possible model of human motor neuron disease. Subsequent pathologic studies, however, revealed that this animal instead represented a hereditary peripheral neuropathy (Hirano 1977).

References

Goldman JE (1983) The association of actin with Hirano bodies. J Neuropathol Exp Neurol 42: 146-152

Hirano A (1977) Fine structural changes in the mutant hamster with hind leg paralysis. Acta Neuropathol (Berl) 39: 225-230

Hirano A (1978a) A possible mechanism of demyelination in the Syrian hamster with hind leg paralysis. Lab Invest 38: 115-121

Hirano A (1978b) Changes of the neuronal endoplasmic reticulum in the peripheral nervous system in mutant hamsters with hind leg paralysis and normal controls. J Neuropathol Exp Neurol 37: 75-84

Hirano A (1980) Further observations on peripheral neuropathy in the Syrian hamster with hind leg paralysis. Acta Neuropathol (Berl) 50: 187-192

Hirano A (1981) A guide to neuropathology. Igaku-Shoin, New York

Hirano A (1983) Reaction of the periaxonal space to some pathologic processes. Prog Neuropathol 5: 99-112

Hirano A, Dembitzer HM (1976) Eosinophilic rod-like structures in myelinated fibers of hamster spinal roots. Neuropathol Appl Neurobiol 2: 225-232

Hirano A, Dembitzer HM (1981) The periaxonal space in an experimental model of neuropathy: the mutant Syrian hamster with hing leg paralysis. J Neurocytol 10: 261-269

Homburger F, Bajusz E (1970) New models of human disease in Syrian hamsters. JAMA 212: 604-610

Jacobs JM, Cavanagh JB (1972) Aggregations of filaments in Schwann cells of spinal roots of the normal rat. J Neurocytol 1: 161-167

Lampert PW, Garrett RS (1971) Mechanism of demyelination in tellurium neuropathy. Electron microscopic observations. Lab Invest 25: 380-388

Ludwin SK, Johnson ES (1981) Evidence for a "dying back" gliopathy in demyelinating disease. Ann Neurol 9: 301-305

Maya K, Inoue K, Hirano A (1981) Pathological findings in the peripheral nervous system of the Syrian hamster with hind leg paralysis. Neurol Med Chir (Tokyo) 15: 36-44

Nixon CW, Connelly ME (1968) Hind leg paralysis: a new sex-linked mutation in the Syrian hamster. J Hered 59: 276-278

Pannese E (1969) Unusual membrane-particle complexes within nerve cells of the spinal ganglia. J Ultrastruct Res 29: 334-342

Peterson C, Suzuki K, Kress Y, Goldman JE (1985) Microfilament lattices (Hirano bodies) in brindled mice. J Neuropathol Exp Neurol 44: 326

Schochet SS Jr, Lampert PW, Lindenerg R (1968) Fine structure of the Pick and Hirano bodies in a case of Pick's disease. Acta Neuropathol (Berl) 11: 330-337

Spencer PS, Thomas PK (1974) Ultrastructural studies of the dying-back process. II. The sequestration and removal by Schwann cells and oligodendrocytes of organelles from normal and diseased axons. J Neurocytol 3: 763-783

Aberrant Synaptic Development in Mutant "Weaver" Mice

Asao Hirano and Masayuki Shintaku

Synonyms. "Weaver" mouse; murine mutant "weaver."

Gross Appearance

The cerebellum of the weaver mouse is abnormally small and is about one-fourth the size of the cerebellum in the normal littermates (Sidman et al. 1965).

Microscopic Features

The basic cytoarchitecture of the cerebellar cortex is disorganized in the adult weaver mouse, and it is difficult to distinguish between the various cortical layers (Fig. 239 a, b). The molecular layer is abnormally thin, and in the internal granule cell layer, the granule cells are remarkably depleted. The remaining granule cells appear normal, and no evidence of degeneration or necrosis is found. The alignment of Purkinje's cells is markedly deranged, and their dendritic arborization is severely distorted. Basket fibers and climbing fibers are seen around Purkinje's cells (Sidman et al. 1965). Proliferation of Bergmann's astrocytes is also observed. The cerebellar white matter and cerebellar nuclei do not undergo remarkable pathologic change.

Ultrastructure

In the control littermates, the molecular layer consists of a great number of compactly arranged

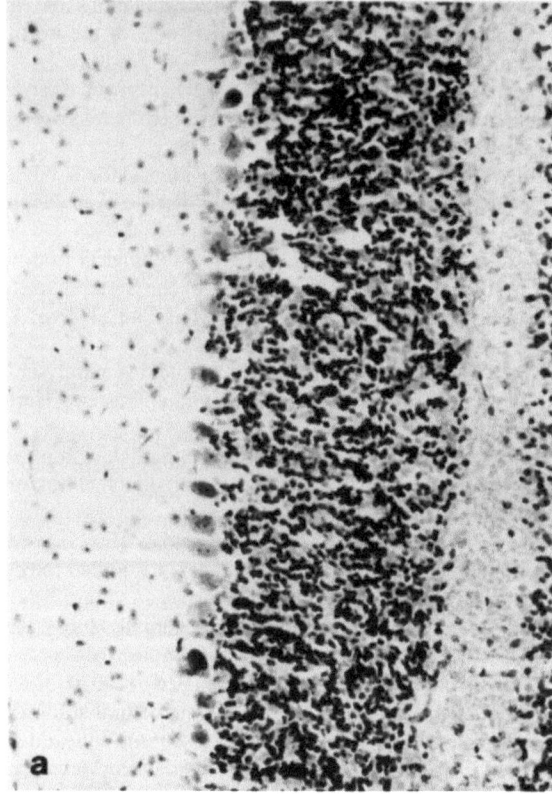

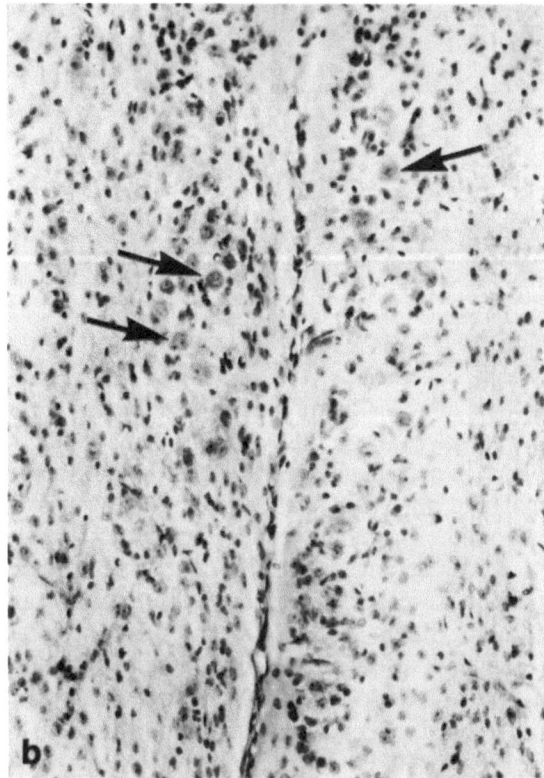

cell processes, most of which are either parallel fibers or Purkinje-cell dendrites and their attached dendritic spines (Fig. 240). Astrocytic processes are not particularly prominent at low magnification but they invest the synapses, soma, and dendrites of Purkinje's cells.

In the adult weaver mouse, the most striking feature is the virtual absence of the small-caliber parallel fibers and the axons of the internal granule cells (Fig. 241) (Hirano and Dembitzer 1973). In the molecular layer, cytoplasmic processes of astrocytes fill the spaces between the remaining neuronal elements. These cytoplasmic processes do not have the abundant glial fibers, glycogen granules, and other indicators of reactive changes seen in long-standing astrocytic gliosis.

On the other hand, dendritic spines of Purkinje's cells are quite common (Fig. 242). These are usually unassociated with any presynaptic elements. Instead, they are invested by swollen cytoplasmic processes of astrocytes. The fundamental fine structure of the dendritic spine is identical to that of the normal cerebellum, except that the average diameter of the spines in the weaver is smaller than that of the normal cerebellum. They have postmembranous densities at the surface apposing the astrocytic process, and, interestingly enough, the extracellular space between the spine and the apposing astrocytic surface is widened (ca. 20 nm) and even contains electron-dense cleft material. The apposing astrocytic processes have no junctional specializations at these sites.

Various cytochemical examinations including ethanolic phosphotungustic acid impregnation and bismuth iodide impregnation methods fail to reveal any differences between these "unattached" dendritic spines in the weaver cerebellum and the spines in the normal control (Hirano and Dembitzer 1973). A freeze-fracture study al-

Fig. 239 a, b. Cerebellum of the normal (**a**) and weaver (**b**) mouse. Note severe paucity of granule cells and thinness of the molecular layer in the weaver cerebellum. Purkinje's cells (a few of them are indicated by *arrows*) are well preserved, but their alignment is deranged. H and E, × 50

Fig. 240 *(above).* The molecular layer of the cerebellum of ▶ a 15-day-old normal mouse. Cross sections of many slender parallel fibers containing a few microtubules are seen. Some of the parallel fibers are expanded and form synapses with dendritic spines of Purkinje's cells. Astrocytic cytoplasm invests the synapses and neuronal processes. TEM, × 33 000

Fig. 241 *(below).* The molecular layer of the cerebellum of a 24-day-old weaver mouse. Parallel fibers are almost completely absent, and "unattached" dendritic spines are seen which are invested by expanded, sole astrocytic cytoplasm. Postmembranous densities are evident in some unattached spines *(arrows).* TEM, × 30 000

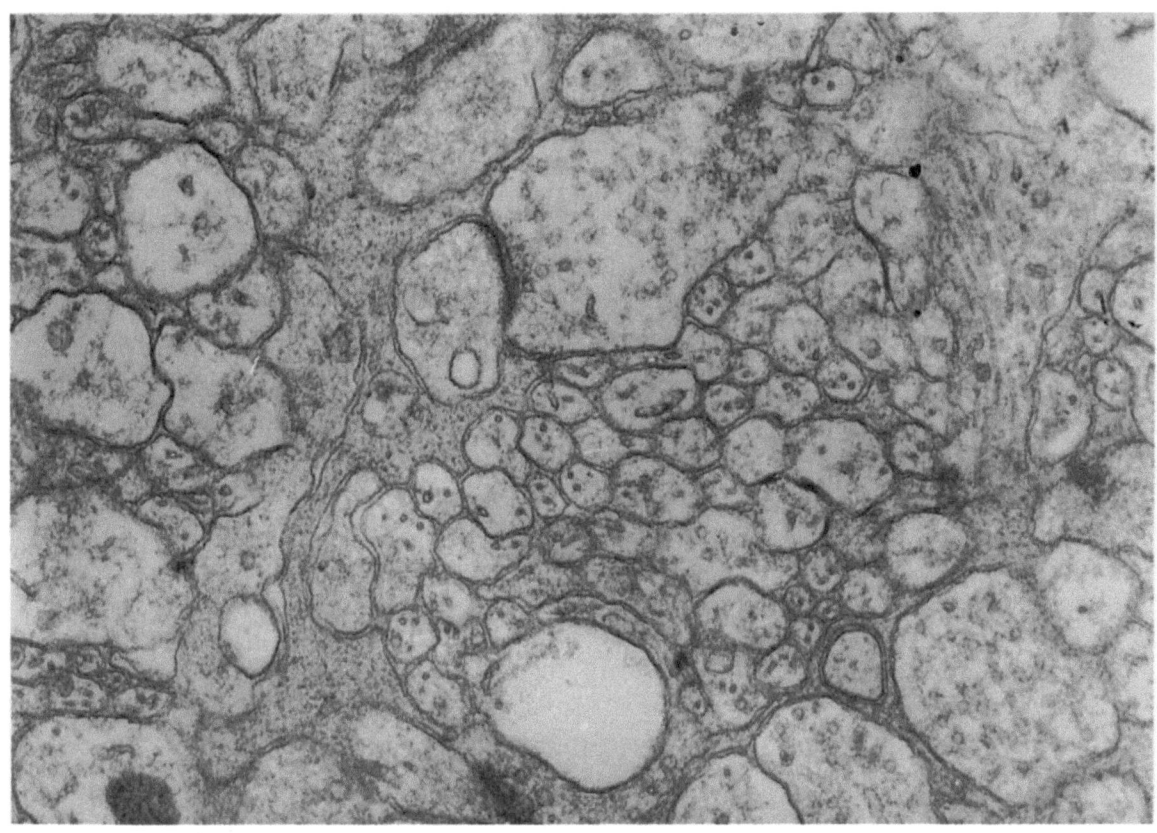

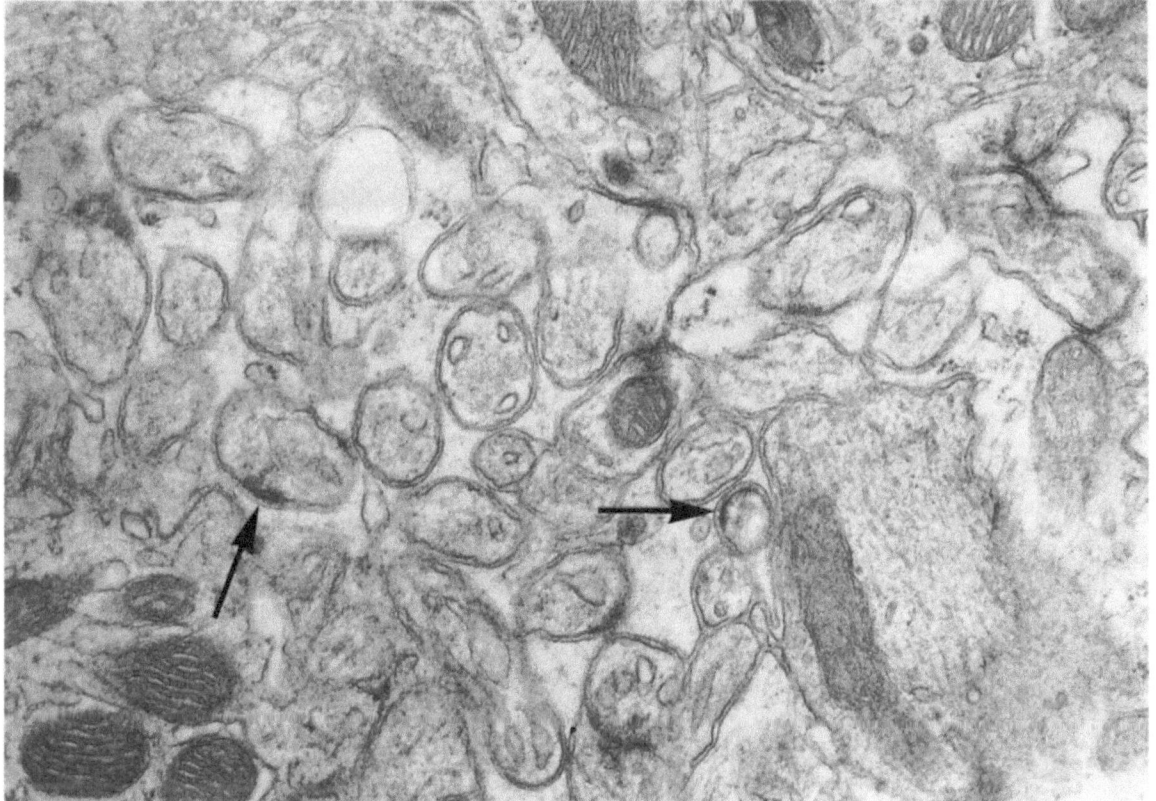

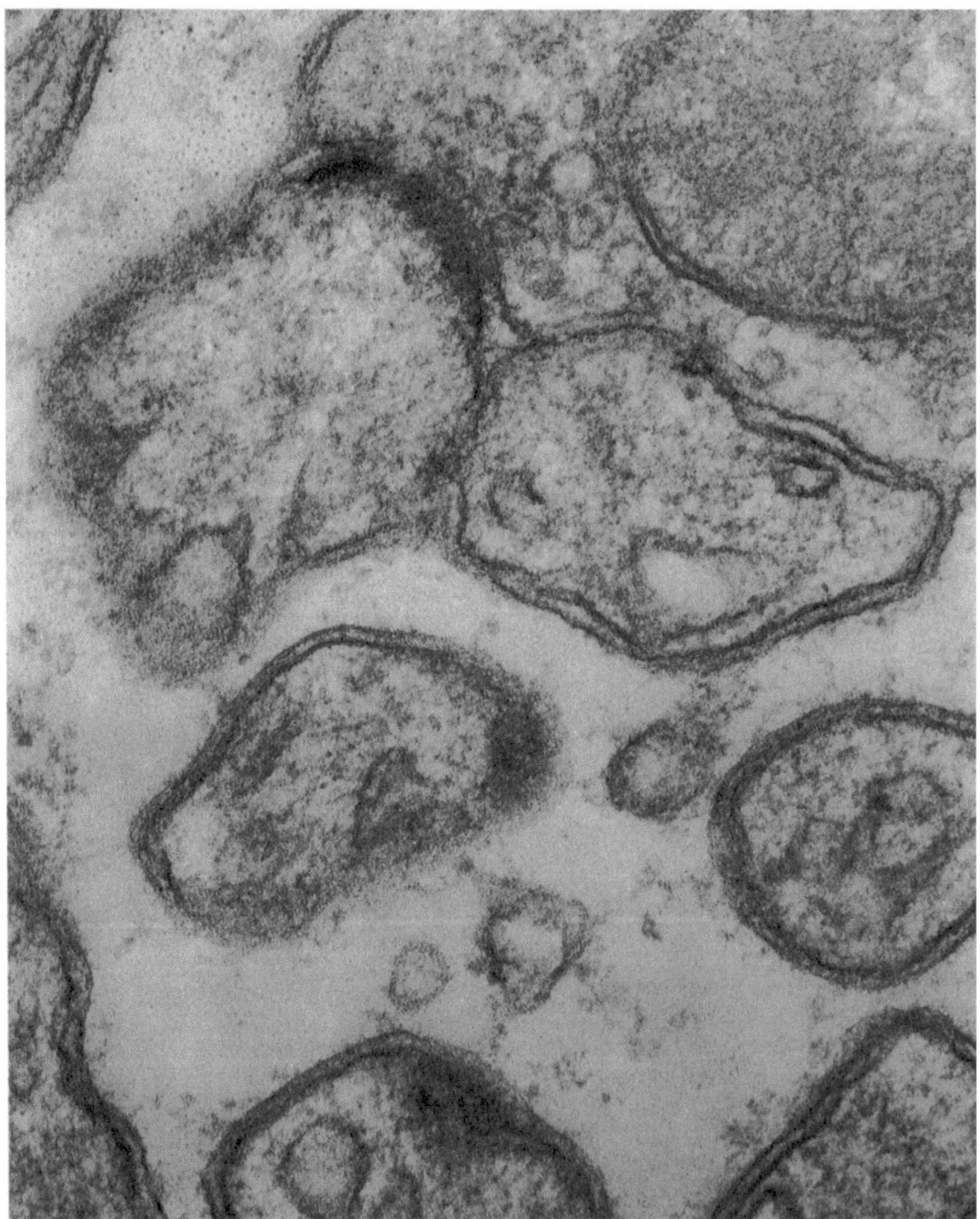

Fig. 242. Higher magnification of the unattached spines of the Purkinje's cells of a 24-day-old weaver mouse. Note postmembranous densities and dense material in the extracellular spaces between the spines and surrounding astrocytes. One synapse between a parallel fiber ending and a dendritic spine is seen *(upper left)*. TEM, × 108 000

so indicates that the dendritic spines of the weaver mouse are morphologically identical to those of normal mouse. Aggregations of 10-nm particles are seen in the postsynaptic region of the outer fracture surface (B-surface) of the unattached dendritic spines as seen in normal dendritic spines (Hanna et al. 1976).

In the youngest weaver mice that we examined (11 or 14 days after birth), numerous unattached dendritic spines were present (Hirano and Dembitzer 1974). These were found even at levels very close to the external granule cell layer. External granule cells were present, but fewer in number than in the control. Numerous examples of degenerating granule cells were seen. Parallel fibers were quite rare in most areas, and no degeneration of presynaptic elements arising from the few parallel fibers was observed. Climbing fibers, on the other hand, were well developed and attached to spines on the main dendrites as well as on the soma of the Purkinje's cells.

The morphologic features of the initial development of both the somatic and dendritic spines of Purkinje's cells in the weaver mouse, which form synapses with climbing fibers, is essentially the same as that in the normal littermates (Hirano et al. 1977b). These somatic spines seem to develop from slender filopodia-like processes and make synaptic contact with the climbing fibers. The synapses finally disappear from the cell body and presumably take up their permanent residence on the dendrites.

Biologic Features

Natural History and Etiology. The murine mutant weaver was discovered in the C57BL/6J strain of mice. The clinical signs manifest themselves at about 8–10 days after birth and include unstable, ataxic gait, fine rapid tremor of the trunk and extremities, and loss of coordination (Sidman et al. 1965). These signs do not appear to progress with age. This disorder was demonstrated to be transmitted as an autosomal recessive trait by a single gene (proposed symbol *wv*).

Pathogenesis. The elucidation of the morphology of synaptic development has been one of the major areas of research in neuropathology (Hirano and Zimmerman 1973; Hirano and Dembitzer 1975b), and various models of synaptogenesis have been presented (Hirano 1979). Throughout all these studies, it has been assumed that contact between the two neuronal elements is needed be-

fore any synaptic specialization occurs, and this assumption has actually been confirmed in many instances (Hirano 1979). However, by observations made on the cerebellum of the weaver, as well as on a number of other models to be discussed, this assumption has been challenged.

When unattached pre- or postsynaptic terminals were found in various conditions, it was traditionally assumed that the complete synapse had originally formed, and that later one of the two synaptic mates degenerated leaving the other behind (Hirano 1979). In the case of the weaver mouse, the interpretation that the granule cells had formed synapses early in development and these degenerated later, leaving behind the unattached dendritic spines, is untenable because granule cell destruction occurs prior to their migration inward to form the internal granule cell layer (Sidman et al. 1965). Study on the young weaver mouse confirmed the degeneration of the external granule cells and the presence of unattached spines (Hirano and Dembitzer 1974), but degeneration of presynaptic elements arising from the parallel fibers was not observed.

The exact process and mechanism of formation of the unattached dendritic spines still remains to be clarified. However, it can be safely concluded that the dendritic spines of Purkinje's cells do not seem to require a "one-to-one" induction of a presynaptic element for the establishment of a specialized postsynaptic apparatus (Rakic and Sidman 1973).

Comparison with Other Conditions

Experimental Animals

Cycasin-Induced Cerebellar Alteration. Hirano et al. (1969) first reported the appearance of cerebellar symptoms after administration of cycasin, the toxic agent of the cycad seed, to mice and hamsters within 24 h after birth. Pathologic examination revealed necrosis of the external granule cells of the cerebellum and subsequent severe cerebellar deformity.

Ultrastructural studies made of mice which were injected with cycasin subcutaneously within 24 h after birth and sacrificed 25 days later reveal a severe depletion of the granule cells and preservation of Purkinje's cells (Hirano et al. 1972). Purkinje's cells have well-developed dendrites bearing typical dendritic spines, including conspicuous postsynaptic membrane thickenings. These spines are devoid of presynaptic terminals (unattached spine) and are embedded in a matrix of astrocytic cytoplasm. No degenerative changes of the presynaptic elements are observed. These ultrastructural features are essentially identical to those seen in the weaver cerebellum.

Cerebellar Alterations Induced by Virus and X-ray Irradiation. Herndon et al. (1971) observed Purkinje-cell dendritic spines devoid of afferent contacts after inoculating neonatal ferrets with feline panleukopenia virus. These spines, which were designated "de-afferented spines" are similar to the "unattached" spines later observed in the weaver mouse. A similar alteration has also been observed in the mouse cerebellum after X-irradiation during the neonatal period (Altman and Anderson 1972).

Thus, at least four apparently unrelated etiologic agents, namely, a genetic mutation, a specific chemical agent, a virus, and X-irradiation, have been shown to lead to substantially the same aberrant development of the synapses. The common mode of action in all cases is the destruction of the cerebellar granule cell in the germinal layer. That is, the granule cells are destroyed prior to the formation of synapses with the Purkinje-cell dendritic spines.

"Staggerer" Mouse. The "staggerer" mouse is another murine mutant which undergoes severe maldevelopment of the cerebellum. The primary genetic defect in the staggerer lies in the delay of maturation of the Purkinje's cells which are unable to form dendritic spines at a time when granule cells and parallel fibers are abundant (Landis and Sidman 1974). Ultrastructural studies reveal that in the staggerer mouse the Purkinje's cells are devoid of dendritic spines and no synaptic contact is established between the parallel fibers and dendritic spines (Hirano and Dembitzer 1975a). The only processes reminiscent of spines are seen on the Purkinje-cell soma, and these somatic spines form synapses with climbing fibers. In spite of the delayed maturation of the postsynaptic elements, the parallel fibers form well-developed unattached presynaptic terminals complete with synaptic vesicles (Sotelo 1973). As the staggerer mouse matures, the granule cells and parallel fibers degenerate leaving the Purkinje's cells behind. At this stage, a small number of spines begin to emerge on the dendritic surface of the Purkinje's cells. Astrocytic proliferation becomes very pronounced, and the cytoplasmic processes of these astrocytes undergo extensive sheet-like expansion and are sometimes arranged in concentric lamellae

around the neuronal cells and processes (Hirano and Dembitzer 1976).

These pathologic processes in the staggerer mouse represent an apparently opposite situation to that seen in the weaver mouse and in the experimental conditions described above. In the staggerer mutant, the presynaptic terminals of the granule cells are capable of development without the direct influence of postsynaptic mates, just as the Purkinje-cell dendritic spines can develop without presynaptic elements in the weaver mouse.

Human Diseases

Granule Cell Type Cerebellar Degeneration. The granule cell type of cerebellar degeneration is a rare degenerative disorder of unknown etiology. In this disorder, the cerebellum is abnormally small due to a severe paucity of granule cells, while Purkinje's cells are comparatively well preserved. In an ultrastructural study of such a case, a large number of unattached dendritic spines of the Purkinje's cells were found (Hirano et al. 1973). These unattached spines were provided with the postmembranous densities and were embedded in a matrix of astrocytic cytoplasm. These findings are remarkably similar to those of the weaver cerebellum.

Menkes' Kinky Hair Disease. Menkes' kinky hair disease (X-chromosome-linked copper malabsorption) is a sex-linked, hereditary disorder which is manifested by seizures, developmental retardation, and characteristic changes of the hair. Copper deficiency due to malabsorption of dietary copper is the basis of this rare disease. Neuropathologic examination discloses extensive degenerative changes of the brain, most prominent in the thalamus (Iwata et al. 1979a) and cerebellum (Iwata et al. 1979b). In the cerebellum, both the granule cells and Purkinje's cells are severely reduced in number, and the remaining Purkinje's cells show characteristic changes. These consist of an elaboration of somatic sprouts and abnormal arborization of the dendritic tree (Purpura et al. 1976; Iwata et al. 1979b).

An ultrastructural study of the cerebellar cortex revealed a severe reduction of the number of granule cells and a large number of somatic spines as well as dendritic spines of Purkinje's cells, some of which were unattached to presynaptic endings. These unattached spines showed postmembranous densities and were invested by astrocytic processes (Hirano et al. 1977a).

Cerebellar Neuroblastoma. In a case of cerebellar neuroblastoma arising in an 18-month-old boy (Shin et al. 1978), the tumor was composed of closely packed small cells which were arranged in rows separated by fibrillary material. Electron microscopy revealed that these tumor cells had parallel cylindrical processes which contained small, clear presynaptic vesicles (Hirano and Shin 1979). These findings indicate that the presynaptic elements can also develop without the immediate influence of a postsynaptic mate. An essentially similar process has been observed in the young staggerer mouse (see above).

Addendum

Although we have confined ourselves to the aberrant synaptic development in the cerebellum of the weaver mouse, some recent investigations have revealed another intriguing neuropathologic change in this mutant. Schmidt et al. (1982) found neuronal loss in the substantia nigra, which was associated with a reduced concentration of dopamine in various areas of the brain and a decrease of tyrosine hydroxylase (TH) activity in the striatum. A selective decrease in the number of TH-positive neurons was demonstrated in the substantia nigra (Triarhou et al. 1986; Gupta et al. 1987). These results indicate that the weaver mouse has a specific developmental failure in the dopaminergic system. Dopaminergic neurons from ventral mesencephalic anlagen of a genetically normal embryo transplanted into the brain of adult weaver mice were found to survive and innervate the host neostriatum (Triarhou et al. 1986).

References

Altman J, Anderson WJ (1972) Experimental reorganization of the cerebellar cortex. I. Morphological effects of elimination of microneurons with prolonged X-irradiation started at birth. J Comp Neurol 146: 355–406

Gupta M, Felten DL, Ghetti B (1987) Selective loss of monoaminergic neurons in weaver mutant mice - an immunocytochemical study. Brain Res 402: 379–382

Hanna RB, Hirano A, Pappas GD (1976) Membrane specializations of dendritic spines and glia in the weaver mouse cerebellum. A freeze-fracture study. J Cell Biol 68: 403–410

Herndon RM, Margolis G, Kilham L (1971) The synaptic organization of the malformed cerebellum induced by perinatal infection with the feline panleukopenia virus (PLV). II. The Purkinje cell and its afferents. J Neuropathol Exp Neurol 30: 557–570

Hirano A (1979) On the independent development of the pre- and postsynaptic terminals. Prog Neuropathol 4: 79–99

Hirano A, Dembitzer HM (1973) Cerebellar alterations in the weaver mouse. J Cell Biol 56: 478–486

Hirano A, Dembitzer HM (1974) Observations on the development of the weaver mouse cerebellum. J Neuropathol Exp Neurol 33: 354–364

Hirano A, Dembitzer HM (1975a) The fine structure of staggerer cerebellum. J Neuropathol Exp Neurol 34: 1–11

Hirano A, Dembitzer HM (1975b) Aberrant development of the Purkinje cell dendritic spine. Adv Neurol 12: 353–360

Hirano A, Dembitzer HM (1976) The fine structure of astrocytes in the adult staggerer. J Neuropathol Exp Neurol 35: 63–74

Hirano A, Shin WY (1979) Unattached presynaptic terminals in a cerebellar neuroblastoma in the human. Neuropathol Appl Neurobiol 5: 63–70

Hirano A, Zimmerman HM (1973) Aberrant synaptic development. A review. Arch Neurol 28: 359–366

Hirano A, Dembitzer HM, Jones M (1972) An electron microscopic study of cycasin-induced cerebellar alterations. J Neuropathol Exp Neurol 31: 113–125

Hirano A, Dembitzer HM, Ghatak NR, Fan KJ, Zimmerman HM (1973) On the relationship between human and experimental granule cell type cerebellar degeneration. J Neuropathol Exp Neurol 32: 493–502

Hirano A, Llena JF, French JH, Ghatak NR (1977a) Fine structure of the cerebellar cortex in Menkes kinky-hair disease. X-chromosome-linked copper malabsorption. Arch Neurol 34: 52–56

Hirano A, Dembitzer HM, Yoon CH (1977b) Development of Purkinje cell somatic spines in the weaver mouse. Acta Neuropathol (Berl) 40: 85–90

Hirano I, Shibuya C, Hayashi K (1969) Induction of a cerebellar disorder with cycasin in newborn mice and hamsters. Proc Soc Exp Biol Med 131: 593–599

Iwata M, Hirano A, French JH (1979a) Thalamic degeneration in X-chromosome-linked copper malabsorption. Ann Neurol 5: 359–366

Iwata M, Hirano A, French JH (1979b) Degeneration of the cerebellar system in X-chromosome-linked copper malabsorption. Ann Neurol 5: 542–549

Landis DMD, Sidman RL (1974) Cerebellar cortical development in the staggerer mouse. J Neuropathol Exp Neurol 33: 180

Purpura DP, Hirano A, French JH (1976) Polydendritic Purkinje cells in X-chromosome-linked copper malabsorption. A Golgi study. Brain Res 117: 125–129

Rakic P, Sidman RL (1973) Organization of cerebellar cortex secondary to deficit of granule cells in weaver mutant mice. J Comp Neurol 152: 133–162

Schmidt MJ, Sawyer BD, Perry KW, Fuller FR, Foreman MM, Ghetti B (1982) Dopamine deficiency in the weaver mutant mouse. J Neurosci 2: 376–380

Shin WY, Laufer H, Lee YC, Aftalion B, Hirano A, Zimmerman HM (1978) Fine structure of a cerebellar neuroblastoma. Acta Neuropathol (Berl) 42: 11–13

Sidman RL, Green MC, Appel SH (1965) Catalog of the neurological mutants of the mouse. Harvard University Press, Cambridge

Sotelo C (1973) Permanence and fate of paramembranous synaptic specializations in "mutant" and experimental animals. Brain Res 62: 345–351

Triarhou LC, Low WC, Ghetti B (1986) Transplantation of ventral mesencephalic anlagen to hosts with genetic nigrostriatal dopamine deficiency. Proc Natl Acad Sci USA 83: 8789–8793

Subject Index*

---

* Page numbers in **boldface** indicate the principal discussion; Figures are designated by the letter "f" following the
page number; Tables are found on page numbers followed by the letter "t".